THE CARBOHYDRATE ADDICT'S HEALTHY HEART PROGRAM

BREAK YOUR CARBO-INSULIN CONNECTION TO HEART DISEASE

RICHARD F. HELLER, M.S., Ph.D.

RACHAEL F. HELLER, M.A., M.Ph., Ph.D.

FREDERIC J. VAGNINI, M.D., F.A.C.S.

BALLANTINE BOOKS • NEW YORK

A Ballantine Book
Published by The Ballantine Publishing Group

Copyright © 1999 by Dr. Richard Ferdinand Heller and Dr. Rachael F. Heller

All rights reserved under International and Pan-American Copyright Conventions. Published in the United States by The Ballantine Publishing Group, a division of Random House, Inc., New York, and simultaneously in Canada by Random House of Canada Limited, Toronto.

Ballantine Books and colophon are registered trademarks of Random House, Inc.

www.randomhouse.com/BB/

Library of Congress Catalog Card Number: 00-107756

ISBN 0-345-42612-6

Cover photograph by Scott Hime

Manufactured in the United States of America

First Edition: September 1999
First Trade Paperback Edition: November 2000

10 9 8 7 6 5 4 3 2 1

**Listen to the people who have benefited from
*The Carbohydrate Addict's Healthy Heart Program***

"My energy level has increased considerably. I now exercise four to five times a week and (gasp!) actually enjoy it! Before, I was always tired and lethargic—now I feel like a new person. Plus my cholesterol has gone from 218 to 150."

—LINDA SHERMAN
Alexandria, Virginia

"I started six months ago at 181 pounds. Today I am 154! I feel good about myself and know I will continue to feel this way. This program is just too easy!"

—LILIAN HOLLAND
Valencia, California

"Since I began this program, my cholesterol levels have gone from 200 to 147. My blood sugar levels are normal again and my doctor is simply amazed."

—BARBARA SCHERER
Bonn, Germany

"It is amazing to me that I do not suffer cravings or hunger on this program. This will be my one and only way of eating from now on. I recommend this program to my friends and family and to anyone who asks me."

—ALBERT LIOY
San Diego, California

**Selected by the Book-of-the-Month Club
A Featured Alternate of the Quality Paperback Book Club
Selected by the One Spirit Book Club**

OTHER BOOKS BY DRS. RICHARD AND RACHAEL HELLER:

The Carbohydrate Addict's Lifespan Program

The Carbohydrate Addict's Diet

The Carbohydrate Addict's Healthy for Life Plan

The Carbohydrate Addict's Program for Success

Carbohydrate-Addicted Kids

The Carbohydrate Addict's Calorie Counter

The Carbohydrate Addict's Carbohydrate Counter

The Carbohydrate Addict's Fat Counter

The Carbohydrate Addict's Gram Counter

The Carbohydrate Addict's Cookbook

Visit the Hellers at their Web site at:
www.carbohydrateaddicts.com

TO EVERY CARBOHYDRATE ADDICT
WHOSE HEART HAS BEEN MADE VULNERABLE
ON SO MANY LEVELS

DISCLAIMER

The information in this book reflects the authors' experiences and is not intended to replace medical advice. It is not the authors' intent to diagnose or prescribe. The intent is only to offer information to help you cooperate with your physician in your mutual quest for optimal health. Only your physician can determine whether or not this program is appropriate for you. Before embarking on this or any other program, consult your physician. In addition to getting regular checkups and supervision, you should discuss any questions or symptoms with your physician. In the event you use this information without your physician's approval, you are prescribing for yourself, and the publisher and authors assume no responsibility.

As with any program, one size cannot fit all, and your program should be individualized in conjunction with your physician. It is important that together you develop your own specific program based on his or her advice and your own particular requirements and preferences, so that you may derive the best benefit from this program.

Do not mix and match guidelines from this program with recommendations from other plans. Be guided by your personal physician; let him or her help you and make important suggestions. Bring this book to your physician's office. Have your physician read it, and understand the program, and advise you. As in all matters, your physician's recommendations should be paramount.

Chromium may reduce the need for insulin or other diabetic treatments. Therefore, diabetics, in particular, should be closely monitored by their physicians.

This program is not intended for pregnant or nursing women or for children or teens. Their needs are so specialized that they cannot be addressed here.

The dialogue, quotes, biographical facts, and anecdotes recounted in this book are actual and true to life. They come from hundreds of interviews. No individual has been directly quoted or described unless specific written permission was obtained. All names used in this book, other than those of scientific researchers, have been changed to protect anonymity.

Notice: The terms *Reward Meal*®, *The Carbohydrate Addict's Diet*®, *The Carbohydrate Addict's Healthy Heart Program*®, and derivatives and abbreviations are registered and service trademarks owned by Drs. Richard and Rachael Heller and cannot be used without their written permission.

CONTENTS

Don't Buy This Book!   xi

Carbohydrate Addiction Defined   xiii

The American Heart Association Guidelines
and The Carbohydrate Addict's Healthy Heart Program   xiii

Introduction: A New and Kinder Medicine   3

PART I. THE HEART OF THE MATTER: YOUR PERSONAL HEART HEALTH PROFILE

1. Three Wishes for a Second Chance   21
2. The Insulin Connection: Getting to the Heart of the Matter   48
3. High Blood Pressure, Weight Gain, Blood Fats, and Diabetes: Taking Insulin to Heart   65
4. Are You a Carbohydrate Addict at Risk?   99

PART II. TAKING IT TO HEART: THE BASIC PLAN—A PROGRAM OF BALANCE

5. The Carbohydrate Addict's Healthy Heart Program: Step 1: Balanced Nutrition   119

6. The Carbohydrate Addict's Healthy Heart Program:
   Step 2: Balanced Supplementation   152

7. The Carbohydrate Addict's Healthy Heart Program:
   Step 3: Balanced Activity Options   187

PART III. HEART HEALTH ENHANCERS—FOR TODAY AND TOMORROW

8. Heart Health–Enhancing Options—For Life   197

9. On the Horizon: Emerging Warriors in the Battle
   for Heart Health   219

10. Heart and Soul: The Mysterious Power of Prayer   235

11. Helping Hands: You Are Not Alone   246

PART IV. RECIPES FOR SUCCESS

12. Eating Hearty, Part I: Low-Carbohydrate Recipes   257

13. Eating Hearty, Part II: High-Carbohydrate,
    Reward Meal Recipes   279

    APPENDIX: Incorporating Low-Fat, Low-Saturated Fat,
    Low-Salt, and Other Health Agency Dietary
    Recommendations into Your Program   307

    REFERENCES   313

    INDEX   339

ACKNOWLEDGMENTS

We wish to express our deep appreciation to:

Mel Berger of the William Morris Agency, by far the finest agent and adviser in the world. His thoughtful and incisive advice, common sense, creativity, years of experience, caring, and hard work make him the best agent and the best friend anyone could ever have.

Cathy Repetti, our editor, for her interest, concern, keen mind, and commitment to bringing out the best in her authors.

Scott Miller, Mel Berger's most capable and industrious assistant, whose trusted reliability and concern have been unfailing.

In addition, Drs. Richard and Rachael Heller would like to acknowledge:

Leslie St. Louis, M.D., for his integrity, wide range of knowledge, generous concern, and very wise counsel.

Douglas E. Hertford, M.D., for his interest, sincerity, and expert advice.

Martin W. Weber, who is always there when needed and whose interest and ability to ask the right questions at the right time (and have the right answers as well) have proved invaluable and unerringly on target.

Irwin Neus, D.D.S.; his capable and sage office coordinator, Adrienne Belanoff; and his wonderful staff, whose interest, support, sage comments, and contributions are always valued.

Deborah Nicolai and Jonathan Martin Heller (in order of appearance in this world), who bring joy and laughter into our lives.

Maggie Boulineau and her superb staff at the Comfort Inn in Lake Buena Vista, Florida, for making us a wonderful home away from home on our frequent visits to Walt Disney World, where we both work and play hard.

Apple Computer Company and its support staff, for the development, care, and "feeding" of our powerful, user-friendly PowerBooks and Power Macs. Thanks to Apple's hard work, these invaluable tools have facilitated our work and enriched our lives.

In addition, Dr. Frederic Vagnini would like to acknowledge:

My wonderful wife, Mary Ann, the mother of my beautiful daughters, Grace and Clare.

My dear sisters, Anne and Grace, who have always been beside me and behind me with help and encouragement. Anne's support has been invaluable, and Grace, a Catholic nun for thirty-five years, has never let me forget the amazing power of prayer.

Susan Hill, R.N., R.V.T., who, among other capacities, has served as director of nursing at The Cardiovascular Wellness Centers, director of my Non-Invasive Cardiology Laboratory, and fellow researcher. Her keen intelligence, capability, and commitment have made a world of difference.

Maria Santoro, my director of clinical nutrition and weight loss, who understands the needs of patients as well as the latest in nutritional research. Her sage advice and caring involvement have healed, helped, and offered hope.

Goeffrey Proud and Joanne Dolinar, coeditors of the *Cardiovascular Wellness Newsletter*, for their fine writing and commitment to communicating the very latest in heart health research.

Keith Frankel and Ed Frankel, owners of Garden State Nutritionals, who have helped me to develop, formulate, and produce cutting-edge, twenty-first-century cardiac and insulin-regulating products.

My committed and capable staff at The Cardiovascular Wellness Centers, whose devotion to our patients is incomparable. Special thanks to my administrator, Johanna Frick, and her daughters, Suzanne and Debbie.

Don't Buy This Book!

This is not a one-size-fits-all plan for heart health. This is a special program designed specifically for the carbohydrate addict, the person who experiences intense and recurring cravings for starches, snack foods, junk foods, and sweets, and who, often without ever knowing it, has a hormonal imbalance that can lead to weight and eating struggles, diabetes, high blood pressure, blood fat problems, atherosclerosis, and if not corrected, to heart disease as well.

If you have picked up this book because you identify with the term *carbohydrate addict*, if you sometimes lose control over your eating no matter how hard you try, if you feel that healthwise you are sometimes your own worst enemy, and if you wish that you could find a deprivation-free program designed especially to fit your needs—a sane, sensible, back-to-basics program in keeping with the dietary guidelines of the American Heart Association and other major health agency dietary recommendations*—read on. A wonderful journey of discovery and freedom awaits you.

On the other hand, if you are pretty sure that you are *not* addicted to starches, snack foods, junk foods, or sweets, if you don't find that these foods trigger you to eat far too much or far more often than you intended, if you don't feel that your cravings are sabotaging your efforts to get and stay healthy, don't buy this book.

The Carbohydrate Addict's Healthy Heart Program has been designed to do one thing and do it very well: to help balance insulin levels and reduce the insulin resistance that leads to carbohydrate cravings, easy weight gain, high blood pressure, abnormal blood fats, adult-onset diabetes, and heart disease. In that one goal lies an abundance of wellness and health for the carbohydrate addict who, often without knowing it, suffers from Insulin Resistance Syndrome (also known as Syndrome X).**

On this program, as insulin levels balance and insulin resistance drops, blood pressure, blood sugar, and blood fat levels normalize; cravings disappear; and excess weight drops off (and stays off) naturally. Carbohydrate addicts who follow this program look better and feel better, and their doctors say they are healthier, showing greater improvement in heart health indicators than they ever thought possible—all without struggle or sacrifice.

So if you think you may be addicted to high-carbohydrate foods; if starches, snack foods, junk foods, or sweets have at times overpowered you; if you've lost control when you have truly tried your best—then you've come to the right program. Welcome home. We have a wonderful world of exciting change waiting just for you.

On the other hand, if you're not a carbohydrate addict, we want you to know that although none of the guidelines or recommendations in this Program should cause you harm, still, the Program is not intended for you.

Carbohydrate addicts have been shamed and blamed for too long. This is their time, their chance to claim the health and happiness they deserve. So please understand why we must be blunt and say that if you are *not* a carbohydrate addict, don't buy this book.

°The U.S. Department of Health and Human Services' *Dietary Guidelines for Americans*, 4th ed. (The U.S. Department of Agriculture); The American Heart Association's guidelines, *Eating Plan for Healthy Americans;* and The American Cancer Society's *1996 Guidelines on Diet, Nutrition, and Cancer Prevention.*

°°High blood pressure, adult-onset diabetes, excess weight (in particular, abdominal obesity), atherosclerosis, and heart disease form a cluster of diseases that are often referred to as heart disease risk factors and that, in combination, may be referred to as Syndrome X, Metabolic Syndrome, The Deadly Quartet, Insulin Resistance Syndrome, or the Diseases of Civilization.

Carbohydrate Addiction Defined

Carbohydrate addiction is a physical imbalance that leads to a compelling hunger, craving, or desire for high-carbohydrate foods—an escalating, recurring need or drive for starches, snack foods, junk foods, or sweets.

High-carbohydrate foods include, but are not limited to: bread, bagels, cake, cereal, chocolate, cookies, crackers, Danish, fruit and fruit juice, ice cream, potato chips, pasta, potatoes, pretzels, rice, pie, popcorn, and sugar-sweetened beverages.

In addition, carbohydrate act-alikes—sugar substitutes, alcoholic beverages, and monosodium glutamate (as well as free glutamates)—may trigger intense or recurring carbohydrate cravings, weight gain, or insulin-related health problems, including high blood pressure, risk-related blood fats, adult-onset diabetes, atherosclerosis, and heart disease.

As many as 75 percent of those who are overweight and have high blood pressure or risk-related blood fats are carbohydrate-addicted. Though many people may suspect there is a physical imbalance that is causing them to crave carbohydrates and gain weight easily, and that triggers or exacerbates many of their health problems, the underlying cause of their cravings and their weight and health struggles often goes undiagnosed and untreated.

The American Heart Association Guidelines and The Carbohydrate Addict's Healthy Heart Program

The Carbohydrate Addict's Healthy Heart Program is not a fad diet. It is a balanced, back-to-basics, scientifically based program that can help you correct the insulin imbalance that leads you to crave high-carbohydrate foods and can contribute to the development of heart disease. Best of all, this program can help break insulin's stranglehold on your heart health for life.

The guidelines of this program are in keeping with the current recommendations of the American Heart Association, the American Cancer Society, and the U.S. Department of Agriculture's Department of Health and Human Services.*

(continued)

Reports from these well-respected agencies offer guidelines to aid in the prevention of, among other disorders, adult-onset diabetes, obesity, cancer, high blood pressure, stroke, atherosclerosis, and heart disease. Suggestions for incorporating these agencies' dietary guidelines into your program can be found throughout this book as well as in "Incorporating Low-Fat, Low–Saturated Fat, Low-Salt, and Other Health Agency Dietary Recommendations into Your Program," on pages 307–312.

It is important to remember that only your physician can determine which health agency dietary guidelines are appropriate for you and how best to incorporate them. Before including any recommendation in your eating plan, be certain to consult your doctor.

*The U.S. Department of Health and Human Services' *Dietary Guidelines for Americans*, 4th ed. (U.S. Department of Agriculture); the American Heart Association's guidelines, *Eating Plan for Healthy Americans;* and the American Cancer Society's *1996 Guidelines on Diet, Nutrition, and Cancer Prevention.*

THE CARBOHYDRATE ADDICT'S
HEALTHY HEART PROGRAM

INTRODUCTION:
A NEW AND KINDER MEDICINE

There was a time when we ate food simply because it tasted good and gave us pleasure.

There was a time when we walked just for the enjoyment of it, and when we were done, we felt relaxed and happy.

There was a time when we viewed our bodies as givers of pleasure and life, and we felt good and secure knowing that our bodies could be trusted and relied upon.

There was a time when our doctors, and medical science in general, were held responsible for finding the source of our physical ailments, and it was expected, their job was to cure us as well.

Now, it seems, a most amazing transformation has taken place. Food is viewed as medicine, chosen for its ability to ward off an impending state of ill health rather than for the pleasure or satisfaction it gives. We keep our bodies under strict surveillance, and act as if they harbor some untrustworthy beast waiting to attack us from within—one that requires a strong hand and a disciplinarian's watchful eye. Activity, now in the form of regimented exercise, has become arduous and demanding. Pleasure has been replaced by a self-righteous sense of sacrifice and society's confirmation that by giving up all things enjoyable, we offer proof of our goodness, dedication, and self-discipline.

Each media message reinforces our sacred responsibility to fight, at all costs, the physical changes associated with growing older gracefully. In virtually every little action—or lack thereof—we live in judgment both of one another and of ourselves. In the end, in a frenzied quest for a longer life, we have lost some of the pleasure and joy that once filled our days and which made life worth living, too.

Even in illness, there is no respite. The media carry the message that according to the evaluations and statistics of some faceless group of scientists, it is we who are responsible for our own health and for our ill health as well. Although the burden of our physical well-being can be linked in part and to some degree to our own actions and choices, in the extreme this kind of thinking frees the medical establishment of virtually all accountability. Logically, this kind of responsibility shifting makes us into the presumed-guilty perpetrators of crimes against ourselves. It is time to stop blaming the victim.

> The physician is now called on to supply us with quick-fix solutions that may never cure the source of the problem.

The physician who was at one time our confidant and friend in healing, the person on whom we could rely to understand our problems, is today often called on to do little more than supply us with the magic pills—quick-fix solutions that promise to extricate us from our medical quagmire of symptoms without ever remedying the cause of the problem.

Though it is clearly not the desire of either, patient and doctor alike seem to be caught in some gladiatorlike arena in which neither can meet the other's demands. All too often, we as patients are made to feel that we are to blame for getting sick in the first place. We get the message, especially in the area of heart health, that we were given a perfect body to begin with, and had we not abused it, it would not be giving us problems now.

We are told that we should be able to stick to eating and exercise regimens that, given the many other demands with which we are trying to cope, are virtually impossible to incorporate into a normal lifestyle program or leave little time or freedom for the luxury of some simple, basic pleasures. To make matters worse, we are often made to feel guilty for taking up a physician's most valuable time when all that is required is "a little self-discipline," all too often in the form of our simple and unquestioning compliance and self-sacrifice.

> Our concerns go unaddressed, our needs unmet.
> We feel as if we are always to blame
> for our own health problems.

Our concerns go unaddressed, our needs unmet, and when we are unable to achieve ideal health, we are seen as "our own worst enemy," for in the end, we have moved into an age in which we are being told, "Patient, heal thyself."

All too often, our doctors find themselves consigned to the role of priests, hearing our confessions, judging our most private actions and inactions, then offering penances by which we might redeem both ourselves and our health. We find it difficult to go to them for help without fearing their scrutiny and chastisement, and finally, acting as if we were children, we may withhold from our own physicians the very truths that might otherwise set us free.

Nowhere is this struggle more intense than in the area of heart health, and for none is heart health more elusive and failure more prevalent than for those who suffer from the hormonal imbalance that leads to an addiction to carbohydrates. With cravings that virtually overpower them, the carbohydrate addicts have little chance of being successful with traditional weight-loss or health-enhancing eating programs. Their biology literally sets them up for failure, and instead of their intense cravings' being treated as evidence of the physical problem it is, these victims are blamed and shamed by friends, family, media; by the medical establishment at large; and even by themselves.

> Something is very wrong with this entire scenario.
> It is time for a change—
> for a new and kinder medicine.

Something is very wrong with this entire scenario. It is time for a change—for a new and kinder medicine, one more like the medical treatment we received when many of us were kids, a type of medical care that offers help instead of blame, support instead of judgment, information rather than condemnation, understanding, empathy, and the facts and simple strategies that can be used by real people, in real life, to make a real difference in their heart health—without deprivation, struggle, self-blame, or sacrifice.

In the pages that follow, you will learn about some of the most exciting and promising approaches to heart health that we have found to be especially important to the carbohydrate addict. Taken from Eastern and Western disciplines alike, from both traditional and evidence-based complementary approaches, from holistic to high tech, these remarkable advances will offer you a world of powerful alternatives you might otherwise never have discovered.

The information and recommendations you will find in these pages may surprise you. They will offer you a front-row view of the newest approaches, scientific findings, and programs that are emerging on the cutting edge of heart health research especially relevant to the carbohydrate addict.

Medical breakthroughs can take decades to filter down into common practice; many languish in unread medical journals, forgotten forever on some library shelves—potentially lifesaving discoveries that simply get lost among other, more profitable discoveries or are squelched because of vested economic interests. Some research results differ from current medical practice, and though the treatments they would support are as effective as standard protocol, if not better, they are disregarded or squelched. Even worse, they may be unfairly ridiculed by the media, whose advertising dollars may dictate which stories are given credence and which are not.

As always, you must check with your personal physician on all health-related matters. If your doctor is unaware of the research that we have included, he or she will find more than two hundred references in the back of the book to support and explain these treatments and findings. If at all possible, we encourage you to open a dialogue with your doctor, to help him or her understand your needs and preferences, and to work together on deciding the course of your future health care. Remember, the best health care is negotiated, not dictated.

In Chapter 11 you will find essential information on the ways in which, long after you have read this book, you can keep current with the wide world of heart health options available to you. Bring the alternative approaches you discover to your doctor's attention and discuss the real-life implications of all that you have learned. As a carbohydrate addict, it is vital for you to have a physician with whom you can discuss heart health care options specifically appropriate to your physical and lifestyle needs. After all, when it comes to your health, as with so many things, if you do not speak up on your own behalf, who will?

BACK TO BASICS

This, then, is not another if-you-just-did-what-you-know-is-right-you-wouldn't-be-killing-yourself health book. This is a down-to-earth, back-to-basics survival guide that will help you discover current, state-of-the-art medical breakthroughs that can help you reduce your risk for insulin-related heart disease, get healthy, and stay healthy—without blame, shame, or impossible demands.

> We will help you determine your probable risk
> for insulin-related heart problems
> and identify which simple, struggle-free steps
> can help you—without deprivation.

This book will help you to understand why you crave carbohydrates more intensely than do nonaddicted people, why your cravings are an important sign that your body is in a state of imbalance, and the ways in which restoring your body's hormonal balance can help you regain and preserve your optimal heart health. In the pages that follow, we will help you determine your probable risk for insulin-related heart problems and identify which simple, struggle-free steps can help you reduce that risk—without deprivation.

The book you now hold in your hands was written in celebration—a sharing of the most up-to-date heart health research findings available to bring you both health *and* happiness. The recommendations you will find here are simple and fun, and are designed not only to make you feel good and look good but to help you stay healthy as well. Standard, one-size-fits-all programs usually require you to make sacrifices that are impractical or genuinely not doable in the long run, especially for the carbohydrate addict. Most programs ask you to live by the numbers: counting calories or fat grams, dealing cards, measuring, or figuring percentages. Naturally slim, naturally healthy people don't live by the numbers. Neither can you—at least not for very long—for you, as a carbohydrate addict, have a physical imbalance. That imbalance must be corrected in order for you to achieve an easy and lasting success. We know what causes your addiction, and we know how to correct it.

If you are a carbohydrate addict,[*] this program has been designed es-

---

[*] For help in determining whether you are a carbohydrate addict at risk for insulin-related heart disease, take our quiz in Chapter 4.

pecially for you. It does not ask you to fight overpowering cravings or to live with hunger and deprivation, nor does it require you to follow an exercise regimen that is time-consuming or unlivable. Rather, it has been designed to correct the very hormonal imbalance that has caused your cravings and that can encourage the development of heart disease risk factors. With this program, carbohydrate addicts from around the world have achieved peace of mind, health of body, and joy of spirit—all at the same time.

If you are skeptical, if you find it difficult to believe that something as easy and promising as our program will stop your cravings and reduce your risk for insulin-related heart disease, we recommend the following: try our eating program for three days. You may be in for the biggest surprise of your life. Although we've added an extra day as a buffer zone, most carbohydrate addicts find that within the first forty-eight hours, a dramatic change occurs: their cravings for starches, snack foods, junk foods, and sweets are greatly reduced—some find their carbo hunger virtually eliminated. Energy levels soar, and a sense of well-being and peace may fill you, simply because your body is no longer forced to deal with a hormonal overload it is not equipped to handle.

Although cravings and hunger are generally greatly reduced in a matter of forty-eight hours, other insulin-related heart disease risk factors cannot be expected to reverse in a matter of days. Amazingly, triglyceride levels can be reduced within a matter of weeks (although we ourselves have documented changes within three days).

The nutritional portion of this program alone has been shown to move abnormally high blood sugar levels toward normal within a few weeks or less,* and depending on your body's metabolism and response to the program, as the weeks pass, triglyceride and cholesterol levels (total, HDL, and LDL levels) and insulin levels should all move toward normal as well. But the first and most dramatic change you will experience will be the elimination or reduction of your cravings—and *that* you can see within a matter of days!

Many have said that the lack of struggle is the true miracle of the program. Each day on the program makes it easier and more pleasurable to follow, so that with each passing day, your health-enhancing choices become a way of life.

* If you are a type II (adult-onset) diabetic on The Carbohydrate Addict's Healthy Heart Program, with—and only with—your physician's guidance, you may be able to or need to reduce your insulin-related medications (oral or injectable). Never change these medications or the dosage without your doctor's approval. Always do so only with your physician's consent and monitoring.

> Many of the guidelines that follow
> can help prevent, correct, or even reverse
> your risk for insulin-related heart disease.

SIMPLE STEPS TO EASE YOUR WAY

The medical breakthroughs that you will read about in the chapters to come are based on the work of hundreds of the world's most respected scientists. We have also incorporated the research that we ourselves have directed and knowledge gained from decades of clinical practice.

Many of the recommendations and guidelines that follow can help prevent, correct, or reverse the effects of the hormonal imbalance that causes the cravings and weight gain that many carbohydrate addicts struggle with every day of their lives and that lie at the core of a carbohydrate addict's increased risk for high blood pressure, adult-onset diabetes, excess weight (in particular, abdominal obesity), atherosclerosis, and heart disease. This cluster of diseases constitutes a group of disorders often referred to as heart disease risk factors. They may, in combination, be referred to as Syndrome X, Metabolic Syndrome, The Deadly Quartet, Insulin Resistance Syndrome, The 4-H Syndrome, or The Diseases of Civilization. The cluster is also common to polycystic ovarian syndrome (PCOS).

For more than a decade in our research and clinical practice alike, we have investigated a single cause that underlies all of these heart disease risk factors—a hormonal imbalance known by a wide variety of different names, including hyperinsulinemia, Profactor-H, and insulin (implying excess levels of insulin).

We refer to it as *hyperinsulinemia* because that is the term currently used by the American Heart Association to describe the excess release of insulin that we have found to have such a powerful effect on the heart health of the carbohydrate addict. The body's response to hyperinsulinemia, its way of protecting itself against the high levels of insulin—by literally shutting down the "gates" through which insulin and blood sugar enter and nourish muscle, nerves, organs, and other tissues—is often referred to by medical researchers as *insulin resistance*. Since this term is remarkably easy to understand (in contrast to the usual Latin jargon that fills the medical journals), we will continue to use it throughout this book, as we do in our lectures, grand rounds, research reports, and findings as well.

> For many, hyperinsulinemia (excess insulin) and insulin resistance lie at the base of high blood pressure, adult-onset diabetes, excess weight gain, and risk-related blood fats.

As appropriate, we will define in more detail these two important terms, *hyperinsulinemia* and *insulin resistance*. Chances are, you will become very comfortable with these terms and use them often as you discover how, as a carbohydrate addict, much of your health and happiness depends on a balance of both insulin and blood sugar.

For now, rest assured that all of the exciting new breakthroughs that await you will be described in understandable English rather than in medical mumbo jumbo. You will discover why you crave high-carbohydrate foods (like starches, snack foods, junk foods, and sweets) more intensely than do other people, why typical low-fat diets may not work for you, and why you may be genetically programmed to gain weight easily and/or to have an increased risk for heart disease. Most important, you will learn what you can do to reverse these hunger- and health-related problems simultaneously. Among all the other exciting things you will discover, you will learn how to communicate to others why your body is different from theirs and what you are doing to "normalize" your body—without self-sacrifice and without deprivation.

So sit back and relax as we guide you each step of the way on this amazing journey of freedom, promise, and discovery.

THE HIDDEN CONNECTION

The discovery of hyperinsulinemia's (excess insulin's) powerful effects on health answers many questions that have puzzled scientists and physicians for decades:

- Why do some people do all the "right things" and still get heart disease?
- Why do some people do all the "wrong things" and remain free of heart disease?
- Why can some people eat high-fat foods and still maintain normal blood fat levels?
- Why do some people have a difficult time controlling their eating, while others seem to do so naturally, with little effort?

INTRODUCTION: A NEW AND KINDER MEDICINE

- Why do some people gain weight so much more easily than others?
- What is the link between stress and illness? What can be done to break that link?
- Why are so few of us able to follow our physician's health recommendations consistently (even though we know they are for our own good)?
- Why do so many so-called healthy diets actually fail to prevent heart disease in so many people?

With the discovery of the insulin link to heart disease and to heart disease risk factors, answers to these questions are now emerging—and bringing with them lifesaving changes in medical care and heart disease prevention.

Over the decades the demands of our research, teaching, and patient responsibilities have required all three of us to keep up with the latest scientific discoveries—to be able, at a moment's notice, to access the findings of scientists from around the world. It is not an easy task, even for the three of us working together, but each of us has special areas of interest, knowledge, and skills. In the end, working as a team has most certainly paid off.

It was not until we made comparisons of improved health in patients and research participants and integrated the latest research findings from several different medical specialties that we came to understand the insulin link to heart disease.

A SURPRISING CHANGE OF HEART
DRS. RICHARD AND RACHAEL HELLER

We didn't anticipate it; it wasn't in the plans—personally or professionally—but life has a funny way of turning your expectations upside down, and when it happens for the good, you have to grab on to it with both hands and enjoy the ride.

When we began our research program, our sole intent was to discover and correct the physical imbalance that caused some people to crave high-carbohydrate foods to the point where they would lose control of their eating. We knew that many carbohydrate addicts also seemed to gain weight more easily and had a harder time keeping it off.

From our personal experience as well as from our research, we suspected that the hormone insulin would prove to be the culprit and that in *some* people, eating high-carbohydrate foods such as starches, snack foods, junk foods, and sweets often, throughout the day, led to *hyperinsulinemia* (excess levels of insulin in the blood). Since insulin was already known to stimulate appetite and make food taste better, it was not surprising to find that those research participants who seemed particularly "sensitive" to carbohydrates often released too much insulin when they ate these foods and, as a result, found themselves overpowered by their bodies' cravings for more of the same foods.

During our first few years of research at Mt. Sinai School of Medicine in New York, we set ourselves to the task of documenting the carbohydrate-insulin-craving link and worked hard to get the evidence that would explain to the scientific community at large the secondary impact of insulin on weight gain in these same research participants.

> Hyperinsulinemia and insulin resistance are not rare conditions. Researchers estimate that more people have these problems than do not.

In a short time, however, we realized that the excess release of insulin we were witnessing appeared to affect far more people than we had anticipated: up to 75 percent of the overweight and many normal-weight individuals as well appeared to have the physical imbalance that was causing them to intensely and repeatedly crave high-carbohydrate foods.

Our findings along with the work of other scientists soon revealed that hyperinsulinemia appeared to affect the majority of Americans—in fact, a far greater number of people seemed to have this "excess of insulin" than did not. What we found even more startling was the fact that many people had no idea they were releasing far too much insulin and so were completely unaware of the impact it was having on their health and their lives.

Soon it became increasingly clear that whereas some people who had a hyperinsulinemic response to high-carbohydrate foods experienced the telltale cravings that are the hallmark of this imbalance, others showed no outward signs of having this hormonal imbalance at all. We were concerned about these "hidden" carbohydrate addicts as well. With no sign or clue, their physical well-being—in particular, their heart health—might be in the same grave jeopardy as those who knew they had this physical imbalance and were aware of its health-threatening potential. We were unsure as to what to do and where to go, though we were certain of one thing: we could not do all of the research alone.

Fortunately, at the same time, other scientists were also beginning to report the power of this silent killer. Research results were soon pointing to the conclusion that millions of people were destined for poor health and, in some cases, needlessly dying from the harmful changes brought on by excess insulin levels—an imbalance that very few, if any, ever suspected they might have.

For most of our lives, the three of us had unknowingly suffered the weight and health problems that came from hyperinsulinemia, and together we had devoted our joint professional careers to conquering this medical mystery. Almost from the start, the results indicated we might very well be successful in all that we had envisioned—and more.

Simply by reducing their insulin levels, up to 80 percent of our research participants were able to reach their goal weight and maintain their weight loss without struggle. This accomplishment was, in itself, our dream come true. But then something unexpected—and wonderful—happened. Report after report began to pour in, each one documenting that along with weight loss, there were unmistakable improvements in health and well-being. Our readers and research participants now totaled more than half a million, and more and more letters arrived every day.

We heard it over and over again, from readers, research participants, research scientists, nutritionists, and physicians: along with the weight loss came wonderful and unexpected improvements in health and well-being, especially in the area of heart disease risk factors:

- Blood pressure levels that had been dangerously high for years were approaching normal.
- Total cholesterol levels had decreased by as much as 25 to 60 percent.
- Good cholesterol (HDL) levels were rising.
- Undesirable cholesterol (LDL) levels were falling.
- Dangerous, though less publicized, triglyceride levels plummeted.
- Blood-clotting abnormalities, important aspects of arteriosclerosis and heart disease, normalized.
- Energy levels and motivation to exercise greatly improved.
- Many adult-onset diabetics showed even greater improvements, including better blood sugar control, and, in some cases, with their doctors' monitoring and guidance, they were able to greatly reduce insulin therapy or stop it altogether.

Each letter seemed a testimony to the fact that by both their own and others' standards, our research participants and our readers as well were not only feeling better and looking better; they were getting better, too! Blood tests and physicians' reports confirmed that day by day they were reducing, or in many cases reversing, their risk for insulin-related heart disease and, best of all, in so doing, they were greatly improving their chances of living long, happy, productive, and healthy lives.

We tried not to get too caught up in the excitement (although it was difficult). At first we assumed that the unexpected bonus of heart health experienced by our readers and research participants was due to their loss of weight. Many of them had lost twenty-five, fifty, and, in some cases even a hundred or more pounds. Still, not all of the people on our program were overweight. Some chose to follow our guidelines because they were tired of struggling to keep their weight within normal limits and enjoyed the freedom from cravings our program provided. These research participants and readers had little or no weight to lose; yet as they continued on the program, they reported the same heart health benefits as others who had lost far more weight. Since even these normal-weight research participants and readers were showing significantly lower levels of risk, weight loss could not be assumed to account for their new and welcome health improvements.

So we searched for a different factor, a common denominator that all of our people, overweight and normal-weight alike, shared—one that might explain the improvements seen in both groups. We knew that it couldn't be age or sex or ethnic group or socioeconomic level. Our readers and research participants came from every background and from every walk of life. We knew that we weren't the cause of the change—not directly, anyway—for the vast majority of reports came from medical professionals as well as readers who had never met us!

In the end, one such phone call forced us to admit to ourselves that the obvious common denominator had lain before us all along but was so simple, so amazingly obvious, that we could barely imagine that it held so crucial a key to heart health.

A MESSAGE FROM THE HEART
DR. FREDERIC VAGNINI

My job is simple; my task is clear. I am a cardiovascular surgeon. I am also a medical specialist in the field of cardiovascular health and disease. Whenever possible, I use my expertise in my medical specialty so that patients need never require help from my surgical specialty.

With the exception of my surgical skills, for decades, the only weapon I had in my arsenal for preventing and reversing heart disease was black-and-white and, unfortunately, not always read all over. Research was the sword on which I counted to cut through the fog of misinformation that surrounded heart health care in this country more than three decades ago. Although media medical reports proclaimed that modern medicine was winning the war on heart disease, I was in touch with the real-life pain and struggle of those for whom current recommendations were simply not working.

> Traditional medicine was not exactly failing my patients, but it was not always helping them to succeed either.

Some of my patients were simply unable to stick to demanding and unforgiving eating restrictions and exercise requirements; others were unable to tolerate the side effects of certain medications or of multiple drug interactions. Although most of my patients did their absolute best, still, they were not doing as well as they and I thought they should. Traditional medical approaches were not exactly failing them, but they were not always helping them to succeed either.

I knew that each new scientific finding could hold the ultimate "key" to my patients' heart health and, in some cases, could mean the difference between life and death. Each piece of research required time and thought and more research, but in the end, no one could ask for a better payback than seeing the research literally breathe life into those who needed it.

From the heart-related benefits of antioxidants to the then revolutionary research in dietary fiber and saturated fats and the discovery of the importance of a new variety of vitamins, amino acids, and minerals, each new finding opened doors of opportunity for heart disease risk reduction. As I saw the wonders that these supplements—in combination with diet and other lifestyle changes—could achieve, I knew it was essential to get this information to as many people as possible.

These were the days when most physicians dealt with heart disease after the fact. *Preventive medicine* was a brand-new term and, as with so many things in this field, was treated with some suspicion. Perhaps some of these physicians had not seen the compelling research that I had; perhaps they had not seen the amazing changes I had witnessed as one after another of my patients turned their lives and health around; perhaps some were too set in their ways. Whatever the reason, it didn't matter.

I had seen the power that my patients had to avoid the heart problems that so many physicians believed to be inevitable, and I wasn't giving up without a fight. I preached my risk-reduction gospel wherever I could. Listeners to my *Heart Show* on WABC and, later, WOR radio, dubbed me "The Prevention Doctor."

At the time it was meant as just an affectionate nickname, but as preventive medicine's power to save lives has become recognized and respected, it is a name that I continue to wear proudly and try very hard to live up to.

Over the years I found that by combining my traditional medical training in conventional heart disease treatment with the wide world of alternative and complementary medicine, I was able to choose from a whole array of complementary approaches to best suit the needs of my listeners and patients.

> My anger grew as I witnessed, firsthand,
> that too many of my patients were
> losing their battle with heart disease
> through no fault of their own.

At times, current medications—alone or in combination—seemed the best strategy. Although some of the vast array of drugs available and sometimes pressed on patients offered them much-needed help, too many drugs had too many side effects, and for some, the problems they encountered far outweighed the benefits. I came to see many of my stalwart patients as the quiet heroes they were. My anger grew as I witnessed, firsthand, that too many people were losing their battle with heart disease through no fault of their own. For some, the vitamins and other supplements were sandbags unable to keep back the rising river of heart disease.

I was caught on a treadmill of conscience. My patients as well as listeners to my radio show and those who tuned in each weekend to watch me on *Fox Weekend on Health* knew me and trusted me; many counted on me to bring them alternatives to traditional treatments that were failing them. Others relied on my evaluations of new drugs and nutritional supplements and knew that I would give them my honest opinion of the pros and cons of each new treatment, drug, supplement, operation, or protocol. Still, with many of the strategies nothing seemed to fit together and explain why heart disease occurred in some; for others these approaches were clearly not enough. And I couldn't figure out why.

Nobody seemed able to fit together the pieces of the puzzle so that those behaviors we call "risk factors" and "lifestyle considerations" made any real sense in terms of predicting and preventing heart disease. So in 1993, when I first learned about the Hellers' insulin-balancing eating program, I found an effective, livable solution that not only provided an answer to my patients' prayers but, in addition, as you will see, proved to be the answer to my own prayers as well.

> **The Hellers' insulin-balancing program made good sense, good science, and good medicine.**

The Hellers' insulin-balancing program made good sense, good science, and good medicine. It explained and complemented what I already knew about preventive medicine and added a further key component of insulin balance and reduction of insulin resistance. Their eating program literally changed my life, and of paramount importance to me, it has also done the same for so many of my patients.

As you will read in the coming pages, I lost more than ninety pounds and have continued to keep my weight off for almost a decade—with none of the typical sacrifice that I and my patients had experienced on so many other "weight-loss" or "health-enhancement" programs. Today I look and feel as I wish I had twenty years ago (more about that in the next chapter), and what is more, I see the same kind of changes in my patients, too.

> **I lost more than ninety pounds and watched as my heart disease risk factors disappeared.**

As my own blood tests and those of my patients confirmed, for those on the Hellers' eating program, a significant reduction in insulin-related heart disease risk factors is the rule rather than the exception. But when I combined the Hellers' program with my own repertoire of heart health–enhancing strategies, I was in for a real surprise. In combination, the Hellers' eating program and my prevention and treatment approaches achieved the greatest improvement in heart health I had ever witnessed.

The reason for my patients' astounding success was that many of my heart health–enhancing strategies corrected or prevented, directly or indirectly, the very insulin overload that the Hellers recognized and addressed in their program. Indeed, without knowing it, we were approaching the same issues in heart disease and heart health from two different but complementary positions. Taken alone, each of our approaches worked well. Combined, each multiplied the effectiveness of the other, many times over.

After a simple phone call to the Hellers to tell them of the astounding success I was witnessing, we were a team, sharing information and inspiring one another. It was as if we had each been waiting for this opportunity to work together. As the saying goes, a burden shared is lighter, whereas joy shared is greater. Each new discovery and connection sent us to the phone so that we could share our excitement with one another as the newest "piece" fit into the emerging heart health puzzle and brought us one step closer to a complete understanding of this vast and complex picture medicine calls "heart health."

The book you hold in your hands is the result of that work—the whole puzzle, assembled and laid out, with the whole picture clear and visible for all to see. *The Carbohydrate Addict's Healthy Heart Program* is the product of hard work and commitment and countless late nights spent reading and taking notes and reading some more. It is in great part as well the gift of hundreds and hundreds of patients and research participants who were willing to share their experiences so that others might benefit from their failures, their insights, and their ultimate successes.

The insulin-balancing eating component of this program alone has been used by more than 1.5 million people on three continents. The entire Carbohydrate Addict's Healthy Heart Program, however, holds an even greater promise of success by providing a breakthrough approach for the prevention and potential reversal of heart disease and its many risk factors.

This, then, is our sincerest wish, from Drs. Richard and Rachael Heller and myself: May this program bring to you, as it has to each of us and to our research participants and patients alike, a new and kinder medicine, a simple solution to your fears and concerns that brings with it the precious gift of health—and life.

PART ONE

THE HEART OF THE MATTER

YOUR PERSONAL

HEART HEALTH PROFILE

1

THREE WISHES FOR A SECOND CHANCE

Chance favors the prepared mind. —*Louis Pasteur*

In the game of life, it was the bottom of the ninth, and the three of us were about to strike out: out of hope, out of luck, and out of time. But we did not strike out. Instead, we turned our lives around and took back our health (together with our energy, sanity, and joy).

In the pages to come, you will learn about the scientific discovery that literally gave us back our lives. You will learn, too, how you can break free from insulin's powerful potential for heart disease—and stay free.

First, come join us as we share our stories with you, for our discovery comes not only from mountains of scientific literature, books, and test tubes but from the difficult lessons that life has provided us as well.

SO PERFECT A PURPOSE:
DR. RACHAEL HELLER'S STORY

I believe that things happen for a reason or, at least, that with the right attitude something good can come out of even the worst of experiences. I never really stopped believing this, although, for many years, when the challenges were hard and I was very young, I could have argued the other side quite well.

I don't have the simple childhood memories that so many people have of friends and playing games, of parties and adventures, and of a whole wide world to discover and explore. I remember sadness and pain and a permeating truth that seemed to shape my every action and every thought.

> **In a child's world of wanting to belong,
> I lived with the unforgiving fact that I was different.**

In a child's world of wanting to belong, I lived with the unforgiving fact that I was different: I was fat. And every interaction—from my brother's unrelenting teasing to my classmates' ridicule to strangers' disapproving stares—told me in word and look that being fat was a very bad thing and, what was worse, that I was to blame.

My parents, though thin in their youth, fought a losing battle with their weight as they approached their late thirties. By the time that each had reached forty, there were clear signs of oncoming heart problems. My mother's blood pressure was out of control, and both my parents showed the telltale signs of diabetes. Within a few short years, my father's blood pressure was far above normal. My mother had suffered three heart attacks, and we lived with an oxygen tank in the closet. I slept lightly, listening for any signs of her distress. In the blink of an eye, within four short years, they were both gone—my father at fifty-two, my mother at fifty-five.

My older brother, fearful of becoming overweight and suffering the same ill health as my parents, chose what he considered an acceptable alternative, but within a short time he was as addicted to diet pills as he had been to junk foods and sweets. When he added other addictions to his repertoire, his immune system failed. He never saw his fortieth birthday, losing a long and terrible battle to a rare form of leukemia that preyed on his already-compromised body.

> **Before I was out of my twenties,
> both my parents and my older brother had died.
> I was young, alone, sick, fat, and desperately poor.**

I was young and alone, and most of all, I was sick and fat as well. I had no money, no real friends, and no one to whom I could turn. I had just been witness to what could be likened to a terrible automobile accident, and although I wanted desperately to avoid the collision myself, nothing I did seemed to make any difference. I had dreams of being behind the wheel of an old car, and though I saw it heading for a crash, I could not make the brakes respond. I stomped my foot on the brake pedal, I tried desperately to turn the wheel, I even tried to open the door and jump out, but nothing I did had any effect. And I awoke in terror to find that my nightmare was simply a reflection of my waking reality.

Some people say that, although they had been chubby as kids, they never suffered any health-related problems until they hit middle age. Not me. At twelve years of age, I was hospitalized for stroke-level hypertension. My blood pressure was 220/120, and I was twice my normal weight. Though not yet in my teens, I had already become a "high-risk patient." My menstrual periods had stopped, and my belly, sides, back, shoulders, and arms were already scarred with deep-purple stretch marks.

> As a teenager, when I should have been concerned
> with friends and dresses and parties,
> I was trying to cope with staying alive.

Long before I ever kissed a boy, I had become familiar with terms like *hypertension, stroke,* and *coronary artery disease*—warnings, said the doctors, of things to come. I had become knowledgeable about death and illness before I knew anything about life and love. At a time when I should have been concerned with friends and dresses and parties, I was trying to cope with staying alive.

Upon discharge from the hospital, I was given no medication and virtually no help. "Lose weight and bring down that blood pressure," cautioned one doctor, "or you'll never . . ." Embarrassed, he looked up into my young face, ruffled my hair, and walking down the hall, called back, "Take care now, hear?"

Knowing of no other alternatives, I did what I saw adults do then and what many still do today. I continued the same practices that had proved unsuccessful in the first place, promising myself that this time I would try harder.

I tried harder and harder and harder, but the results never improved. At fourteen they hospitalized me again, this time trying to determine the cause of headaches, foggy thinking, and an odd assortment of seemingly unrelated symptoms such as panic attacks and sweating. I was addicted to diet pills by this time and used the hospital stay as a chance to break the drugs' hold on me. Still, my doctors were intent on finding a cause for my neurological problems. Had they but checked my insulin and blood sugar levels after I ate high-carbohydrate foods, they would have uncovered the blood sugar swings that were causing these classic hypoglycemic responses. Instead, they did a multitude of brain scans and EEGs and were never able to find proof of the petit mal epilepsy they believed to be responsible for my symptoms.

Back at home, the torrent of teasing, ridicule, and humiliation that filled my every waking moment was unspeakable, and had I been able to do anything—anything—about it at all, I would have. And though doctors told my parents that I obviously didn't want to lose weight or I would have done so, they were terribly wrong.

> To me, a typical adolescence would *not* have been a time of turmoil and distress. It was my fondest wish.

I know now that, like my parents and brother before me, I was the unfortunate victim of a physical imbalance that caused me to gain weight easily and to crave starches, snack foods, junk foods, and sweets with an intensity that I could hold off for only so long. My body ached for these high-carbohydrate foods, it screamed for them, and though at times I literally cried as I ate them, I could not stop myself. Sometimes I would eat them until I was sick, then fall into a semistupor of sleep or walk around in a kind of drugged fog.

My weight climbed, and the state of my health plummeted. By seventeen I weighed more than three hundred pounds. My blood pressure remained dangerously high, and my heart was unable to handle the strain. By my midteens I had developed an irregular heartbeat and a murmur; a young heart that should have been healthy and strong was literally being torn apart from within. Now any exertion brought heart pain. It was not long before I was diagnosed with adult-onset diabetes. In high school I spent most of my senior year at home, though I'm not sure whether I really felt ill or just wanted to avoid my classmates' unrelenting abuse.

The irony of this horrendous state of affairs is that I had done everything in my power to lose weight and get healthy. At nine years of age, I had a weekly appointment with a weight-loss doctor. I was a veteran of diets and diet pills by the time I was eleven. A year later I knew the calorie count of every food in the supermarket. From diet pills to diet pops, from cellulose cookies to calorie counting, I had tried them all before I had even hit my teens. Nothing worked.

With each new weight-loss approach, the story was the same. I would boost my motivation, talk myself into action and commitment, and be successful for a few days or a few weeks. Then, sooner or later, the cravings would return, and I would find myself out of control. With each attempt I became more frustrated, angry with myself, fatter, and sicker. I was clearly in a lose-lose situation with regard to just about everything. I couldn't give up, and it made no sense to keep trying. But keep trying I did—every new book, new approach, new diet. I would try it, and though with each new attempt I felt my enthusiasm wane, I still gave it my best. In the long run, I always failed. Then I'd wait until I couldn't stand it any longer, and I would try something new.

> Every new diet, book, product—I would try it.
> In the long run, I always failed.
> Then I'd wait until I couldn't stand it any longer,
> and I would try something new.
> In the end, the only thing I lost was my health.

On commercial weight-loss programs, I watched my weight go down—then up again. I repeated this frustrating and disheartening process six or eight times over. I tried Atkins (becoming very ill by following his entry program for too long), hypnosis, Metrecal, behavioral therapy—you name it, I tried it. I drank it, measured it, weighed it, and exchanged it. Whatever it took, I tried it. But nothing took the weight off and kept it off. I founded the Philadelphia chapters of Overeaters Anonymous. I even tried water fasts (once for forty-two days while I continued working and going to school). But it was the same old story we all know too well.

In the end, the only thing I lost was my health. The years slipped by, marked mostly by which weight-loss program I was currently following. By the time I was in my thirties, my health had become seriously impaired. My heartbeat was irregular, and I had already suffered at least one episode of tachycardia (in which the heart literally beats out of control and no longer productively pumps blood). My high blood pressure was wearing down my cardiovascular system, and it was only a matter of time before my heart simply gave out.

> By the time I was thirty-five,
> my triglyceride level was three times normal,
> I was twice my normal weight,
> and my body was literally collapsing.

At that time blood pressure medication was not something that was typically given to people my age, so each new visit to the doctor brought only more blame and shame and yet another preprinted diet sheet. With the advent of routine blood fat testing, a triglyceride level of more than 350 (more than three times the ideal level) left both me and my doctor speechless.

At thirty-five the rest of my body started to show the effects of the high blood fats, blood sugar swings, and excess weight. I was in pain almost all the time; my feet and knees were collapsing under the pressure. The blood sugar swings left me in a fog for hours. I was irritable and unhappy and devoid of hope. A cold and searing pain clutched my heart whenever I exerted myself at all. My heart was enlarged, and the lining that surrounded it was inflamed. My life was slipping away, like grains of sand between my fingers, without ever having been lived, and somehow, for some reason, though I really tried my best, everyone said I was responsible for this dismal situation.

> My body seemed to be some kind of "fat machine,"
> making blood fats and body fat by the carload.
> Then my salvation came in a phone call.

Like my parents and brother before me, I was well on my way to an early death. With each doctor's visit or hospital discharge, I was cautioned to watch my weight and my diet, but I had tried that over and over again, and though I nodded in agreement, and though I knew I could be a very determined and strong person in other areas of my life, deep down I knew that no diet ever had, or ever would, work for me. Still, though I just didn't know what else to do, I could not let myself give up.

My exercise regimen was exhausting. Had I seen results, I would have stuck with it, but I ached all over each time I finished a session, and I was just too tired to keep it up. For all the discomfort, it simply didn't seem to make that much of a difference.

My body seemed to be some kind of "fat-making machine," turning all the food I ate into fat instead of burning some of it as energy. Even when I mustered every bit of strength and forced myself to hold on and not give in, I seemed to gain weight on the same amount of food that caused others to shed pounds. And to make matters worse, as my body fat increased, so did the levels of fat in my blood. I was desperate, watching myself spiraling into a pit, knowing I was to blame for my own failure, but unable to pull out of the tailspin.

My salvation came in the form of a phone call—one of those unimportant things that seems like a simple annoyance at the time but, in retrospect, becomes a turning point in your life.

The ringing phone shook me from my sleep, and the X-ray technician informed me that my early-morning appointment had been changed to four in the afternoon. "Now don't forget, you can't eat anything between now and then. Liquids like coffee or tea are okay, but nothing to eat."

> At nearly 270 pounds, the thought of not eating all day threw me into a panic.

At nearly 270 pounds, the thought of not eating all day threw me into a panic, but I could figure no way out. Steeling myself to the task, I headed for work and, I thought, a day of torture. I was director of student services at a private school, and although my day would normally have been filled with counseling sessions and meetings, the postponement of my X ray left me with a day free to catch up on my paperwork. Still, the thought of the long hours ahead, without food or diversion, made the day stretch endlessly before me. Amazingly, the hours passed quickly, and even more surprising, I was far less hungry than usual. Coffee break time came and went. I worked right through lunch. I barely thought of food. My energy remained high, and my ability to concentrate seemed better. My usual midafternoon slump failed to appear, and as I headed out to my X-ray appointment, I experienced a sense of well-being that I could not remember ever having felt before.

I arrived at my appointment in wonderful spirits. As I entered the hospital for the X ray, I was aware of feeling somehow liberated from the clouded thinking and cravings and tiredness that had filled me for so long. Despite this, I had brought along two French crullers, tucked away in a brown paper bag, ready to revive and nourish me in the dressing room after my X ray.

The X ray completed, I headed out for a well-earned dinner, my crullers still in the bag, uneaten and unneeded. Dinner was wonderful. I don't think I had ever tasted so marvelous a meal, before or since. As a reward, I ordered everything I wanted: soup, salad, bread and lots of butter, pasta, veal parmigiana, and coffee. Though I was more than satisfied, I slowly relished my crullers on the way home. I was satisfied in body but not in mind, as I chastised myself for ruining a wonderful day of fasting with a meal that would surely put on the pounds.

But I was in for a surprise. The next morning my weight had dropped by two pounds. I checked and rechecked—moved the scale around the bathroom floor as I usually did in a vain attempt to bring the numbers down. Now I was trying to get the scale to balance at a higher weight so that I could make sense out of what it was saying. Try as I might, however, my weight remained two pounds lower than the day before. Water weight, I told myself. It will be back in a day or two.

Still, something in me, a well-trained scientist combined with a bit of a gambler at heart, dared me to try it again, and taking up the challenge turned out to be the chance of a lifetime.

The next day went almost as easily as the first, except for the games my mind began playing with me. I told myself that I couldn't skip breakfast and lunch again (though I knew I had done it so easily the day before). I felt great, but the voices in my head kept chipping away at my confidence. I compromised by getting a cup of coffee and two more crullers to be put away as my after-dinner treat. I promised myself the best dinner ever, though deep inside I wondered whether I might not give in and have those crullers before the end of the day.

The afternoon flew by, and before I could torture myself with the question of "to cruller or not to cruller," it was time to leave work. I wanted to enjoy dinner in the privacy of my own home, so assuming I would add some special goodies I had waiting at home, I stopped by my favorite pizza restaurant and ordered a giant pizza slice (a small pie in its own right), half of one of the large submarine sandwiches, and a Greek salad, all of which I proceeded to take home. The meal was delicious! I ate it all, though at the end I struggled to get everything down. That had never happened before! And, try as I might, I could not face the chips and cookies that awaited me on the shelves. I could barely eat one of my crullers, and as I sat and thought about my reduced appetite, I wondered whether it could in some way be connected to not eating all day.

I considered that perhaps my stomach had shrunk. I wasn't sure how accurate that was from a biological standpoint, and I also knew it wouldn't explain my lack of hunger and the increased clarity in thinking I had experienced all day. My typical headaches were gone, and even the discomfort in my chest had vanished. Most amazing of all was the satisfaction that I felt after the meal. I felt more complete than I had ever remembered feeling after eating. It was wonderful.

The next morning—the third day—brought even more confirmation. I didn't wake up hungry as I normally would after a big dinner, and as unbelievable as it was to me, I had lost another pound. I didn't know what was causing it, but I was on a roll, and nothing could have convinced me to stop what I was doing.

> Nothing made sense.
> I was doing everything they said was wrong,
> but I felt better and was less hungry
> than I had ever remembered feeling.

Afraid to change a thing, I followed the same eating plan for several weeks, with similar results. I continued to lose two to three pounds each week, and my cravings were literally gone! I felt better than I had in years, and for the first time in as long as I could remember, I had renewed hope and—I was almost afraid to think it—a way out.

And what a way out it was. As the weeks passed, I began to test foods to see whether some could be added as breakfast or lunch foods without bringing on the cravings and weight gain that had ruled my life for so long. I was afraid to meddle with something that was working so well, but if I could, I wanted the freedom and pleasure of eating more than one meal a day (no matter how good that single meal might be). Slowly and methodically, I discovered a wide array of high-fiber and protein-rich foods that satisfied me, kept me free of cravings, and still enabled me to enjoy what I had come to refer to as my "reward meal." And I was losing weight all the while.

> My weight, blood pressure, and blood fat levels
> dropped so dramatically
> that my doctor didn't believe the results.

At the time I didn't understand why it worked. All I cared about was the fact that it did work. I lost more than 150 pounds over the next eighteen months (later I lost another 15 pounds without even trying!), and I kept it off—struggle-free—for more than fourteen years. With each passing day, it seemed that I was growing healthier as well. My blood pressure was so much better than at my last visit that my doctor thought something was wrong with his blood pressure cuff!

My blood tests showed such great changes in my triglyceride levels that he questioned the accuracy of the report. With repeated testing my doctor was at a loss to explain the wonderful results. I wasn't. It all made sense to me: whatever had been driving me, pushing me to crave high-carbohydrate foods, was gone, and everything else seemed to be righting itself as well.

> **I know with an unshakable certainty that the most difficult of experiences may hold a perfect purpose.**

Our bodies are amazingly resilient. When we stop hurting them, they stop hurting us. The long battles that had filled my thoughts and dreams were over. Gradually, in the months that followed, my heart murmur disappeared, and my heartbeat became regular and strong. My headaches disappeared, as did my panic attacks and mood swings. Even my knees and feet stopped hurting. With each passing day, I grew stronger and more confident, healthier and happier. Life was good, and though I hardly dared to believe it, my personal nightmare was over.

In time I met the man who was to become my loving husband, partner, coauthor, and colleague. Together we would discover the scientific basis for this simple but effective way of eating that had set me free and would soon do the same for more than 1.5 million others.

Still, when I look back in wonder at all that has gone before, I know with an unshakable certainty that, although we may be tempted to deny it in hard times, and despite the fact that we may never understand it all, the most difficult of experiences may hold within them so perfect a purpose and answers long sought.

THE DOMINO EFFECT:
DR. RICHARD HELLER'S STORY

I was racing against the clock. "Can you keep it up?" the technician asked. "Are you okay?" I smiled to myself. My feet seemed to move on their own. I could barely feel the moving belt of the treadmill below me. My body seemed to be running with virtually no effort. What would have been an exhausting and torturous exertion in the past was now a confidence-building challenge.

"How old did you say you were?" the technician queried, checking his chart once again. "Jeez," he exclaimed to the young man he was training. "He's way past 100 percent capacity. This guy's got the heart of someone half his age."

My story is simple, but for me, it has its own quiet wonder. I was a chubby, happy, healthy child; a stocky teenager; and a strapping young man. I was strong and healthy, and I loved feeling fit. I would have thought that all my jogging, swimming, and general physical activities would have kept me naturally slim, but they didn't. Though I didn't like to admit it, keeping my weight in line was a bit of a struggle. It seemed I was in a never-ending battle to maintain control over my expanding waist and my "love handles." Still, except for a few extra pounds, I was young and healthy. I assumed I would always be that way.

> My parents had been active and healthy.
> I was active and healthy as well.
> And, I assumed, I always would be.

I came from what is often referred to as "good stock." My parents had been healthy all their lives, too, or at least their rare visits to doctors had never revealed any obvious problems.

I excelled in competitive swimming in college, and had I not come to the sport in my early twenties (too late to compete actively), I was told that I would have been Olympic material. All through my thirties, although a little stocky, I was the picture of good health. I jogged fifty to sixty miles a week and told everyone that I just loved the good feeling that running gave me. The truth be told, my early-morning runs had more to do with keeping my weight down than my feelings up. Often when I was jogging, I wondered why I was out torturing myself.

My father had been strong, healthy, and powerful all his life. As he approached middle age, the pounds came on slowly, and almost without our noticing it, my once-slim father had quite a bit of a tummy. It never seemed important, and though, from time to time, we would tease him about his expanding waistline or his increasing love of snack foods and sweets, we never realized these were indications that he was in the early stages of diabetes and heart risk–related problems.

Within a few short years, he suffered a heart attack followed almost immediately by a stroke. He died in a matter of days. I was away at the time, and my mother refused to allow the tragic news to interrupt my "well-earned vacation." She was a very practical woman and told me that since my brother was with her to take care of everything, my coming home early would serve no purpose other than to ruin a much-deserved rest that I desperately needed.

In the end, I never got a chance to say good-bye to my father, and in many ways, not being there for his funeral allowed me to pretend in my mind that he was still alive. On some level I never came to grips with the fact that the generational buffer that had stood between me and my own mortality was gone.

My mother had buried her grief by the time I returned and hardly ever spoke of it to me. When I visited, it was as if my dad were at work or out visiting a friend. His clothes remained as they had always been, arranged neatly in closets and drawers, his bed untouched. It was easier for both of us to act as if nothing had happened. She missed him, she would say, and on occasion she would cry. I would hold her, but at the same time, neither of us ever forced the other to face the finality of his leaving.

By not fully experiencing my father's death, I allowed myself to deny my own mortality as well, and one by one, I began to allow small but significant signs in my body to go unnoticed—signs that I should have known were lining up like dominoes ready to fall, one after another, until the entire row collapsed, taking my health, and perhaps my life, down with it.

> **As I reached my early forties, everything seemed to fall apart.**

As I reached my early forties, however, everything seemed to fall apart. Time was passing, and I was showing signs of declining strength, health, and well-being. Within the university, even a full professor's monetary compensations are rather meager when there is a family involved. In order to earn more money, I took on part-time teaching positions one by one, in addition to my full-time teaching load. It was not uncommon for me to teach classes at two or three colleges outside the university while continuing my full-time duties. Though my ex-wife's income was desperately needed to support her desired lifestyle, she had quit her teaching position to return to school, leaving yet another financial gap for me to fill. Still, above all, I took pride in being a good husband and father and, without complaint, took on most of the child-care responsibilities as well. I worked like a maniac and felt like superman.

> I was a super father and super husband, and I couldn't afford to stop and heed the signs of approaching disaster.

My typical work day began at 6:30 in the morning preparing for lectures or marking papers that might have remained ungraded from the night before, and I continued with teaching, mentoring, research, and committee responsibilities throughout the day without a break until midnight (when I finished the laundry and packed the kids' sandwiches—including little jokes and love notes that they always expected—for the next day).

In addition to my insane full- and part-time workloads, I loved the role of Mr. Mom. I made hot dinners for the family, prepared cool lectures for my students, and lived a decidedly lukewarm existence. Relatives, friends, and colleagues looked upon me with awe. My power was undeniable, my ability legendary . . . but I didn't stop to heed the signs of approaching disaster. It was like standing on a railroad track oblivious to the oncoming train racing toward me from behind.

By the time I literally dropped into my bed at night, I was so tired that I truly could not think. I was so exhausted, I simply didn't care about anything. Like a hamster on some kind of crazy exercise wheel, I couldn't seem to stop. During the day, I grabbed whatever was quickest to eat in order to keep up my energy, and as the meals and snacks-on-the-run took their toll, my expanding waist became a full-fledged belly. My tummy was more than a bit bigger than my father's had been, but I never allowed myself to see that the pattern of the father was repeating itself in the son.

Day after day, month after month, year after year, the dominoes of stress, tiredness, poor eating, worry, lack of sleep, lack of pleasure and joy, each in its own time and to its own degree, began to form a perfect line, ready for the first touch or breeze to begin the almost inevitable sequence of collapse.

> The signs of oncoming heart problems were lining up, like dominoes ready to fall.

It all started with the surprise anniversary party that I had been planning. It looked as if it was going to come off perfectly, but in the end, I was the one who was in for a surprise. All the plans I had made were coming together wonderfully, and I knew my wife didn't suspect a thing. She had been sent away to boarding schools as a young girl and never really had a birthday party. We married when she was very young, and with the children coming so soon, all of our attention went to them. I very much wanted to give her this anniversary party as a special gift of love and appreciation.

> There was always more to do and no time to get it done. As hard as I tried, I just couldn't seem to get it all under control.

It was one of those precious moments of joy, the kind you never forget, the kind you think happen only in some romantic movie. But this one I was going to make come true. Still, one thing marred the excitement: I had been having pains in my chest for at least a week, and though I told myself that they were just "muscle cramps," I couldn't deny what I knew to be the typical signs of an impending heart problem. One at a time, the dominoes were becoming less stable.

The night of the party, I could barely drive home. My body was screaming for rest. I had been grabbing food on the run, even more than usual. I simply didn't have enough time to do everything. My daughters had sore throats that week, and each got sick at a different time; two unplanned trips to the doctor pushed my already impossible schedule past endurance.

It all started around five in the afternoon on the day of the party. I had finished shopping for food for the week and for the party, the laundry was done, and I had just picked up my daughters from their friend's house. I told myself that the only things on the agenda were a quick bath and dinner for the kids so that I could get them ready for bed before the guests arrived.

The kids were quieter than usual, and instead of being thankful, I was concerned that they might be getting sick again. I wasn't feeling so well myself. Although I longed for sleep, I knew I had a very special party to host, so I steeled myself for the long evening ahead. My eyes desperately wanted to close, and I battled continually to keep them open.

Earlier in the week I had fought off some chest pain, waited it out, and willed it to be gone. I simply didn't have the time and energy to deal with it. Now, as I felt the ache return deep in my chest, I brushed it aside and went back to all the things still undone.

> **I fought off the chest pain, waited it out, and willed it to be gone. I simply didn't have the time to deal with it.**

Our guests arrived in good spirits, and the evening looked as if it was going to be a solid success, but as I reached down to pick up my youngest daughter to carry her off to bed, a giant fist closed around my chest. I couldn't breathe, I couldn't move, I could barely stay focused. I was struck by the thought of being carried out on an ambulance litter as friends stood silently by. "What a surprise that would make," I thought wryly.

For a while I had considered raising the amount of my life insurance coverage. Now, all I could do was blame myself for putting it off. I was going to die, and I should have taken better care of my family.

I will never know how I managed to do it, but somehow I forced myself to continue to smile and say all the right things. I have a high threshold for pain. I've had root canals performed without benefit of anesthetic. For better or worse, this inborn gift helped me keep up my facade. Late in the evening, the grip on my chest loosened a bit, but even as it faded, I could still feel the deep soreness that reminded me that all was not well. The dominoes had rocked violently, but they hadn't tumbled down, and I was grateful for that.

When the guests had departed, I dragged myself to the bedroom, barely able to think or talk. I promised my wife that I would clean up in the morning and was asleep in an instant. The next day was filled with post-party cleanup and a zoo trip I had promised my daughters. My wife was meeting a friend at her school library, so I told myself I didn't have time to go to the doctor. Besides, the pain had subsided—for the time being at least.

Over the next few weeks, the tightness in my chest returned again and again. I started getting used to it; I felt it more often than not. I had myself convinced that it was just a muscle strain from picking up my daughters or sitting in a bad position or one of those rib muscles that takes quite a while to heal. A few days after the party, when I finally got around to applying for an increase in life insurance, I realized that I would have to get a physical exam, and I panicked. I didn't think I could ever pass, and I was really scared.

I talked it over with my good buddy, and he told me what I wanted to hear. Although we clearly should have known better, together we convinced each other that I had some sort of virus or that I had pulled a muscle. "After all," my friend concluded, "you're too young to be having a heart attack." The dominoes had begun to teeter dangerously, but I simply looked the other way.

I decided to hold off on applying for the extra insurance until I was in better shape, not wanting them to mistake my "muscle pull" for "something more serious," and deep in the most incredible case of denial, went on with my life. But the pain did not go away. It not only continued, it grew worse. I had to admit that I needed help. Wanting to keep it from my wife, I chose a doctor at random out of the phone book and went to see him.

Luck was with me. The doctor was good, and he was blunt. "You're exhausted, and you're treating your body like hell," he said. "Your blood pressure is dangerously high, and I'm willing to bet your cholesterol is through the ceiling." When my blood tests came back, they more than confirmed his predictions. I had been eating poorly, gaining weight, and running my body into the ground. "If you don't make some major changes," he cautioned me, "you'll never see those kids grow up."

> I was taking care of everyone but myself.
> I was helping raise kids whom I might never see grow up.
> But I was set on denying it all.

My doctor was caring but minced no words, and I will always be grateful for the time and interest he gave me that day—and in the days to come. "If your children or your wife needed good food or rest or exercise, you would stop everything else and see that they got it. You'd probably even do it for your dog, but for yourself . . ." I didn't need to own a dog to get the message, and he didn't need to finish his sentence. His competent and caring hand had reached down and steadied the teetering dominoes.

A veteran of many years of medical practice, this fine physician did not rely on an EKG that had failed to reveal any notable heart problem. He felt sure that the pain in my chest was serious, and he trusted his own instincts.

> Though nothing was improving,
> I went back to the doctor for regular checkups.
> Somehow, seeing him made me feel safe.

"The recurring pain is an important sign," he concluded. "How much more evidence do you need before you'll believe that your body is trying to tell you something?"

Still, some of us just need to learn the hard way. Not only didn't the pain tell me something, I took the opposite tack and started jogging again. I was up at dawn straining and pushing my body beyond endurance. I ran about six miles each day, and in the interests of getting "healthier," I gave in and started taking the time to eat the hot meals that I prepared for the family. I started to cut down on snacking and focused on trying to eat "balanced meals," never knowing that for me and my carbohydrate sensitivity, they were not the healthful meals I thought them to be.

I kept my medical visits a secret; I promised myself that when I was "all better," I would explain everything. I went back to my doctor for periodic checkups, having convinced myself that as long as I returned to see him on a regular basis, I would be safe. I changed a few things here and there, got a bit more sleep, ate an occasional salad for lunch, but this haphazard approach didn't work, and nothing about my health showed any sign of improvement.

Lab tests revealed that my cholesterol and triglyceride levels were getting higher (we didn't know much about HDL and LDL cholesterol then). My blood pressure was out of control, but I didn't want to take any drugs. I regarded them as Band-Aids to cover up the problem. I wanted something to correct the cause of the problem, but I didn't know where to turn. During a single doctor's appointment, my blood pressure would peak at dangerous levels, then return to near normal within a few minutes. "Not a good sign," my doctor remarked in his usual understated manner. I know now how serious a sign that was.

> The low-fat diet was driving me crazy.
> I never felt satisfied.
> And even though I tried,
> my blood fat levels were getting worse!

I was in my late forties by then, and if I had been objective, I would have had to admit that my weight was rising by leaps and bounds. Although I had stopped weighing myself when I hit the 215-pound mark, my weight gain had clearly continued unabated.

The extra weight and added years began to take their toll on my knees. Jogging was no longer a good idea, and after my second knee injury, my doctor strongly recommended that I give it up indefinitely.

For the first time, reality set in. I was really scared. Until then, I had been able to keep my weight in check (somewhat) by staying active, and I was afraid that without the balance provided by exercise, my weight would skyrocket.

For many years, relatives, family, and friends bore witness to my enormous appetite. When I was a kid, they didn't call me the "human garbage can" for nothing. I finally turned to a low-fat eating plan but wasn't able to stick to it consistently. The restrictions were driving me crazy, and I was always hungry. To make matters worse, my blood fat level was so high that I had counted on my jogging and my active lifestyle to balance it all out. I felt sure that those were all that stood between me and a heart attack. Cholesterol-lowering medications were pretty new then, and I felt, as I do now, that if I could control my problems with exercise, that was a far better choice. With the exercise now gone, I had nowhere left to turn. Finally, after all their warnings, the dominoes began to tumble.

> **I started keeping track of all the foods that made me hungry— and every single one was high in carbohydrates.**

I perform really well under pressure. That's when I do some of my best thinking and surprise even myself. I flashed on a solution: I'd handle the health problems the way I handled a room that needed to be cleaned up. When I felt overwhelmed with the cleanup task ahead, I would stretch out my hand and pick up the first thing I touched. Then I would put it away. And so I would continue, over and over again, until everything was in order. In this case the first thing I "touched" was my weight. At the time, it didn't seem much of a way to handle one's overall health care, but my weight was the first thing that came to mind when I thought of what needed to be changed—and am I glad it did.

In the weeks that followed, I used my scientific training in search of clues that would help me in my battle. I started off by eating only when I

> **When I carbo-loaded only once a day, and had low-carbohydrate foods at my other meals, my weight dropped, and my chest pains disappeared. And my cravings were gone!**

was hungry. That sounded as if it should work, but it didn't stop me from overeating. It seemed as if I would just get on a carbo-eating cycle and never stop being hungry. Still, I took careful note of which foods increased both my hunger and my tiredness.

To the trained scientist in me, it was obvious that large meals containing high-carbohydrate foods—such as starches, snack foods, fruits, and sweets—were often followed by hunger, cravings, and a sort of drugged feeling. This would lead me to a snack of—you guessed it—high-carbohydrate foods, particularly sugary ones.

I had been told to "carbo-load" when I jogged, but when I carbo-loaded, I felt bloated and tired. I started thinking of myself as "carbohydrate-sensitive" and noticed that when I carbo-loaded only *once* a day, and then ate high-fiber, low-fat, low-carbohydrate meals during the rest of the day, I felt better than I had in a long, long time.

When I started to follow this program consistently, my weight dropped, and my chest pains disappeared. I felt great and began to look healthier and younger than I had when I was jogging. The more improvement I saw, the more motivated I became. I read up on the powerful impact of stress reduction on the improvement of heart health and added it to my routine. I even began to take time for myself, and it felt good!

The program that I had hoped would help me lose some weight was making me healthier as well. By the time I made it back to my doctor, I had lost nearly twenty pounds. It had been only a little more than two months, but my blood pressure was better than he had ever seen it. My new blood tests confirmed what I had hoped for: my weight-loss program was also improving my overall health.

To some it might not have made sense. Though my diet was not extremely low in fat, the fats in my blood were dropping. Though my diet did not restrict my salt intake, my blood pressure was dropping to normal limits. I was eating the food I loved, in the more-than-generous portions that I adored, but I was losing weight. Neither my doctor nor I could deny it: whatever I was doing was working, and I was doing it without struggle.

> I no longer felt like a failure.
> My health and my life had become precious to me
> in a way that I had never before let myself admit.

I no longer felt like a failure, blaming myself for obviously suicidal tendencies. I was simply a man who had not yet discovered the right health-promoting nutritional program. This new program was obviously the one that I had been searching for but had always eluded me, until now. My health and my life had become precious to me in a way that I had never before let myself admit. For so long, I had denied how much I wanted to be healthy and free to enjoy my life. Now it looked as if I finally knew how.

Shortly after my marriage ended, I found Rachael. It was literally love at first sight. Not only did each of us find a soul mate, but we found, in addition, that we were not alone in the very discoveries that had saved each of our lives. Working together we found that thousands of scientists had already uncovered the hormonal imbalance and made the connections that had led to my slow and steady weight gain and deteriorating health over the years as well as to Rachael's lifelong weight and health struggles. This same imbalance, the overrelease of insulin, led to the ill health that had accompanied and followed our weight gain and that would, in all probability, have led to our unnecessarily early deaths.

Independently and alone, each in our own way, we had discovered the program that you now hold in your hands and that has stood the test of time. Today I am far healthier than I was fifteen years ago. I take no medication and have the strength and health that men half my age would envy.

> Now I no longer live in fear, self-blame, shame, or frustration.
> Each new day is a gift—
> one that grows in the sharing.

I am grateful and happy, and although this may sound odd, I treat this program as I would treat a good friend. The benefits and blessings it has brought have repaid tenfold every little bit of energy I have contributed. It has given me back my very life, and I will never, ever take it for granted. I no longer live in fear, self-blame, shame, or frustration. Each new day is a gift—one that grows in the sharing.

IN MYSTERIOUS WAYS:
DR. FREDERIC VAGNINI'S STORY

I am a religious man. Most people find the fact that I am a doctor who believes so strongly in my religion a bit unusual at first. It makes perfect sense to me, however, for I am witness to the miracle of God's work every day.

I have held the evidence of a greater power in my hands, in the beating heart of a child that had, against all odds, managed to keep pumping blood into that little body long after it should have given up. I have been witness to that which goes beyond the physical: an old man who holds on with every ounce of strength within him until his wife can make it to his side to say good-bye, then with a kiss, a smile, and the squeeze of a hand, passes on; the will and determination of a mother who, refusing to abandon her children, wins out over her illness. As this doctor's pronouncements were mocked, I smiled and was humbled.

> I have been privileged to do God's work
> for more than three decades.
> Though science is a precious and powerful tool,
> I try never to forget who makes it all possible.

I have been privileged to do God's work for more than three decades, and though science is a precious and powerful tool, I try never to forget who makes it all possible. It is no wonder, then, that in the worst of times I turn to my higher power for guidance and help. Often I ask for help in the service of others, but on this one cold night in February, seven years ago, it was for myself, my wife, and my daughters that I prayed.

It was almost seven o'clock by the time the office was empty. My patients were gone by six, and after a bit of catching up, my nurses and assistants were on their way. I had called home to say hello to my girls and to tell my wife that once again I would not be home for dinner. I had some correspondence to catch up on, forms to complete, lab tests to review, and several patients to visit in the hospital. It was going to be another long night, and there was nothing that could be done about it.

I tried to begin, but I couldn't seem to get organized; my thinking was not focused, and each sentence I tried to compose was a struggle. It had grown dark, and through my window I could see big, white snowflakes beginning to fall. I smiled. Tomorrow was Saturday, and if the snow was deep enough, I could clear some time to take my oldest girl sledding in the afternoon. She had been sleeping with her Christmas sled in her room, waiting for the snowfall, and I could almost hear her wonderful laugh as she raced over the snow for the first time.

Reluctantly, my mind turned to the long evening ahead, and I decided that a little caffeine would fortify me. My thoughts turned to some doughnuts that I hoped might be left over from the big box I usually brought in for my staff each morning (mostly as an excuse for my own indulgence). Tackling the pile of papers at hand, my eyes were drawn to a lab report precariously poised atop the mound. Unlike the other lab reports, it was not accompanied by a patient file, as was my procedure. The great number of "flags" caught my eyes. Flags are abnormal blood readings that the lab places in a separate column for easy reference by the physician. This lab report was fraught with them, and they were not good. Triglycerides were three times normal; the cholesterol was high, and the proportion of good and bad levels of distribution forecast upcoming heart problems.

> I had been running from my own awareness
> of my deteriorating heart health.
> I pushed my chair back from my desk,
> just as I wanted to push myself away from the truth.

I could feel my usual lecture forming in my mind as I reached to identify the patient so that I could phone him or her and relate the bad news. Then came the shock. The patient was me, and the forecast of doom I had just witnessed was for none other than myself. I had been running from my own awareness of my deteriorating heart health. I pushed my chair back from my desk, just as I wanted to push myself away from the truth.

Looking out my window, I let my mind wander until I imagined my own grave beneath a white covering of snow. Like Scrooge in *A Christmas Carol*, I felt as if I were privy to seeing the days ahead, and I didn't like the story. I put my head down to think and rest. It was then that I felt it: a presence, a sense of comfort, a knowledge that I was going to be all right. It filled me and fortified me, and without thought, I began to speak to God. It was not an unfamiliar communication; God and I went way back. I prayed before every heart operation I performed, before I had to present a family with bad news, and before I went to bed each night. My prayers had helped me through the years, and with the channel open and ready, I knew I would find comfort and help.

I asked for guidance that night—guidance in making the right choices to keep myself alive and guidance in making better choices in the future. Taking advice had never been one of my strong points, though now, with reality staring me in the face, my arrogance was gone, and I wanted nothing more than to receive the guidance I so desperately needed. I had to admit, I certainly had not been doing so well following my own advice.

Though I had been slim and well-built in my youth, I gained weight as I settled into a comfortable home life with my wife, Mary Ann. I am a big man, over six feet five inches tall, and the first few pounds I put on never really showed. I was still relatively slim when a triple whammy poured on the pounds.

The first punch came by way of a severe back injury that left me unable to keep up my rigorous exercise regimen. The second punch came with Mary Ann's pregnancy, which gave a whole new definition to the word *snacking*. She couldn't eat large meals, so she subsisted on minimeals during the day and evening. Though she kept her weight under control, I did not. Before I knew it, I was not only eating my meals but keeping her company when she snacked, providing the second punch in my weight-gain knockout. Whereas she was satisfied with a bit of ice cream in the evening, my cravings were triggered by its sweet, rich taste. So by the time she was done snacking, I had just begun. The pounds began to mount, and I grew bigger far more quickly than did she. I remember turning sideways in front of the mirror and thinking that I looked pregnant, too. Although I had once been convinced that I was immune to weight problems, I found I was as vulnerable as anyone.

> I remember turning sideways in front of the mirror and thinking that, like my wife, I looked pregnant.

I came from a family of men and women with adult-onset diabetes. Early deaths were common among my mother's eight brothers, many of whom were overweight or obese and whose children were likewise. Though I did not know it at the time, their excess weight was not their fault. They carried within their genetics a "thrifty gene," which set them up for easy weight gain, adult-onset diabetes, and heart disease. And along with the genetics I had inherited came not only their humor and height but the predisposition for heart disease as well.

> **I was already clearly overweight when I traded in the cigarettes for about forty pounds of fat.**

I will never know whether, given some time after the birth of my first daughter, I would have been able to fight off the cravings successfully and bring down my weight. Instead of concentrating on losing weight, however, I added a second demand that made it even more difficult to take off the pounds: I had promised my wife and myself that I would give up my ten-year two-pack-a-day smoking habit. After my daughter's birth, I traded in the cigarettes for about forty additional pounds of fat. Bit by bit, pound by pound, and almost without realizing it, I had become obese.

Tipping the scales at three hundred and some pounds, more than ninety pounds above my ideal weight, I still managed to convince myself that I could bring my eating and weight back under control if I just tried a little harder. Given my own obvious lack of success, I felt a bit uncomfortable advising patients on weight loss, so I generally avoided the issue as much as possible. Like many doctors, I handed out the typical diet sheets, pretty much knowing that no one could follow these diets for long. Like any good physician, I cautioned patients to follow a sensible eating plan and didn't really have much of an answer when they protested that their cravings drove them to overeat and lose control.

Though at the time I didn't realize I was doing it, I was turning a deaf ear to them and to myself as well, simply because no alternative was available. It wasn't the kind of medicine I wanted to practice, but I suppose it was understandable. The nutritionists with whom I had worked over the years all spouted the same timeworn dogma that did not work for most people but had become the standard for the profession: low-fat foods, exercise, sensible meals. What was not acceptable was the fact that I almost ignored the help and hope that I had before me.

Earlier that day a patient I had been taking care of for years came in for a routine checkup. His weight was down; his blood pressure had dropped to normal for the first time in as long as I had known him; and his spirits were high. He looked great, and as his blood tests were later to confirm, he was healthier than I had seen him in many years. He smiled mischievously as he explained the basis of the program that he was following, then handed me a package that held the Hellers' first book.

> **I prayed for guidance; I should have prayed for humility.
> As often happens, God provided both.**

I wasn't sure whether the gift was intended for my own use or so that I could learn about the program that was responsible for the improvements I saw in him, but I responded with a false enthusiasm and promptly put the book on the bookcase behind my chair. And that's where it stayed as file after file, paper after paper, placed on top, buried it somewhere in the middle of an ever-increasing mound.

There I sat, not three feet from the pile, with no thought of the book or the patient who had been caring and thoughtful enough to bring it to me. Instead, I prayed for guidance from above. Had I known myself as I do now, I would have prayed for the humility to follow any guidance that might come, but as often happens, God provided both.

Thinking that my prayers were to go unanswered, I reached for my lab report and, sliding my rolling chair backward, turned to place it on the bookcase behind me, where I would not need to look at it or deal with it for quite a while. Then something seemingly small happened that changed both my life and the lives of my patients. As my chair rolled backward, it hit the bookcase that held the pile of papers and files awaiting my attention. Out of sight lay the book that held my salvation.

> **The moment I saw the words *carbohydrate addict*,
> I felt the Hellers were talking about me.**

Everything tumbled to the floor. The pile of papers at my feet reminded me of the mess that I was making of my own health. I was annoyed at having to spend more time and energy cleaning up the scattered papers when something caught my eye. The book my patient had given me was now atop the pile, the words *carbohydrate addict* from its title seeming to shout out to me. The moment I saw it, I felt the Hellers were talking about me. A part of me wanted to reach for the book, but I was afraid to move.

The ringing of the phone startled me, and as a drowning man would reach for a lifeline, I grabbed for the receiver. The sweet voice of my wife on the other end of the line was telling me that, given the snow, she was worried and had called to tell me to drive even more carefully than usual. I was so happy to hear her voice, I could barely speak. When she asked if I was okay, I was surprised to find that, indeed, I was. The pain was gone.

> **I had been given a second chance.
> My feelings of guilt and helplessness
> have been replaced with confidence and trust.
> I am healthy and happy and very grateful.**

I looked out the window. The storm was over, within and without. I had been given a second chance, and I knew that in the book that lay before me, I had been given the guidance for which I had prayed. To my continuing astonishment, I grabbed onto it with both hands and have never let go.

Today I am well and happy. More than happy, I am grateful for a way of life that has brought me health along with peace of mind and spirit. My feelings of guilt and helplessness have been replaced with confidence and trust. By all accounts, my blood pressure, blood fats, and other heart health indicators are those of a young man with the best of genes.

> **I have brought the Program into my practice
> as I had taken it into my life.
> It has helped heal my patients as it healed me.**

In the same way that I have brought it into my life, I have carried the Hellers' discovery into my medical practice and, in time, expanded on it. By working side by side with them—and combining their program with my knowledge of cardiovascular testing, nutrient supplementation, pharmaceutical intervention, and my own scientific research—I have been able to provide my patients with a uniquely effective program for heart disease risk prevention and reduction and for heart health restoration as well.

For my patients, intense carbohydrate cravings, weight gain, high blood pressure, abnormal blood fats, adult-onset diabetes, and the Insulin Resistance Syndrome they constitute (or Syndrome X, as it is often known) no longer represent a sentence of progressive illness and suffering, self-blame, and shortened life. Instead, any one of these disorders, or all of them together, present the opportunity for a new start—a whole new beginning that is now filled with help and hope.

I have always been told that God works in mysterious ways. As a child, I thought that truism to be little more than a phrase meant to keep me quiet when I asked too many questions, but now it has a very different and personal meaning to me. I cannot imagine that I would have been open to the help that was offered to me unless, first, I was forced by a power greater than myself to pay attention. So life grabbed me by the neck and shook me hard. When it got my undivided attention, it served up a solution that both saved my life and, today, has given that life a most special purpose and the ability to help others, too.

2

THE INSULIN CONNECTION
GETTING TO THE HEART OF THE MATTER

Everything is clear if the cause be known.—*Louis Pasteur*

Good and bad, day and night, yin and yang. Since time began, the world has been the battleground for two opposing forces. At every moment of every day, a similar combat takes place within your body. The way you look, think, feel, and act depends on the outcome of this never-ending tug-of-war. The stakes are high: your health, your well-being, indeed, your very survival depend on a lasting truce, an essential balance.

Two opposing forces face off in this power struggle for your health. The first combatant is insulin. Insulin affects your every movement and every breath. When most people hear the word *insulin,* they think of diabetes, but insulin's powerful influence can lead to high blood pressure, risk-related blood fat levels, weight gain, atherosclerosis, peripheral vascular disease, and heart disease in a great many people who are not diabetic. When it comes to the nondiabetic, few doctors and fewer patients are aware of insulin's impact on heart health.

> Insulin's powerful influence can lead to weight gain, peripheral vascular disease, risk-related blood fat levels, high blood pressure, atherosclerosis, and heart disease.

THE INSULIN CONNECTION

Insulin's power comes from the fact that it is your body's Saving Hormone. It is a miser in the truest sense of the word, although being the Saving Hormone is no easy task. Insulin must also meet the body's other demands: appeals for energy to enable muscles to maintain their health and do their jobs well, to fuel the nervous system, and to repair the very organs that keep the body going. So although insulin wants nothing more than to store away as much energy as possible, by converting carbohydrates into fat and storing that fat in your fat cells, it must give up some of your body's precious food energy to keep you going.

> Insulin is the Saving Hormone;
> glucagon is the Spending Hormone.
> When these hormones are out of balance,
> they can put your heart health in jeopardy.

The second force in this power struggle is glucagon, your body's Spending Hormone. For some reason, although most people have heard of insulin, few have heard of glucagon. (Perhaps insulin has a better press agent!) Just as insulin directs excess food energy into the fat cells, glucagon's job is to bring that same energy out of the fat cells so that it can be used to repair and fuel your body between meals. It's pretty easy to remember: insulin—in, glucagon—out.

When your body is in good hormonal balance, foodwise, insulin and glucagon complement each other and maintain a perfect harmony. Insulin rises, makes you want to eat, fuels your body a bit, and directs some energy to be put away, in your fat cells, for later. Then insulin levels fall. Glucagon rises, opens the doors to the fat cells, and the energy that is released is burned to keep the body running smoothly. After a time insulin levels rise, and the whole cycle begins again.

There are times, however, when this balance can turn into a battle of hormones that can put your heart health—and your very life—in jeopardy.

Insulin is more powerful than glucagon. We think of it as a bully. When insulin is released into the blood, glucagon diminishes significantly. Glucagon will only return when insulin levels fall.

When you think about it, for survival purposes, insulin's control over glucagon makes perfect sense. In prehistoric times, when a caveman came upon a surplus of food (feast), insulin was needed to help channel as much of the food into storage in the fat cells as possible. Our prehistoric ancestors never knew when they might find food again, and the food that was found was not as energy-rich as it is today, so the body had to be able to put away enough of a reserve to make it through to the next find. Insulin also urged early humans to eat as much of the food as possible so that they could make the most of this life-giving opportunity for nourishment.

On the other hand, when food was not available (famine), glucagon was needed to open up the fat cells and bring out the energy that had been stored away so that it could fuel the muscles and brain and other organs to go out and get nourishment. If no food was available, insulin's craving-inducing and fat-storing ability was not needed.

Bringing in food was the top priority, however, so whenever insulin was released, whenever food was available, survival would dictate that glucagon's job take second place.

> In prehistoric times insulin kept us alive.
> In today's world high levels of insulin
> can literally kill.

In balance, the cycle repeated itself, so that food was stored away during times of plenty and used up during times of need—a perfect give-and-take that kept cavemen and cavewomen healthy, happy, and alive.

In modern times, this hormonal tug-of-war still occurs, but it is now being thrown out of balance, with insulin gaining control. The outcome of this battle can often mean the difference between a long, healthy existence and one plagued by heart problems—or cut short by heart disease.

ON THE TRAIL OF A KILLER

Long before the terms *risk factor* and *lifestyle change* had become a part of everyday life, scientists were investigating and documenting the powerful impact that high levels of insulin and the body's resistance to insulin had on blood pressure, obesity, atherosclerosis, adult-onset diabetes, and heart disease. More than sixty years ago, in the journal *Lancet*, the eminent scientist Dr. H. P. Himsworth first apprised the medical community of the hormonal imbalance that has been identified as chronic reactive hyperinsulinemia (continually high levels of insulin) and insulin resistance. At the time Dr. Himsworth implored both his fellow researchers and physicians to focus their attention and effort on this vital hormonal imbalance.

To Dr. Himsworth and to the scientists and physicians who quickly followed his lead, it was apparent that an imbalance in insulin lay at the base of several devastating diseases. At the time, however, the technology needed to pursue and extend his discovery had not yet been developed, so Dr. Himsworth's insights and predictions remained unappreciated and unaccepted. Himsworth died never knowing that his breakthrough could save millions of lives. The experiments that were needed to bring this insulin breakthrough into medical practice were, in Himsworth's day, simply impossible.

Five decades passed before researchers would acquire the tools to fully explore the consequences of insulin imbalance that Dr. Himsworth first described and that have since been linked to so much needless illness and death. Not until 1988, in an article published in the medical journal *Diabetes* by Dr. G. M. Reaven, did current research confirm and again begin to explore insulin's great impact on human health. In that article Dr. Reaven concluded, "It now seems quite clear that Himsworth was correct, and the point of view he introduced has become well established."

How sad it is that for lack of the necessary technology, five decades of help were lost to those who could have benefited from Dr. Himsworth's life-giving breakthrough in the understanding of hyperinsulinemia's impact on illness and health. The tide of scientific understanding has turned. In the last few years alone, hyperinsulinemia and the insulin resistance it can cause have been identified, researched, and documented by literally thousands of scientists.

In the past, when researchers studied the excess release of insulin, they often used the term *hyperinsulinemia,* meaning "too much insulin." In the beginning physicians and scientists alike thought of hyperinsulinemia as a simple excess of insulin, a not-too-common disorder that had some effect on the body but that was not fully understood. In the last decade, however, there has been a virtual explosion of discoveries connecting hyperinsulinemia and insulin resistance to an extraordinarily wide variety of diseases. Day by day, the reports of discoveries and connections to Insulin Resistance Syndrome, as it is now called, continue to grow.

> **In the last decade there has been a virtual explosion of discoveries connecting hyperinsulinemia and insulin resistance to an extraordinarily wide variety of diseases.**

In 1983 the number of articles describing insulin as the essential link to other diseases was around 300. Fifteen years later more than 15,000 scientific articles have explored and reported this important and potentially lifesaving discovery.

In 1990 Dr. D. C. Simonson reported in the journal *Hormone and Metabolic Research* that insulin and insulin resistance are often found in those who are significantly overweight as well as in those who suffer from high blood pressure, adult-onset diabetes, atherosclerosis, and heart disease. The following year Drs. R. A. DeFronzo and E. Ferrannini confirmed Dr. Simonson's report and added that high levels of insulin had been shown by many scientists to be the link between diabetes and high blood pressure. In addition, they reported that excess insulin levels led to undesirable blood fat levels in normal-weight, healthy individuals; in overweight people without diabetes; and in those with adult-onset diabetes.

> **The major heart disease risk factors are the tips of the iceberg. Hyperinsulinemia and insulin resistance lie at the base.**

"The physician recognizes only the tips of the iceberg," wrote Drs. DeFronzo and Ferrannini. Diseases and risk factors such as diabetes, obesity, high blood pressure, high triglyceride levels, low levels of (good) HDL cholesterol, and atherosclerosis "extrude above the surface, and the complete insulin-resistance syndrome may be missed."

In a powerful conclusion to their article, these respected scientists noted that even without its effects on blood pressure and blood fat levels, high levels of insulin and the resistance it brings can still narrow the arteries that lead to and nourish the heart.

Most physicians have had little or no education in the diagnosis and treatment of Insulin Resistance Syndrome. Although some physicians consider Insulin Resistance Syndrome to be a relatively rare or unusual disorder, Drs. DeFronzo and Ferrannini found that "[i]nsulin resistance is a common disorder, which occurs with high frequency in the general population."

In a different approach to research, Dr. Robert W. Stout reviewed twenty years of scientific studies by more than thirty scientists, including three large population studies that looked at a total of more than 11,000 people. Dr. Stout concluded that high insulin levels stimulate the production of fat in arteries and the production of cholesterol in the body, and that high levels of insulin have been associated with all the major cardiovascular risk factors: hypertension, elevated triglycerides, elevated cholesterol, decreased high-density lipoprotein, and upper-body obesity, among others. Since that time a mountain of evidence has linked high insulin levels and insulin resistance to all of these as well as to heart disease.

In articles published in the top medical research journals around the world, excess levels of insulin and insulin resistance are being reported as the underlying link, the unifying factor, that connects many of the most prevalent and devastating of this country's top killer diseases. Insulin, insulin resistance, and the diseases and risk factors that make up the Insulin Resistance Syndrome have been implicated in *more than half of this country's deaths each year.*

Currently, the finest scholarly journals regularly include groundbreaking research on the effects of the sweeping impact of insulin and insulin resistance. Some of the world's most respected medical and scientific journals and reports—such as the *Surgeon General's Report on Nutrition and Health,* the *New England Journal of Medicine, Lancet, Clinical Nutrition, Annals of the New York Academy of Science,* the *Journal of Clinical Endocrinological Metabolism,* the *Journal of Human Hypertension,* the *American Heart Journal,* and the *Journal of the American Medical Association* (JAMA)—regularly carry articles that document the impact of hyperinsulinemia and insulin resistance.

Today researchers from all over the world have confirmed the importance of insulin to heart health, and the reports continue to mount in record numbers. It is not unusual for scientists to refer to excess levels of insulin and insulin resistance as the "pathogenic link," the invisible illness-causing connection, that has so long been sought in the fight for heart health and long life.

What seems odd to us, however, is the media's apparent unwillingness to report to their viewers, readers, and listeners the results of so many documented, verified, and long-term scientific studies regarding insulin's powerful connection to heart disease.

> The American Heart Association heralded the news:
> high levels of insulin had been found to be
> "the most statistically significant predictor of heart attack risk"
> —equal to or better than cholesterol levels.
> Yet television, radio, and newspapers
> have virtually ignored the news.

Recently the American Heart Association (AHA) issued a press release announcing the discovery of an important new heart disease risk factor—high levels of insulin. The report went on to explain that as reported in the American Heart Association's medical journal, *Circulation*, "[o]ver 22 years of follow-up, the predictive power of insulin levels was of the same magnitude as that of cholesterol levels." The AHA added that during the scientific study itself, "when compared to other risk factors, insulin levels were the most statistically significant predictor of heart attack risk."

> One wonders why so important a breakthrough,
> one that holds such a powerful potential for saving lives,
> remains unreported in the news.

Yet though the AHA's press releases usually are given top priority in the news, only one of the major television network news shows presented this revolutionary health information to the public, and only a handful of newspapers ever mentioned it. The news articles and the single television news spot on this critical discovery were of minimal length and barely touched on its importance.

One wonders why so important a breakthrough, one that holds such a powerful potential for saving lives, remains unreported in the news. Though these and similar findings have been repeatedly confirmed and verified, they are neither publicized nor acknowledged. Physicians, nutritionists, and the public alike remain unaware of insulin's connection to heart disease, and it is for this very reason that this book was written.

INSULIN RESISTANCE SYNDROME:
PUTTING THE PIECES TOGETHER

Imagine for a moment that you are putting together a jigsaw puzzle consisting of a picture you have never seen. The only clues you have are contained in the pieces that lie scattered before you and the fragments of image that each piece holds. In order to put the puzzle together, chances are you would start by searching out the most recognizable shapes—most likely those with straight edges; then, after assembling the outside border, you would look for pieces that would connect to those already in place. You would work inward, connecting one piece to another until a picture began to emerge.

Scientists follow the same process when they seek the cause and cure of a disease or disorder. First, they look at what they already know and see whether it forms a frame or border into which the other pieces of the puzzle fit. In the case of heart disease, excess levels of insulin certainly formed a side or two of the puzzle, but some of the framework remained unexplained. Scattered pieces—such as adult-onset diabetes, high blood pressure, risk-related levels of blood fats, and obesity—were known to be part of the heart disease puzzle, but their connection remained unclear. Researchers did not understand, for instance, why high blood pressure accompanied weight gain and low blood sugar swings in some people, whereas it accompanied weight loss and high levels of blood sugar in other people. Scientists were pretty certain that insulin was the link and that atherosclerosis and heart disease were often the end point. Still, how it all fit together remained a mystery.

The solution came in the discovery of insulin resistance, the body's way of protecting itself against high levels of insulin and the excess blood sugar that excess insulin attempts to usher into cells. If exposed to too much insulin for too long, the cells of the brain and other vital organs like the muscles and liver would shut the doors (receptor sites) that usually allow insulin and its companion, blood sugar, to enter. Scientists gave this protective process the name "insulin resistance," and cells that shut their doors to insulin and blood sugar are termed "insulin resistant."

The understanding that different cells throughout the body shut down after different amounts of exposure to high levels of insulin held the key to understanding the variety of changes that scientists were witnessing.

The concept was simple but fascinating, and it made a great deal of sense. Suppose, for a moment, that you were facing a flood of water about to enter your home. If you had your most precious possessions in one room, you might run to close the door to that room first. Then, in sequence, you would probably close off and protect each room depending on the value that its contents held for you. This differential protection was what scientists observed in the shutting down of different cells all over the body in response to a flood of insulin.

> If you are a carbohydrate addict,*
> chances are you have experienced
> at least one of these stages firsthand.

*For help in determining whether you are a carbohydrate addict at risk for insulin-related heart disease, take our quiz in Chapter 4.

Today, each of the stages in the progression of Insulin Resistance Syndrome has been described and studied, and though you might not be a scientist, if you are addicted to carbohydrates, chances are you have experienced some of these stages firsthand. The cells in your brain and the rest of the nervous system appear to be the first to become insulin resistant. In order to protect you from a flood of insulin, your body simply closes these cells down (that is, it makes them resistant to insulin). Unfortunately, when the doors to the cells in your brain and nervous system close to insulin, they also close to the blood sugar that insulin ushers in and that would normally nourish them.

In this first stage of Insulin Resistance Syndrome, you may find that within two hours after eating high-carbohydrate foods, you feel light-headed, irritable, or unable to concentrate.° In addition to craving high-carbohydrate foods, you may gain weight easily as an increased quantity of the food energy (transformed into blood sugar) is channeled through the liver, turned into blood fat, then stored in your fat cells.

If hyperinsulinemia continues, a second stage of Insulin Resistance Syndrome may occur, and the postmeal cravings, tiredness, light-headedness, irritability, or inability to concentrate that you felt before may become more noticeable. Your muscles, liver, and other organs will likewise begin to block insulin's entry and, in doing so, will also close off their ability to get nourishment from blood sugar. As muscles experience a decrease in blood sugar fueling, you may experience a decrease in your desire or willingness to be active or to exercise. You might feel less inclined to do very much except what is absolutely necessary. If you do feel motivated to be active or find you must be active, you may lose your desire to continue activity or find that you tire easily.

In this second stage of Insulin Resistance Syndrome, weight gain is almost inevitable, as food energy (in the form of blood sugar transformed into blood fat) is channeled increasingly into the fat cells for storage. In addition to weight problems, in particular abdominal obesity, the second stage of Insulin Resistance Syndrome can herald a wide variety of noticeable heart disease risk factors, including an increase in risk-related blood fats, increases in blood pressure levels, and more.

During both the first and second stages, insulin is able to continue to usher some blood sugar into the cells of many organs, but if no corrective action is taken, these cells will grow more and more insulin resistant,

---

°Signs and symptoms vary from individual to individual. In addition, any single symptom may have a wide variety of causes. As always, check with your physician regarding the cause of any neurological problem.

Progression of Insulin Resistance Syndrome: Stages 1–4

If carbohydrate addicts do not take corrective action or get treatment, they will often move through a series of progressive and predictable stages in which heart disease risk factors increase in number and severity. In combination these risk factors form a cluster of disorders that scientists and physicians refer to by a variety of names, including: Insulin Resistance Syndrome, Syndrome-X, 4-H Syndrome, Metabolic Syndrome, The Deadly Quartet, and The Diseases of Civilization.

The following stages illustrate the progression for the population at large. Individual signs and symptoms may vary and may place a carbohydrate addict at, between, or across any stage of Insulin Resistance Syndrome. Insulin-related risk factors are not necessarily confined to individual stages.

Stage	BLOOD INSULIN LEVELS At Fasting	BLOOD INSULIN LEVELS After Challenge°	BLOOD GLUCOSE LEVELS At Fasting	BLOOD GLUCOSE LEVELS After Challenge°	Additional Insulin-Related Heart Disease Risk Factors°°
1	Normal	Elevated	Normal	Normal	Carbo cravings and/or easy weight gain, possible mild insulin resistance
2	Normal or elevated	Elevated	Normal	Normal	Carbo cravings and/or easy weight gain, mild or moderate abdominal obesity, mild changes in blood fat levels, mildly elevated blood pressure, early atherosclerotic changes, mild or moderate insulin resistance
3	Normal or elevated	Elevated	Normal	Low†	Carbo cravings and/or easy weight gain, moderate abdominal obesity, moderate changes in blood fat levels, moderately elevated blood pressure, moderate atherosclerotic changes, moderate or marked insulin resistance, hypoglycemia (low blood sugar swings), glucose intolerance (prediabetes), increased risk for heart disease

(continued)

Progression of Insulin Resistance Syndrome: Stages 1–4 (continued)

Stage	BLOOD INSULIN LEVELS At Fasting	BLOOD INSULIN LEVELS After Challenge°	BLOOD GLUCOSE LEVELS At Fasting	BLOOD GLUCOSE LEVELS After Challenge°	Additional Insulin-Related Heart Disease Risk Factors°°
4	Usually elevated	Elevated	Usually elevated	Elevated	Carbo cravings and/or easy weight gain, moderate or marked abdominal obesity, marked changes in blood fat levels, markedly elevated blood pressure, advanced atherosclerotic changes, marked insulin resistance, high and low blood sugar swings, adult-onset diabetes, strong potential for heart disease

°Two to three hours after consuming a glucose-rich drink, as per standard oral glucose tolerance tests.

°°Potential insulin-related risk factors progress at different rates depending on genetics and lifestyle factors. These descriptions provide examples of possible progressive states. Uric acid levels as well as levels of fibrinogen (the blood-clotting factor) may increase with stage progression. Energy levels may drop. Progression is also common to women with polycystic ovarian syndrome (PCOS) and may be accompanied by disturbances in the menstrual cycle, androgen and other hormonal imbalances, hirsutism (excess facial or body hair), and/or infertility. As always, confer with your physician for recommendations and guidance.

†Blood sugar levels at two to three hours after glucose challenge may be lower than those at fasting.

closing the doors (or sites) through which blood sugar had previously entered. Now insulin and the blood sugar that accompanies it become trapped in the bloodstream. The liver, sensitive to these high levels of insulin and blood sugar in the bloodstream, transforms the excess blood sugar into blood fat so that it can be removed from the blood, and the blood sugar (now in the form of fat) is stored in the fat cells. In the first two stages of Insulin Resistance Syndrome, then, as insulin resistance grows, insulin has transformed your body into a fat-making machine. As the cells of many organs throughout your body become insulin resistant, your fat cells become the preferred storage site for blood sugar.

In the third stage of Insulin Resistance Syndrome, brain-related low blood sugar swings can become severe, and your muscles may literally be starving for nourishment. At this stage you may experience extreme mood swings, irritability, inability to concentrate, tiredness, muscle shakes, depression, headaches, and foggy thinking. You may gain weight more easily than you ever thought possible and find that your craving for starches, snack foods, junk foods, and sweets has become uncontrollable. Much of the weight you gain may be deposited as abdominal or tummy fat. Most likely, you find that you prefer frequent snacks rather than typical mealtimes, and when you do snack or eat a meal, you may continue to eat even though you are uncomfortable and/or no longer enjoying the food.

> **In the fourth stage of Insulin Resistance Syndrome, blood sugar is trapped in the bloodstream. This is the start of adult-onset diabetes.**

Chances are, as you enter the fourth stage of Insulin Resistance Syndrome, you will no longer be able to ignore or deny the physical changes that have sprung from your body's insulin imbalance. At this stage even your fat cells can become insulin resistant and close down to insulin and to the blood sugar/blood fat it brings along with it. Many of the symptoms you experienced at earlier stages in the progression reach a peak in the fourth stage, with the significant exception of low blood sugar and weight gain.

Two of the signs of Insulin Resistance Syndrome, rising blood sugar levels and weight gain, reverse in the fourth stage. At this final level, even fat cells close down. Now insulin, blood sugar, and blood fat are caught with no place to go. They cannot leave the bloodstream and remain blocked there. So in this final stage, rather than channeling the energy into fat cells, leading to weight gain, your body may no longer be able to channel energy into your fat cells, and your weight may suddenly drop a bit (though usually not to normal levels).

In the same way, the low blood sugar swings that you might have experienced when blood sugar and blood fat were being channeled into your fat cells in the third stage will disappear and be replaced by high levels of blood sugar. At this point, as blood sugar is trapped in your bloodstream, unable to enter the organs or to be converted and then stored as fat in your fat cells, you may be said to have adult-onset diabetes.°

THE MIGHTY THRIFTY GENE

Two powerful forces come together to put the Insulin Resistance Syndrome progression in motion—one is unchangeable, the second is not. Fortunately, by changing the second factor, you can stop and reverse Insulin Resistance Syndrome at any stage.

The first force necessary to set the Insulin Resistance Syndrome progression in motion is your body's inborn response to high-carbohydrate foods. Just as people react differently to loud music or bright lights, just as some people release more adrenaline than do others when they are scared, so some people release more of the hormone insulin when they eat starches, snack foods, junk foods, or sweets.

> **If you inherited a "thrifty gene," your body is likely to overrelease insulin when you eat high-carbohydrate foods.**

Scientists have thought that the amount of insulin you release is determined in great part by your genes, in particular by the presence of a "thrifty gene." If you inherited a thrifty gene, it was thought, your body would be far more likely to overrelease insulin when you ate high-carbohydrate foods, and the more frequently you ate them, we believed, the more insulin you would release.

In 1993 the dream of a breakthrough discovery came true. In a landmark article, Dr. D. E. Comings and his research team identified the D2 dopamine receptor gene (DRD2) as the major gene leading to carbohy-

---

°Adult-onset diabetes is often mistakenly described as the result of not having enough insulin. Whereas too little insulin is the earmark of juvenile diabetes (IDDM, type I), more often than not, initially adult-onset diabetics (NIDDM, type II) have so much insulin that their bodies close down to it (insulin resistance). So, although they have more than enough insulin, their bodies cannot use it. The insulin injections they may be given are meant to force insulin into the cells, past the insulin resistance. Other oral medications may make their bodies less insulin resistant so that their bodies can make use of the insulin they have. Over time, the pancreas may become exhausted and stop making insulin.

drate cravings and obesity. Within a year Dr. E. P. Noble and his team confirmed this same obesity-related genetic variation and established its connection to obesity as well as to adult-onset diabetes.

Today ongoing research has confirmed and continues to expand on these illuminating findings. If you have the thrifty gene, now identified and referred to as the "carbohydrate-craving gene," you are more likely to (1) crave starches, snack foods, junk foods, and sweets; (2) gain weight easily; and (3) overrelease insulin when you frequently eat high-carbohydrate foods.

It is unfortunate that so many carbohydrate addicts and the medical profession at large have never been informed of the powerful biological basis for carbohydrate addiction and obesity and the many heart-related problems to which they lead. It is equally unfortunate that no blood tests are readily available to diagnose this disorder through genetic testing. The good news is that although you cannot change your genes, your genetics need not determine your destiny.

THE VITAL CARBOHYDRATE CONNECTION

Biology is not destiny. In order to progress through the stages of Insulin Resistance Syndrome, in addition to having a thrifty gene, a second influence is usually present, and if you can avoid it, you can help avoid the powerful, progressive, and potentially devastating actions of hyperinsulinemia.

This second factor, the frequent intake of high-carbohydrate foods, can be avoided without giving up high-carbohydrate foods altogether. If you love your starches, snack foods, junk foods, and sweets, you can still enjoy them; you just can't have them all day long.

> Even though you have a carbohydrate addict's genes,
> you can block your progression
> through the stages of Insulin Resistance Syndrome.

High-carbohydrate foods stimulate the production and release of insulin. Even before you swallow the very food you have put into your mouth, your body starts releasing this hormone. Some people start releasing insulin when they see, smell, or even think about high-carbohydrate food. Although genetics plays a part in how much insulin you will tend to release, a much bigger influence comes from how often you eat high-carbo foods leading to the excessive release of insulin. If you eat a plate of pasta and some garlic bread, for instance, and then eat a piece of cake two hours later, you will release more insulin than you would have released had you eaten the pasta, bread, and cake at one sitting.

If high-carbohydrate meals and snacks are frequent, the body releases greater and greater amounts of insulin over time. If the body is allowed to recover some twelve to twenty hours after a carbohydrate load, it will tend to normalize insulin release. Herein lies the saving grace for all of us who are carbohydrate addicts—what allows us to eat high-carbohydrate foods without overreleasing insulin and thereby avoid the typical carbohydrate addict's march toward weight gain, high blood pressure, diabetes, and heart disease.

Nature has provided carbohydrate addicts with a genetic safety mechanism that allows them to eat high-carbohydrate foods without triggering an insulin overload. Scientists have discovered that frequency of carbohydrate consumption can play as important a role in how much insulin is released in the body as the genes with which you are born. It follows the rule of supply and demand. The more often you eat high-carbohydrate foods, the more insulin you produce. In the same way, the less often you eat high-carbohydrate foods, the less insulin you will release when you do eat them—as long as there is a period of recovery from the high-carbohydrate meal.

Changes in supply to fit the demand are typical of many reactions that occur in the body. The more often you use a muscle, for instance, the stronger it gets. The more often you eat, the more saliva you will make. And the more often you eat high-carbohydrate foods, the more insulin you will release. So if your goal is to keep your insulin levels normal and your heart healthy, even though your genetics set you up with the tendency to release insulin easily, you can overcome the impact of high-carbohydrate foods simply by reducing the number of times that you eat them each day.

> **High-carbohydrate foods stimulate insulin release,
> but you can have the foods you love *every day*
> while greatly improving your chances
> for good heart health and long life.**

You *can* have the high-carbohydrate foods you love so much every day while greatly improving your chances for good heart health and long life. Other foods and additives play a part as well, and in the pages that follow,

> ## The Invisible Insulin Connection
>
> **QUESTION:** What do all these risk factors have in common?
> - Smoking
> - Foods high in saturated fat, salt, or sugar
> - Low activity/exercise levels
> - Physical or psychological stress
> - Increased age
> - Insulin Resistance Syndrome (Syndrome X)
> - High blood pressure
> - Excess weight
> - Risk-related blood fat levels:
> - High triglycerides
> - Low (good) high-density lipoprotein, or HDL
> - High (bad) low-density lipoprotein, or LDL
> - High fibrinogen
>
> **ANSWER:** If you said they all lead to heart disease, you are only partly right. They all lead to or are caused by high levels of insulin and insulin resistance. Insulin and insulin resistance form the powerful and invisible connection to heart disease. This dynamic duo creates the only link ever identified to every major heart disease risk factor.
>
> Now that you know what can cause heart disease, we'll show you how you can help stop it—dead in its tracks.

you will also learn why some low-fat foods and sugar substitutes may be the wrong choice for you. For now, rest assured that there is much you can do to change your genetic "destiny" without giving up the pleasures that can make a long and healthy life worthwhile. As you will soon learn, you can have your cake and your health as well.

WHERE CREDIT IS DUE

Had we tried, thirty or forty years ago, to unravel the insulin connection to heart disease, it would have been impossible. The discoveries that you read about in the preceding pages and the scientific basis for the program that you will be reading about in the pages to come are the result of untold years of research and clinical practice by countless biologists, chemists, physiologists, endocrinologists, cell biologists, and nutrition researchers in the world's most prestigious medical schools and universities. No one person or group of scientists was responsible. The important thing is that the knowledge is now available to those who need it and can benefit from it.

Over the last decade the hard work of many excellent researchers has constructed, piece by piece, the scientific foundation upon which we have based the program that you now hold in your hands. As you read on, you will learn how Insulin Resistance Syndrome can shape your life and impact your heart health. You will meet some of the people who have found health and freedom and have used it to help spouses, parents, siblings, and friends.

> On this program you'll find that the old
> "no pain, no gain" philosophy
> is a bunch of muck!
> You do *not* have to suffer to be healthy.

On this program the old "no pain, no gain" philosophy is simply untrue! You do *not* have to give up the creature comforts, pleasures, and joys of life in hopes of gaining ideal heart health and longevity. Your genetics do not dictate your destiny. And you can indeed avoid the heart-related illnesses that may have plagued your parents and grandparents.

You will enjoy all the food that gives you pleasure, the leisure that you love, and the freedom and health that are your birthright. Enhanced heart health is not necessarily a reward that comes only with self-sacrifice and deprivation. Your health and well-being are gifts that are yours for the taking. You have a right to claim them and to enjoy them—for life!

> Your health and well-being are gifts
> that are yours for the taking.
> You have a right to claim them and enjoy them—for life.

3

HIGH BLOOD PRESSURE, WEIGHT GAIN, BLOOD FATS, AND DIABETES

TAKING INSULIN TO HEART

For every disease there is a cause; for every cause, a cure.
—*Dr. Henry E. Sigerist*

Turn on the evening news, open your daily paper, flip through your favorite magazine and you can't miss it. Each day brings a new discovery in a never-ending line of risk factors for heart disease. It has become a veritable scientific free-for-all in which the findings from unconnected and unverified research studies are taken out of context for the primary purpose of drawing readers and viewers. Scientists who own the patents on the drugs they are studying, food and drug manufacturers who support the very research that attests to the merits of their products, scientists who accept great sums of money in exchange for putting their names on research they have never seen—all are given equal coverage alongside legitimate, credible, uncompromised scientific study.

> **Hyperinsulinemia is the single underlying factor that links all the independent risk factors for heart disease.**

No longer can the public be expected to be able to discern fact from fiction, hype from help, nor science from sell. Unfortunately, within this oversaturated arena, legitimate and vital research may be lost forever.

Yet among all the ephemeral scientific "discoveries," many of them backed by powerful vested interests and big advertising money, that appear on daily newscasts, then vanish without a trace, the one discovery that remains steadfast is that hyperinsulinemia is the single underlying factor that links all the independent risk factors for heart disease.

THE DEADLY QUARTET

They have been called The Deadly Quartet: high blood pressure, obesity, risk-related blood fats, and adult-onset diabetes. They are as powerful as they are dangerous; alone or together they can change your life—or cut it short. Separately they have been linked to a hundred different causes, but only one underlying imbalance has been shown to cause them all, and when that one cause is removed, The Deadly Quartet literally disappears.

Hyperinsulinemia is the one factor, the primary cause, or profactor, that can—either by itself or in combination with the insulin resistance it produces—cause high blood pressure, obesity, risk-related blood fats, and adult-onset diabetes as well as virtually all the other recognized risk factors for heart disease. From smoking to lack of exercise, stress to aging, saturated fats to excess weight gain, hyperinsulinemia is the "pathogenic link," the connection to disease, that makes sense of it all. Only hyperinsulinemia can be identified as the culprit in the development of every one of these potent predictors of heart disease.

The good news is, however, that although an insulin imbalance has been confirmed as the fundamental cause of so much ill health and suffering, insulin balance holds the key to freedom from these very same problems. If you or someone you love is significantly overweight or has high blood pressure, risk-related blood fats, or adult-onset diabetes, you are going to be astounded by what you are about to discover. This knowledge can quite literally mean the difference between life and death.

> **Insulin balance can spell the difference between life and death.**

On the other hand, if none of the disorders that make up The Deadly Quartet has touched either you or anyone you love, then count yourself very lucky. Now is the best time, however, to arm yourself with knowledge, for that is the only effective weapon against this most powerful of enemies.

Imagine for a moment that you are looking at a large, flat surface. You see only the smoothness of its plane, its color and contour, and the shape

HIGH BLOOD PRESSURE, WEIGHT GAIN, BLOOD FATS, AND DIABETES

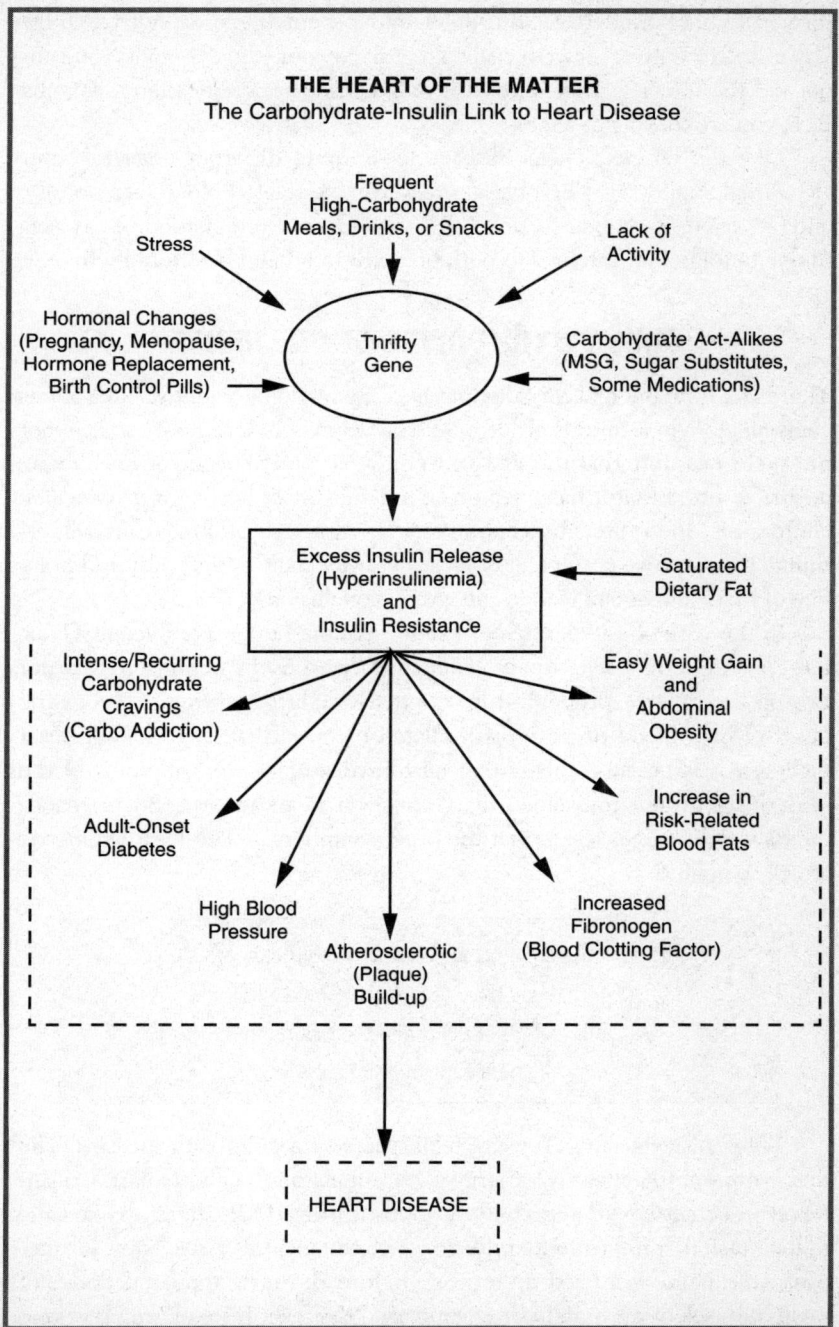

formed by its boundaries. Still, there may be much you do not yet know about it. In fact, you may not realize that from your vantage point, you cannot see the four legs that support it nor realize that rather than a flat surface, you are looking at a table.

Like the tabletop, heart disease looks quite different once the four "legs" that support it—high blood pressure, risk-related blood fats, obesity, and adult-onset diabetes—are fully viewed and understood. It is this understanding that can lead to both peace of mind and health of body.

OBESITY: THE POWER OF PREJUDICE

There is a fundamental mistake that is easily made by scientists and physicians alike. When one disorder or disease comes before another, it is not unusual to assume that the first caused the second. This error in thinking occurs so often that it has been given a name—*post hoc, ergo propter hoc* ("after this, therefore on account of it"). Although at times this way of thinking may prove correct, at other times, especially in the study and practice of medicine, it can lead to the wrong conclusions.

In this case obesity has been wrongly assumed to be The Deadly Quartet's "leader of the pack," the bad influence that must be eliminated in order to stop the others. Although it is true that weight gain often precedes the onset of high blood pressure, risk-related blood fat levels, and adult-onset diabetes, it is far more likely that all four disorders are symptoms of the underlying insulin imbalance that brings on heart disease. So in reality, excess weight gain is a sign that the other members of The Deadly Quartet are close behind.

> Carbohydrate cravings and excess weight gain are signs that you have an insulin imbalance and that other heart disease risk factors can be expected to follow.

Think of it like this: You are taking care of a child with measles. The first symptom to appear is lethargy—a tiredness on the child's part, a disinterest in activity. Next the child develops a fever. Last, there appears the telltale rash that indicates an infection with the measles virus. Now, just because the child was tired or feverish before the rash appeared does not mean the lack of movement or fever caused the rash. Instead, we know that each of these symptoms was related to the same underlying cause, the measles infection. It would seem illogical, even silly, to try to prevent the rash either by making the child active or by washing the child down with cool water in order to bring down the fever.

In the same way, hundreds of scientific studies involving both animals and humans have documented the fact that hyperinsulinemia leads to obesity rather than the reverse. Since, as you will see in more detail, hyperinsulinemia also leads to high blood pressure, risk-related blood fats, and adult-onset diabetes, it makes no sense to blame obesity for the occurrence of these disorders. Instead, if you are going to eliminate the cause of these heart health threats, it is important to recognize that all four disorders spring from the same underlying imbalance.

In both our scientific studies and private practice, when overweight patients and research participants were asked to follow a program designed to reduce insulin levels and insulin resistance—*a program that entailed no restrictions on the amount or portions of food allowed*—the result was easy weight loss, without need for deprivation or struggle, along with natural, positive change in all heart health indicators. Clearly, if reducing insulin levels resolved weight problems, it was the hyperinsulinemia that caused the weight gain in the first place.

This phenomenon has been described by many other researchers, though some continue to get the process backward. These scientists still claim that when people lose weight, they reduce their insulin levels and improve their blood pressure and their blood fat and blood sugar levels. We now understand that the improvements they observe come not from the loss of weight but from the weight-reducing diet that changes carbohydrate intake. Even before a great deal of weight is lost, the changes in carbohydrate intake lowers insulin, which, in turn, leads to many heart health–related improvements. Many low-fat diets reduce total carbohydrate intake or the frequency of carbohydrate intake and, in doing so, reduce insulin levels as well. Reducing saturated fats may offer the additional benefit of removing saturated fat's insulin-releasing power as well.

> Even before a great deal of weight is lost,
> changes in carbohydrate intake lowers insulin,
> which, in turn, leads to many
> heart health–related improvements.

In both animals and humans, when levels of insulin are increased—either naturally or by means of injections or infusions of insulin—weight gain is usually inevitable, even when no additional food is consumed! High insulin levels turn bodies into fat-making machines. Without high levels of insulin, bodies burn up extra calories; in the presence of high insulin levels, bodies make fat even without the intake of additional calories. It is clearly the excess insulin that makes us fat and not the reverse.

Why, then, do we hear the opposite message? Why are we told, over and over, that obesity leads to heart disease rather than the fact that hyperinsulinemia leads to obesity and ultimately to heart disease? In some cases it is a simple misunderstanding or lack of awareness of the available research. In other cases it seems that the prejudice against the obese has spilled over into the area of scientific study and led to errors in thinking. Even worse, those who control the big business of dieting may also have a financial interest in perpetuating untruths that imply that the overweight lack willpower.

Although commercial programs have an abysmal long-term success rate, they continue to propagate the illusion that all it takes is a little willpower to get slim and trim and *healthy*. How different their advertisements would look if, according to all science knows about weight loss, they were forced to say, "Well, most weight gain is really biological, and once you understand the way in which your insulin imbalance turns your body into a fat-making machine, and correct the cause of your cravings and weight gain, you won't need to come back to us." They know that good science is not always good for their business.

> Commercial weight-loss centers and diet drug and food manufacturers know that good science is not always good for their business.

So regardless of whether it's the result of an honest misunderstanding, the power of prejudice, or the vested interests of the diet industry, the wrong message is being perpetuated.

The facts are clear and simple: over time, excess insulin leads to intense carbohydrate cravings and weight gain, then to insulin resistance, high blood pressure, risk-related blood fats, adult-onset diabetes, and heart disease. When you reduce excess insulin levels, you reduce your risk for insulin-related heart problems as well. It is that simple—and that wonderful.

THE UNINTENTIONAL SCAPEGOAT

The unspoken assumption about the overweight is that they eat "too much." If you are overweight, chances are, every diet you go on tries to get you to lose weight by forcing you to eat less. The assumption is that you gained weight because you ate too much to begin with. Yet nothing could be further from the truth. Scientists have shown, over and over again, that the overweight eat no more, and in many cases less, than normal-weight individuals.

> **In many cases the overweight eat less than normal-weight individuals.**

More than three decades ago, scientists discovered that contrary to popular belief, what you ate did *not* necessarily determine what you weighed. They found that some people seemed to be "naturally thin" and seemed to have the ability to overeat without gaining weight. As far back as 1967, Drs. D. S. Miller and P. Mumford documented the fact that some people were able to virtually double their food intake, consuming an extra 8,000–10,000 calories per week, and still lose weight.

In the following year the eminent researcher Dr. E. A. H. Sims along with his colleagues tested the "You are what you eat" hypothesis. They overfed their fifteen research participants up to 3,000 calories per day, with the goal of increasing the subjects' weight by 25 percent. The researchers were surprised to find that 3,000 extra calories per day did not bring about the desired weight gain. These research participants apparently "burned up" the extra calories they took in rather than storing them as excess weight. Two important exceptions were noted, involving one research participant who had been overweight in his youth and another who had a strong history of adult-onset diabetes in his family. Both these subjects did gain weight on the high-caloric diet, and not so coincidentally, both could be expected to have high levels of insulin as well.

Although it is contrary to what people believe—and in some cases want to believe—your weight does not necessarily reflect how much you eat. As far back as 1982, Dr. J. P. Morgan and his colleagues found that those research participants who weighed the most and had the greatest percentage of body fat ate less than those who weighed the least and had the smallest percentage of body fat. Even more amazing was a second finding—that the heaviest research participants ate as little as half as many calories as their slimmer cohorts, yet they maintained the highest weights!

In two different studies, conducted a number of years apart, both Dr. J. V. Durnin and Dr. R. Leibel of Rockefeller Institute reported that even under severe caloric restrictions, the overweight tend to maintain their excess weight levels. Dr. Leibel further discovered that even when overweight and normal-weight women ate the same food and the same number of calories, the overweight remained overweight and the normal-weight stayed at their ideal weight level. In order to lose weight, Dr. Leibel discovered, the overweight women had to eat far less than their normal-weight counterparts.

> Although some people who are overweight think they overeat, often they eat no more than "naturally slim" people.

Although some of those who are overweight may believe that they eat enough to justify their weight level, it appears that their perceptions may be influenced more by their own self-consciousness and self-condemnation than by fact. Dr. Morgan's research as well as other studies strongly indicate that something other than food intake has a powerful influence on how much we weigh and how the weight is stored. Many of us have suspected as much from our own personal experience, but it was important, as well, to have reputable scientific research confirm our perceptions.

Yet old beliefs die hard. Despite the fact that scientists have documented that weight gain is attributable to far more than the sum total of the calories we consume minus the number of calories we expend, many health professionals, the media, and most of the public—even those who have experienced this phenomenon themselves—have a hard time accepting these documented research findings.

> You are no more to blame for being overweight than you are for the color of your eyes.
> There is, however, a great deal you can do.

If you are overweight or tend to gain weight easily and are also addicted to carbohydrates, it is vital for you to understand that your body responds differently to high-carbohydrate foods than do the bodies of those who do not exhibit these tendencies. It is your body's response to these foods, especially when they are eaten frequently, that leads to the excess release of insulin that may be keeping you on a weight-loss merry-go-round.

You are no more to blame for being overweight than you are for the color of your eyes. There is, however, a great deal you can do to end your "battle of the bulge" for good. Keep in mind that your excess weight may be the first sign that The Deadly Quartet is in the background beginning its work, which can lead to the development of serious heart problems.

INSULIN AND WEIGHT GAIN

- Why do some people seem to put weight on easily whereas others who eat far more remain slim?
- Why do some people experience intense and recurring food cravings?
- Why does stress make some people hungry?
- Why do some women get premenstrual cravings?
- Why do many women have so much difficulty losing the excess weight they gained during pregnancy?
- Why do so many people gain weight when they stop smoking?
- Why do most people who diet tend to regain all the weight they have lost (and more)?
- Why do some of us, as we grow older, gain weight on the same food that used to keep us at a normal, or near-normal, weight?

These questions have baffled physicians, scientists, and patients alike for years. It was only after the insulin connection to cravings and weight gain was discovered that answers could be found. Hyperinsulinemia and the insulin resistance it causes have been identified in people who gain weight easily, in those who crave carbohydrates on a regular basis and/or when stressed, in women who are pregnant or premenstrual, in those who crave carbohydrates when they stop smoking, and in people who are simply growing older. In some ways, one could say that science has found the essential factor that repeatedly forces some of us to fight the battle of the bulge while others are exempted.

At first, scientists could hardly believe the impact of this "wonder" hormone. More than fifteen years ago, Dr. Paula Geiselman and Dr. David Novin reviewed the experiments done by some of this country's most respected scientists in the field of food intake and weight. They combined their own findings with the best research in the field and found that for some people the very sight, smell, taste, and eating of high-carbohydrate foods can lead to a predictable insulin-related series of events that culminated in weight gain. Other scientists, including Dr. D. C. Simonson of Harvard Medical School, confirmed the importance of insulin-related changes in the hunger–weight gain cycle.

> Today it is a well-recognized fact that those who are overweight release too much insulin after consuming high-carbohydrate foods.

Drs. T. Silverstone and E. Goodall and Yale University's Dr. Judith Rodin, as well as scores of other scientists, have documented the insulin connection to hunger, cravings, and weight gain. Today it is a well-recognized fact that those who are overweight release an excess of insulin after consuming high-carbohydrate foods, and that the excess levels increase the more often these foods are eaten.

TWO ESSENTIAL KEYS
DRS. RICHARD AND RACHAEL HELLER REMEMBER

For more than a decade we have known that the more often you eat high-carbohydrate foods, the greater your release of insulin. In addition, we have discovered that when high-carbohydrate foods are eaten alone, without the balance of other foods, insulin levels also peak and stay high. These two discoveries are crucial to the design of an eating plan that is both easy and effective, a livable program that allows people to enjoy high-carbohydrate foods while reducing insulin levels.

Our breakthrough came when we discovered that reducing the number of times each day that high-carbohydrate foods are eaten and balancing high-carbohydrate foods with protein and high-fiber foods can eliminate the chronic hyperinsulinemia that leads to carbohydrate cravings and weight gain as well as the many heart-related health problems that follow.

> Our breakthrough came when we discovered the importance of the "frequency factor" in high-carbohydrate intake and insulin release.

The discovery of these two keys to insulin balance—frequency (how often each day you eat high-carbohydrate foods) and food balance (what foods you eat with your high-carbohydrate foods)—gave us the blueprint for a program that does not require you to give up the high-carbohydrate foods you need and love in order to reduce your insulin levels. As you will discover, on this program you will still enjoy high-carbohydrate foods every day while simultaneously balancing your insulin release.

At the American Institute of Nutrition's annual meetings in 1993, 1994, and 1995, we presented our research documenting that research participants with insulin-related carbohydrate cravings experienced fewer and less intense cravings and also lost weight without struggle by changing how often they ate high-carbohydrate foods. Carbohydrate addicts were able to lose weight and reduce or eliminate cravings without giving up the foods they loved the most.

Although such widely respected authorities as the surgeon general of the United States have reported that insulin promotes increases in blood fat (and its storage in fat cells), it is amazing that even today many practicing physicians do not yet recognize the overwhelming importance of the role that high insulin levels play in the cause and, most important, the elimination of excess weight.

When it comes to weight gain, hyperinsulinemia packs a triple whammy. High levels of insulin:

- Cause food, in general, to taste especially good
- Make some foods taste very sweet
- Cause recurring cravings for certain foods (carbohydrate addiction)

This is insulin's way of enticing you to take in energy. The high-carbohydrate food you eat is changed into blood sugar and, in the presence of hyperinsulinemia, is then converted into blood fat by your liver. Depending on how much insulin remains in your bloodstream and how resistant to insulin your body's cells have become, the fat in your blood may remain for a while, only to be stored away in the fat cells. Even then, hyperinsulinemia can do damage, for if insulin levels remain high, the fat is locked into your fat cells, making it easy to gain weight but difficult to lose it.

If you are overweight, the amount of food you consume, the kinds of food you desire, even the way your body metabolizes your food are almost certainly linked to the amount of insulin you release. If you have a family history of weight or eating problems, high-carbohydrate foods eaten frequently throughout the day, as well as stress, inadequate nutrient supplementation, and inactivity can have devastating effects on your cardiovascular health, well-being, and longevity. How wonderful that the very program you find in this book, which provides guidelines that were designed to improve your heart health, can reduce your cravings and weight as well.

CUTTING YOUR HIGH BLOOD PRESSURE RISK

If you are one of the more than 58 million people who have been diagnosed with high blood pressure,* you may be far luckier than you think. You may be showing a clear sign that hyperinsulinemia is at work. In many cases high blood pressure is your body's way of telling you that it is out of balance insulinwise, and if you heed this warning signal and take appropriate action, it could literally save your life.

In and of itself, high blood pressure does not always indicate that there is a silent insulin imbalance beginning to wear down your healthy heart. If, however, you have high blood pressure in combination with recurring carbohydrate cravings, weight gain, or undesirable blood fat levels, your blood pressure now becomes a vitally important symptom—the second and undeniable sign that a potentially health-endangering insulin imbalance is progressing in your body. It cannot be considered "just high blood pressure"; it is your body's cry for help, and you must respond.

When people are told they have high blood pressure, most react in one of two ways: either they assume they are in no immediate danger and make some vague promise to get it under control, or recognizing the seriousness of the situation, they make changes they've been told will bring their blood pressure under control, no matter how difficult the sacrifice. In either case most will begin drug therapy and/or reduce the salt and fat content in their diet. Less-than-diligent patients may not be surprised when, over time, they see little or no decrease in their blood pressure levels. After all, they tell themselves, I haven't really been that careful, and you can't expect the pills to do the whole job.

*The term *high blood pressure* refers to the most common form of high blood pressure, generally known in medical and scientific circles as essential, or primary, hypertension. In the past this prevalent form of high blood pressure was so termed because no known cause had been identified; that is, the rise in blood presure was considered to be the primary or essential event. Currently, the terms *primary* or *essential* have been dropped from common usage, and unless otherwise specified, the terms *high blood pressure* and *essential/primary hypertension* are used synonymously. In addition, hyperinsulinemia has now been identified as the primary, or essential, event in the development of this disorder.

When diligent patients who undertake a concerted effort to make changes also see very little improvement in their blood pressure readings, they may become concerned and frustrated. The reason for their failure is rather simple. Traditional recommendations are not necessarily aimed at correcting the cause of the problem; rather, they may be nothing more than attempts to reduce the symptoms.* Unless you remove the cause—in this case high levels of insulin—you may be fighting the problem for the rest of your life.

> With blood pressure, as with all health concerns,
> if you don't correct the cause of the problem,
> the symptom is sure to return (and in many cases grow worse).

Attempting to control your high blood pressure with a low-salt or low-fat diet may be likened to treating a fever with Tylenol: the medication may reduce the symptom for a while, but unless the cause of the underlying problem is corrected, the symptom is sure to return (and grow worse).

It is unfortunate that to this day relatively few patients are being told what scientists have known for many years: hyperinsulinemia is one of the most powerful causes of high blood pressure, and lowering your insulin levels can reduce your blood pressure while helping you lower your chances of heart attack and heart disease.

As far back as 1990, in his excellent review of previous research, Dr. R. W. Stout concluded that high levels of insulin are closely associated with a cluster of cardiovascular risk factors that include not only high blood pressure and undesirable blood fat levels but high levels of sugar in the blood and excess weight as well.

The following year Dr. H. R. Black, of the Yale University School of Medicine, confirmed Dr. Stout's views and added that repeated research studies had made it clear that hyperinsulinemia and insulin resistance form a link to excess weight gain, high blood pressure, and adult-onset diabetes mellitus, three conditions that often herald heart disease. Pointing to the fact that other studies have also reached the same conclusion, Dr. Black appealed to the scientific community to consider hyperinsulinemia a potent cardiovascular risk factor.

Prior to these and other similar studies, high blood pressure was

---

Never change or stop your medication except on your physician's recommendation. Work with your physician in all matters. Self-prescription is clearly not the intent of this book.

assumed to be the *cause* of heart disease. As a greater understanding emerges, many scientists are concluding that high blood pressure is a *symptom* of excess levels of insulin, a sign that hyperinsulinemia is present. So rather than supporting the old view that high blood pressure causes heart disease, new studies are making it clear that hyperinsulinemia itself leads to the development of high blood pressure and often, then, to heart disease.

THREE ROADS, ONE DESTINATION

Hyperinsulinemia leads to high blood pressure in three different ways. First, excess levels of insulin directly stimulate your sympathetic nervous system and cause your heart to beat faster, blood vessels to narrow, and blood pressure levels to rise. If you have a family history of high blood pressure, you are likely to develop chronic (ongoing) high blood pressure in response to high levels of insulin.

Second, hyperinsulinemia helps to regulate salt levels in your blood. The higher your insulin levels, the more salt you retain. The more salt you retain, the more water is kept in your bloodstream. You may find that even though you have been avoiding some of the foods you love in order to reduce your salt intake, insulin has nullified all your efforts. The resulting high blood pressure is dictated by a simple law of physics. Just as forcing more water through a hose will result in greater pressure, when you must force more fluid through the same space because there is extra water in your bloodstream you develop high blood pressure.

The third way in which hyperinsulinemia can lead to high blood pressure is by narrowing the openings in the arteries (called lumens) through which your blood flows. High levels of insulin can stimulate the production of cholesterol in the liver and the buildup of plaque in the walls of arteries. The space for blood flow is decreased, and again, blood pressure rises.

As blood pressure rises from hyperinsulinemia's three effects, the heart must work harder, pumping against greater and greater resistance. The end result is to raise blood pressure even higher.

Although hundreds of scientific reports have confirmed hyperinsulinemia's powerful effect on blood pressure, Harvard Medical School's Dr. L. Landsberg summed up the findings of many of his colleagues when he reported that hyperinsulinemia increases salt retention and stimulation of the heart, kidneys, and blood vessels and, in a follow-up report, noted that high blood pressure in the overweight is an unfortunate "by-product" of excess levels of insulin.

Today scientists from around the world (including Dr. A. M. Sharma and his colleagues from the Free University of Berlin; Dr. K. Landin from the University of Göteborg, Sweden; Dr. E. Feraille and his colleagues from the College de France in Paris; and others) are confirming that excess levels of insulin and the resulting insulin resistance are often high blood pressure's silent villains.

Insulin's powerful and silent actions have led scientists to recognize that high blood pressure is not a physical disorder that stands by itself; rather, it is a *symptom*—a very important symptom—indicating that a powerful underlying insulin imbalance is progressing slowly behind the scenes. Physicians who, despite their busy practices and unending demands, are able to stay current with the newest scientific discoveries no longer view high blood pressure as a problem that must be controlled but rather as one that—by correcting the underlying cause—can and must be eliminated for life.

INSULIN AND RISK-RELATED BLOOD FATS

A revolutionary change in medicine is about to take place, and it will be marching right across your dinner table. In the last decade, since the importance of blood fats to heart disease has been studied extensively, a new and surprising relationship has emerged.

> A revolutionary change in medicine is about to take place, and it will be marching right across your dinner table.

For several years the experts have disagreed, with some claiming that dietary fat raised blood fat levels, some saying that trans fatty acids were the key, others saying that dietary cholesterol was the real villain, and still others showing evidence that high-carbohydrate foods were more detrimental than dietary fat. To add to the confusion, researchers found that four out of five people who followed low-fat diets did not reap the expected health benefits. Who was right? It now appears all of them were right (and to some degree, all of them were wrong).

No one-size-fits-all answer works when it comes to diet and blood fats. It may be that for some all fats are unhealthful, whereas for others cholesterol is the culprit; but for carbohydrate addicts, the key to keeping blood fat levels low has been tied to the type of fat that is consumed and its effect on insulin levels.

The good news is that the answer is simple and practical, and best of all, you don't necessarily have to do away with fat in your diet.* Today a major discovery by several research teams has uncovered the insulin link to dietary fat and risk-related blood fat levels. Now carbohydrate addicts can stop blaming themselves for high triglyceride and cholesterol levels and learn easy steps they can take to help reduce risk-related blood fat levels.

From Dr. K. D. Ward's research in The Normative Aging Study to Dr. A. R. Folsom's study of more than four thousand middle-aged healthy adults to Dr. J. A. Marshall's study of more than a thousand men and women from twenty to seventy-four years of age to Dr. E. J. Mayer's study of nondiabetic women, the findings are the same: saturated dietary fats increase insulin levels, whereas unsaturated fats do not.

Saturated fats and trans fatty acids tend to be solids or semisolids at room temperature, whereas unsaturated fats tend to be oils. Typical sources of saturated fats include butter, shortening, palm oil, coconut oil, and meat fats. Trans fats are found in many margarines and vegetable shortenings and are used in cookies, crackers, and French fries. They may be included as hydrogenated fats in the ingredients listing. Unsaturated fats include the monounsaturated oils (peanut, olive, and canola oils) and the polyunsaturated oils (safflower seed, sunflower seed, corn, and fish oils). (See pages 221–226 for an in-depth discussion of dietary fats and a handy chart of "Simple Fat Facts" and "Fast Fat Facts.")

Even as new research continues to emerge, one of the most powerful and compelling studies has been The Nurses' Health Study, conducted by Dr. Frank B. Hu and his colleagues at Harvard Medical College and Brigham and Women's Hospital and published in late 1997 in the esteemed *New England Journal of Medicine*. Dr. Hu's team studied more than eighty thousand women for fourteen years and found that replacing only 5 percent of energy from dietary saturated fat with energy from unsaturated fat reduced the risk for heart disease by almost half! Quite a benefit for so small a change.

This same landmark study confirmed our own research findings that high-carbohydrate foods appear to lead to far greater heart-related health risks than do foods containing unsaturated fats. Dr. Hu concludes his report

---

*As always, check with your physician and follow his or her recommendations regarding the best eating program for your individual needs.

> **Replacing dietary saturated fat with unsaturated fat cut the risk for heart disease by almost half!**

by noting that in this unusually large and long-term study, replacing saturated fat and trans fatty acids with unsaturated fat is more effective in preventing coronary heart disease in women than reducing overall fat intake.

Studies such as these signal a wave of change in thinking that recognizes the distinct effects that different dietary fats have on the risk of heart disease. Now carbohydrate addicts can be freed from the unnecessary limitations imposed by traditional low-fat diets. For carbohydrate addicts, low-fat diets have proved problematic, to say the least. Low-fat diets, by their nature, encourage the frequent intake of high-carbohydrate foods, which, in turn, increase insulin levels.

Carbohydrate addicts who follow these regimens often experience intense carbohydrate cravings, weight gain, increased blood pressure, increases in risk-related blood fats, and increased risk for insulin-related heart disease. Ironically, the very diet that has, in the past, been prescribed in order to lower blood fat levels, when given to the carbohydrate addict, often backfires, increasing insulin levels, which, in turn, urge the body to produce higher levels of blood fats.

> **The discovery is surprisingly simple: for the carbohydrate addict, total fat is not as important as the *kind* of fat that is eaten.**

The discovery is surprisingly simple: for the carbohydrate addict total fat is not as important as the *kind* of fat that is eaten. Saturated fats lead to hyperinsulinemia, whereas unsaturated fats do not increase insulin levels. If you are a carbohydrate addict, the discovery that saturated fat rather than unsaturated fat leads to hyperinsulinemia reveals a wonderful freedom in your food choices, allowing you to enjoy many of the foods you love while giving you a powerful tool in reducing your risk for insulin-related heart disease. Now you can include olive oil, canola oil, peanut oil, corn oil, and other unsaturated oils in your cooking without feeling that you are cooking up your own heart attack in the process.

A Tiger in a Cage: Peter, Steve, and Matthew's Story
DR. FREDERIC VAGNINI REMEMBERS

Three generations sat across from me in my consulting room. The family resemblance was unmistakable—the same curly chestnut hair, now graying in the older two, the same chiseled chin, and the same piercing blue eyes. Matthew, the youngest, was the first to speak.

"We're worried about my grandfather," he began, and it seemed as if Peter's smile faded a bit at being identified as the patient. "He's not doing well," Matthew continued in his less-than-subtle manner. "He's stopped taking his medicine, and his blood pressure is back up again. He's eating anything he wants, he's putting on weight and not exercising, and anybody can see he's headed right for another heart attack."

Matthew's father, Steve, interrupted his son's presentation and, in a much calmer voice, related his concerns. His father, Peter, he explained, was now sixty-five and had suffered a heart attack when he was only in his early fifties. Although there had been no permanent damage, it had been touch-and-go for a while, and the experience had left the entire family shaken and worried. Over the years, the immediacy of their distress had lessened, though Peter's health had remained something of a concern when considering vacations or the like.

After his heart attack Peter's health had remained stable for several years, and at his physician's suggestion, he had been able to discontinue all medication with no apparent negative impact on his heart health nor any increase in heart disease risk factors. His blood pressure, blood fats, and blood sugar levels had remained stable and within normal limits. Clearly his diet—a diet of his own making that involved basic moderation—had been working well.

Then, about four years ago, something changed. Peter's weight, always a bit of a problem in the past, began to increase. At first the pounds crept up gradually, one or two a month and a couple more after holiday celebrations. Unlike in the past, these added pounds no longer dropped off in the weeks following the festivities. Slowly but surely, over a few years, Peter had gained nearly twenty pounds.

Other heart disease risk factors were increasing as well: his triglyceride levels had nearly doubled, his desirable cholesterol levels had dropped, and the undesirable blood fat levels had increased. His blood pressure had become dangerously high, and his family physician had started him on blood pressure medication along with a diuretic to reduce water retention.

"That's when the problems began," Peter explained, speaking for the first time. "That medicine is terrible. It makes me tired, and . . . I don't know . . . it makes me feel lousy. I get this headache all the time, whether I take the medication or not, and I know it's from the high blood pressure, and I hate it. I'm hungry all the time, too," he continued. "I don't know, not exactly hungry but not satisfied either. I can't explain it. I hate that stuff, the medicine, and I know they think I'm crazy for not taking it," Peter nodded at his son and grandson, "but they're not me."

Matthew and Steve rose to the occasion, each trying to communicate his concern and frustration and each asking me to make Peter "listen to reason."

"I'd rather look for the cause of the problem first," I suggested, and went on to explain that in taking any case history, it was essential whenever possible to determine what change had occurred that might account for the series of heart health–deteriorating events.

"It was the medication," Peter declared. "Pure and simple. That's when all the trouble started."

I quickly reminded him of the key points he had just relayed to me. "First came a slow and steady weight gain," I recounted.

"And a rise in blood pressure," Matthew added. "And that made the doctor put you on blood pressure medicine."

"And now that I think about it," Peter added, "I wasn't feeling so good when he first told me to start taking the medication. You know, sluggish. Sometimes after I'd eat, I'd feel strange—I'd get shaky or feel real tired. But it was nothing compared to how bad I feel now."

I continued on my search for the change that had caused Peter's blood pressure rise and weight gain and prompted his doctor to prescribe the medication. "Can you think of anything that changed in your life about four or five years ago?" I asked.

"No, and that's the crazy thing," Peter answered readily. "Just the opposite. Everything was pretty much the same. In fact, I was doing better, and I should have been getting healthier instead of worse."

"What do you mean when you say you were 'doing better'?"

"Well, I had started eating better, cutting down on my fats and eating a lot more fruits and vegetables. I stopped eating all red meat, and then Steve's wife got after me, and I cut down on the chicken as well. But that's what you're supposed to be doing, isn't it? What's wrong with that?" Peter asked.

"If you substituted a great many sugar-rich foods, all day long, in place of the fats, there could be a great deal wrong with it," I thought, but for the moment I said nothing. First, I wanted to perform a complete physical examination and look at the results of Peter's blood tests and cardiovascular stress test.

Over the next two weeks, I learned a great deal about Peter, and he learned a great deal about himself. He returned once again with his son and grandson, but this time with some interesting observations.

"You know," he began, "you didn't say anything about it at the last visit, but you got me thinking about the food I've been eating, and I started noticing what happened each time I ate. When I ate less meat, I was doing a lot of snacking—I mean a lot—and I felt lousy. Now, it doesn't make sense, because the snacks were low-fat, but that seems to be what was happening. It's crazy, isn't it?"

Based on the results of his physical and other tests, the answer was clear. Peter showed many of the signs of being addicted to carbohydrates: after eating, his insulin levels rose far above normal, his blood sugar levels were too high, and his blood fat levels indicated that he had Type IV hyperlipidemia (blood fat problems), a condition that laboratories have nicknamed "carbohydrate-induced" blood fats. It appeared that the high levels of insulin in Peter's body were turning much of the low-fat, sugary food he was eating into artery-clogging blood fats.

I explained the process to all three men. "Insulin can raise your blood pressure in three ways. First, it stimulates the sympathetic nervous system, causing your heart to beat faster, blood vessels to narrow, and blood pressure levels to rise. Second, insulin helps regulate salt levels in your blood. The more insulin in your bloodstream, the more salt is retained. The more salt, the more water is retained and channeled into the blood. It's a simple law of physics. Forcing more fluid through the same space results in greater pressure—or in this case high blood pressure. Last, insulin can stimulate the production of cholesterol and the buildup of plaque in the walls of arteries. The space for blood flow is decreased, and as would be expected, your blood pressure rises. And of real concern," I added, "as your blood pressure rises from insulin's three effects, your heart has to work harder, pumping against more and more resistance.

"Now, the tie-in," I concluded, "came when you switched to a low-fat diet and cut out red meat and even chicken. That's when you began eating more low-fat snack foods. These foods are high in carbohydrates—in particular, sugar. Because you are carbohydrate-sensitive, the more often you ate high-carbohydrate foods, the more insulin your body released. The more insulin your body released, the higher your blood pressure rose and, because insulin puts your body in a fat-making mode, the more blood fat and body fat your body produced."

I went on to explain that Peter's genetics seemed to predispose his body to release too much insulin when he drank fruit juices and ate sugary snacks. In his case even foods he thought of as "healthy," like cereals and low-fat snacks, were causing insulin surges. When these foods were consumed all day long, his body produced insulin all day long, with results that were apparent.

I suggested that Peter try an experiment. Giving him a list of wholesome low-carbohydrate foods, I asked him to choose foods from the list for all but one of his meals each day. If a food he desired was not on the list, I asked him to save it for one meal each day during which he was free to eat any high-carbohydrate food he desired along with a balance of other low-carbohydrate foods.

"This is not a low-carbohydrate diet," I explained. "This is a low-frequency carbohydrate diet. You can still have high-carbohydrate foods. Only now you'll have them all at the same time along with other foods, in a balanced meal. The rest of your meals will be high-fiber and contain low-fat proteins."

The experiment worked. Within three days Peter telephoned my office.

"I don't know what's happening," he exclaimed. "I feel like my old self again. The headache's gone, and I can tell my blood pressure is much better. My cravings are gone, too; they literally vanished. I almost forgot to eat lunch yesterday. I've been eating fish and chicken . . . and lean meat once in a while and even some dessert."

"And vegetables and salad," I added. "Low-carbohydrate foods at most meals, so you haven't been releasing as much insulin as normal. It sounds like your blood pressure is responding and your blood sugar levels are probably better, too." We chatted a bit, and I made several suggestions that might maximize the effectiveness of Peter's dietary changes.

When I saw Peter, his son, and grandson in my office again, it was several weeks later. "My blood pressure's normal!" Peter announced. "And I feel terrific. If it stays down, my family doctor says I can probably go off medication soon, if that's all right with you," he added.

I nodded my agreement. At my suggestion, in addition to his change in carbohydrate intake, Peter had started an easy walking regimen, about half an hour three times each week. In addition, he had begun taking several important nutritional supplements I had recommended, and the changes seemed to be having the desired effect.

I cautioned Peter that, given his medical history, some medication might be necessary but went on to explain that we would monitor his progress and, in consultation with his family physician, move toward the goal of his being medication-free, as long as it did not compromise his heart health.

Now Matthew, who had been silent at this visit, softly began to tell his tale. "You know, I'm here because I need help, too." His grandfather, father, and I were speechless.

"Well," he continued, "I feel like I'm sitting next to one of those circus wagons with a tiger in the cage, and any moment someone's going to let the tiger out and he's going to attack me. I have watched my grandfather struggle through heart problems all the time I've known him, and I see the same thing beginning to happen to my father. He's starting to put on more weight, and his blood pressure is too high, and as harsh as it sounds, I just don't want to have that to look forward to. I tell myself that I exercise and stay in shape and eat right, but the truth is, I'm not sure that any of it is going to do any good. And grandpop had his heart attack when he wasn't much older than my father." Matthew hesitated, and Steve's face showed that his son's words echoed his own feelings and concerns.

I explained that a similar program might be appropriate for each of them—in Matthew's case helping reduce his risk for insulin-related heart problems, and in Steve's helping to reverse the first signs of insulin's heart risk–raising impact. I added that the Program should be modified to meet their individual physical needs. This answer and reassurance seemed to hearten them all, and we set up an appointment to help both father and son get started on the program.

I was about to broach the subject of balance, of the importance of the spiritual side of heart health, when Peter brought up the topic.

"You know," he began softly, "there's something funny that has happened. I don't exactly know how to explain it, but something else has changed."

We all waited for him to continue.

"Well, when I started feeling the physical change from my new diet come over me, I . . . well, I said a prayer and thanked God. I told Him how grateful I was and asked Him to take care of my family in the same way. And it felt so good, so terrific to be praying again. I haven't really stopped since that day a couple of weeks ago. I don't let a day go by without praying; it's really important to me. I don't know if you pray, Dr. Vagnini," he added, "but it really does something to me way down inside."

"Oh, yes," I thought, "I know." And as I continued my conversation with Peter, I silently thanked God for my life, my profession, and my deep trust in and connection to Him, as well as for leading me to a program that offered health, help, hope, and healing to my patients.

THE CARBOHYDRATE CONNECTION TO INSULIN AND BLOOD SUGAR SWINGS

If you are a carbohydrate addict, it is essential that you understand how your blood sugar levels can be affected by the kinds of food you eat and, most important, how often you eat them.

Most of the things you do each day, you do without thinking. You take a shower, eat breakfast, and dress never considering the degree of coordination and judgment that are involved in the simple performance of these tasks. You naturally put yourself "on automatic," then trust that your body will be able to handle all the challenges with which it is presented. Your most vital life functions, including the regulation of your blood sugar levels, are under your body's unconscious control. You may think you are running your life, but in many ways your body is running it for you.

When all goes well, as you begin to eat, your body releases saliva to help break down your food into simple, absorbable parts. If the food you eat is high-carbohydrate, tastes sweet, or is high in saturated fat,* your body releases insulin into your bloodstream in anticipation of the coming food energy. The food energy that comes from carbohydrates is turned into a simple sugar (glucose), then absorbed into the blood. The more sugary the food, the more quickly it is absorbed. Foods containing complex carbohydrates (starches and soluble fibers) are broken down into simple sugar more slowly and therefore take longer to raise blood sugar levels.

> **Insulin is released when you first see, smell, taste, or even think of high-carbohydrate food.**

The insulin that is released when you first see, smell, taste, or even think of high-carbohydrate food helps to move the blood sugar to different parts of the body, where it is used or stored away. Remember that insulin "opens the doors" to cells so that the blood sugar can bring them energy for growth, repair, and doing the work for which they were designed—for ex-

---

*Although saturated fat is now known to cause high levels of insulin release, this discovery is quite recent. The mechanisms that lead to saturated fat–related hyperinsulinemia and the changes that result from that hyperinsulinemia are not yet understood in detail. At this time, for purposes of explanation, we will concentrate on the well-documented processes involved in carbohydrate ingestion and its effect on blood sugar levels.

ample, contraction of muscles. Insulin then signals the liver and muscle to store away a small portion of extra blood sugar for future use. The major portion of the remaining blood sugar is turned first into blood fat, then stored as fat in the fat cells.

When blood sugar levels begin to drop over time or from activity, the liver makes its small reserve available for the body's use. When the liver's cache has been used, rising levels of glucagon signal the fat cells to open and contribute their stores to the cells that need it for fuel.

Sometimes, things go wrong. In the carbohydrate addict an excess of insulin disrupts this vital hormonal give-and-take. If you are a carbohydrate addict, when you eat high-carbohydrate foods, especially those that contain simple sugars, your body pours far too much insulin into your bloodstream. This excess of insulin upsets the entire balance. The more often high-carbohydrate foods (especially simple sugars) are eaten, the more insulin is released, and the greater the imbalance.

If you have a predisposition for adult-onset diabetes, when you eat high-carbohydrate foods frequently, and when you eat a high proportion of simple sugars (candy, cake, ice cream, cookies, and fruit juice), you may find yourself experiencing many of the signs of low blood sugar within two hours after eating. These symptoms include headache, a foggy kind of thinking, shakiness, extreme tiredness, sweats, or irritability. You may crave something sweet or find yourself surprisingly hungry. You may just feel out of sorts, or if an adrenaline reaction kicks in, your heart may race, and you may get sweaty, and feel as if something were terribly wrong.

Some people describe a sudden low blood sugar drop as a type of fear or panic attack. Although there could be many reasons for these responses and you should always check with your physician to rule out any other cause, if no other reason can be found, you may well be experiencing a *postprandial reactive hypoglycemic response*. In other words, after eating (postprandial), you have a reaction to the high-carbohydrate foods in which your blood sugar drops, causing you to become hypoglycemic.* Hypoglycemia occurs when insulin and the blood sugar it brings are not allowed to enter the cells of the brain and muscles. These insulin-resistant cells leave insulin with little choice but to channel the blood sugar into the fat cells.

---

*Postprandial reactive hypoglycemia is not the same as fasting hypoglycemia, an entirely different condition that stems from an insufficient intake of energy and occurs when the body is inadequately nourished for a prolonged period of time.

> **The more often you eat or drink high-carbohydrate foods or beverages, the greater your insulin release.**

The more frequent the intake of high-carbohydrate food and drink, the higher the levels of insulin release; the higher the insulin release, the greater the drop in blood sugar. The body—sensing that blood sugar is needed by the brain, other organs, and muscles—may release even more insulin in hopes of "breaking through" the resistance and bringing in the nourishment that these cells need.

Yet high levels of insulin lead to intense cravings for the very carbohydrates that led to this imbalance. Each subsequent snack of high-carbohydrate foods or beverages sweetened with sugar substitute can intensify the cycle until the fat cells close down to this insulin "insult," and with no cells to enter, both insulin and blood sugar remained trapped in the blood. The net result: adult-onset diabetes.

For the carbohydrate addict, low blood sugar levels are not the opposite of adult-onset diabetes; they are often the first stage in this addictive, cyclical, progressive, and compelling imbalance.

In our research presented at the annual meeting of the American Institute of Nutrition, we reported that some carbohydrate addicts had such strong reactive hypoglycemic responses to carbohydrates that two hours after eating, their blood sugar levels were almost half of what they were after they had fasted for up to eight hours. For these individuals the more often they ate, the lower their blood sugars fell until these levels "bottomed out."

> **When our carbohydrate addicts ate high-carbohydrate foods often, throughout the day, their blood sugar plummeted until these levels "bottomed out."**

As these carbohydrate addicts' blood sugar levels rose, then fell, they became weaker, hungrier, moodier, and less motivated. The blood tests confirmed what they already knew—that eating actually made some of them feel less "well" than they felt after fasting!

Happily, when these same research participants learned to balance the ways in which they ate high-carbohydrate foods, they found that they could eat the same high-carbohydrate foods without experiencing the low blood sugar–related headaches, weakness, sweats, shakiness, irritability, loss of motivation, or intense cravings with which they had lived for so long.

The Carbohydrate Addict's Healthy Heart Program has been used with success by adult-onset diabetics, particularly in the disorder's early stages, because the program appears to reduce both the excess levels of insulin and the resulting insulin resistance.

If you have adult-onset diabetes, it is important for you to be aware that this program can quickly reduce insulin levels and your body's resistance to insulin. Although this is a most positive aspect of the program, it is important to realize that your need for oral and injectable medications may rapidly and drastically be reduced or eliminated. Adult-onset diabetics must therefore remain under close medical supervision at all times so that their physicians can adjust or discontinue medications as appropriate.

Signs of Reactive Hypoglycemia

Within two hours after eating a full meal:

- Do you feel weak or hungry and find that a snack makes you feel better?
- Do you find it difficult to stay focused? Are you confused?
- Do you find yourself perspiring without reason?
- Does your heart begin to beat rapidly, become irregular, or start to pound?
- Do you feel anxious or fearful without reason?
- Do you feel restless or uneasy?
- Do you often get very tired or unmotivated?
- Do you get a headache?
- Do you feel shaky?
- Do you feel irritable?
- Do you have a strange sense of altered awareness, almost a feeling of observing your own behavior?

If you sometimes have one or more of these signs within two hours after eating, the chances are you are hyperinsulinemic, and most likely insulin resistant as well.

HEALTHY HEARTS: GETTING THERE AND STAYING THERE

Though most people don't want to admit it, there is a great deal of confusion when it comes to heart disease. Patients and research participants ask us in private what they hesitate to ask in public: What is the difference between heart disease and a heart attack? Is heart disease a real disease, or is it something else? What is hardening of the arteries? Do they really get hard? Once plaque forms, does it ever go away? If I have heart disease, can I ever be cured?

The answers we give are simpler than you might think. The heart is a muscle about the size of your fist, and like all muscles, in order to stay healthy, it needs a steady flow of blood both to obtain nourishment and oxygen and to eliminate wastes.

There are at least two different diseases that can be called "heart disease." The first is coronary artery disease, which involves damage to the arteries that lead out of the chambers of the heart and that feed the muscle that forms the wall of the heart. The second disorder, which involves damage to the heart muscle itself, is called coronary heart disease, also known as ischemic heart disease.[*]

Coronary artery disease almost always precedes coronary heart disease. Coronary artery disease is a progressive disease that can be halted, and in many cases reversed, before it leads to coronary heart disease. Because early intervention is always best, it is important to understand each progressive step, how hyperinsulinemia feeds the progression, and the ways in which an insulin-regulating program can halt, and in some cases reverse, this deadly march toward heart disease.

> **Hyperinsulinemia plays a crucial role in the three critical changes that lead to the development of heart disease.**

---

[*]Another, more generalized disorder, cardiovascular disease, involves the narrowing of the blood vessels throughout the body. A blockage in one of these vessels can stop the blood flow and starve the brain or heart of the blood it needs to survive. For ease of reading, heart disease is defined as coronary artery disease, cardiovascular disease, or the damage-related state of coronary heart disease to which they can lead. An additional, less common type of heart disease, valvular heart disease, is not addressed in this book.

Coronary artery disease is a term that describes several different changes that can narrow the arteries to the heart so that the flow of blood to the heart muscle is decreased or in some cases blocked completely. In general, the progression of coronary artery disease can be divided into three critical changes.

CRITICAL CHANGE 1: THICKENING AND NARROWING

The all-important first step in the development of coronary artery disease is a thickening of the inside walls of the arteries that lead to the heart. As fatty streaks appear in the walls of the arteries, the process we call atherosclerosis is said to have begun. As the inside walls thicken, just below the surface, the space through which blood flows to the heart is narrowed.

Most often, narrowing of the arteries is the result of the accumulation of cholesterol and other fats that help to form plaque. Since insulin has the ability to signal the arterial walls to absorb cholesterol from the blood, excess levels of insulin play a key role in the buildup of plaque and the resulting narrowing of the space through which blood flows to the heart.

Sometimes arteries narrow as a result of the body's attempt to repair many tiny vessel injuries. In a process that is still not completely understood, tiny spontaneous hemorrhages can take place, and often in the presence of high levels of insulin, a fibrous plaque may form. If many small areas of injury become calcified, a patient is said to have "hardening of the arteries," or arteriosclerosis.

In addition to cholesterol accumulation and plaque formation, insulin has the ability to stimulate some cells to grow and multiply. When a high level of insulin is present in the bloodstream, the walls of blood vessels are continually bathed with excess insulin, encouraging cells to grow and multiply. As the cells within the walls of the arteries increase in number and size, they, too, reduce the space through which blood can flow to the heart.

CRITICAL CHANGE 2: A DANGEROUS PRODUCT

In the second critical change of coronary artery disease, cholesterol production in the liver is stimulated by high levels of insulin. Very few people realize that 75 percent of the cholesterol in your blood is made by your own body (endogenous cholesterol), whereas only 25 percent comes from the food you eat (exogenous cholesterol).

Even more important is the fact that the cholesterol your body produces is far more dangerous to the health of your heart than that which comes from your diet. As increased levels of insulin-prompted cholesterol flow through your bloodstream, they provide additional material for the formation of plaque in blood vessels. As the cholesterol-enhanced plaque continues to grow, blood flow through the already-narrowed arteries is reduced even further.

CRITICAL CHANGE 3: THE LOSS OF A VITAL PLAQUE FIGHTER

In its third heart-damaging role, hyperinsulinemia reduces the body's ability to destroy a substance called fibrin. Fibrin acts like glue, holding the plaque together. When insulin levels are within the normal range, the body will naturally destroy excess levels of fibrin as they begin to accumulate. The body's natural ability to destroy fibrin and thereby fight plaque buildup is essential to maintaining clear arteries through which blood can flow.

When high levels of insulin are present, however, the body's ability to get rid of fibrin, this plaque-enhancing glue, is reduced. The result is greater plaque buildup, narrowing the space through which blood flows to the heart, as well as an increased chance that blood cells will stick together to form a clot that will be unable to pass through these narrowed vessels.

THE EXPECTED BUT UNFORTUNATE RESULT

As the coronary arteries narrow from plaque formation and as fibrin levels rise, a blood clot is more likely to completely block the blood flow to the heart. Unable to get the nourishment and oxygen that the blood provides, the heart (the muscle itself) can suffer permanent damage—that is, coronary heart disease.

It is easy to visualize the sequence of events. Imagine for a moment that you are drinking fresh-squeezed lemonade through a straw. With each sip, small pieces of lemon begin to accumulate on the inside of the straw. As lemon pieces continue to stick to its walls, the space inside the straw becomes more and more narrow, and less lemonade is able to pass through. You may have to suck harder to get any fluid through, until finally the straw becomes blocked and no lemonade can pass through at all.

With blood vessels being narrowed by the combination of three different insulin-related actions, the heart's blood supply can be sharply decreased or, worse, cut off.

At this point the heart will often react to the lack of oxygen. Sometimes, though not always, there may be sharp pain or an irregular heartbeat as the vital muscle suffers damage. This is what we so commonly refer to as a heart attack. Men and women may experience a variety of different symptoms, including nausea, the loss of sensation in an arm or a hand, and many other seemingly unrelated symptoms. In a silent heart attack, however, there appear to be no symptoms whatsoever.

When a decrease in blood flow to the heart (partial or complete) causes damage to the heart itself, coronary artery disease is said to have led to coronary heart disease. Like an unmistakable fingerprint left on the trigger of a gun, hyperinsulinemia has left evidence of its deadly presence in arteries that have been blocked or narrowed by plaque and the formation of a deadly blood clot (embolism). Cut off from its oxygen-bearing blood supply, the heart is strangled, and the area that receives no life-giving blood literally dies.

If a heart has suffered damage from lack of oxygen, it appears that the injury cannot be undone. In time, however, other, healthier parts of the heart may take over.

Still, the best course of treatment is prevention: prevention of the onset of coronary artery disease, prevention of its progression, and prevention of a reoccurrence if any damage has already been done. For the carbohydrate addict, a key to all three preventive measures lies in the elimination of hyperinsulinemia.

A DECADE OF ENLIGHTENMENT

Although the concept of insulin sensitivity and insulin resistance was first introduced into the medical literature more than fifty years ago, as Dr. D. C. Simonson of Harvard University's School of Medicine has noted, only during the past decade have the causes and the powerful life-threatening consequences of this imbalance begun to be clarified, especially in relation to the part it plays in the development of heart disease.

At this time research by some of the finest physicians and scientists from around the world (including Dr. A. C. Grimaldi of the Service de Diabetologie of the Pitie-Salpetriere of Paris; Dr. S. Del Prato of the University of Padova, Italy; Dr. H. Beck-Nielsen, chief physician of Odense University Hospital, Denmark; Dr. H. Lithell of Uppsala University, Sweden; and Dr. R. W. Stout of The Queens University of Belfast, Northern Ireland; as well as some of this country's most renowned researchers, including Dr. R. A. DeFronzo and Dr. E. Ferrannini of the Health Science

Center of the University of Texas and Dr. A. Garg and his associates at the Southwestern Medical Center in Dallas) continues to confirm and further describe the link between excess insulin production and its attendant insulin resistance and heart disease and its attendant risk factors.

> Research from around the world continues to confirm the link between heart disease and excess insulin levels.
> Reducing your insulin levels appears to be a most vital key to maintaining a strong and healthy heart.

And the research continues to be compiled. Even as you read this page, researchers from around the world are confirming and reconfirming the message they want the scientific and medical world to know: reducing your insulin levels and insulin sensitivity appears to be a most vital key to maintaining a strong and healthy heart.

The Carbohydrate Addict's BASIC Plan and its Heart Health–Enhancing Options have been designed with one goal in mind: to offer you a simple and effective lifestyle plan that will help you normalize your insulin levels and reduce or eliminate your insulin resistance. At the same time, they can provide you with a rewarding, struggle-free, and deprivation-free way of life. One without the other is, after all, not worth the trade-off.

HYPERINSULINEMIA'S CHANGING FACES

For many decades, heart disease has been called a "multifactorial" disorder, that is, coming from many factors. Traditional risk factors for heart disease have included a family history of heart disease as well as a personal history of high blood pressure, risk-related blood fats, excess body fat, adult-onset diabetes, inactivity, stress, and smoking.

Each of these risk factors was known to contribute in some way to the development of heart disease. The part that each factor played, however, remained a mystery. With the discovery of the insulin link, the connection became apparent.

It may take a bit of time before details of the insulin connection to heart disease risk factors make their way into your doctor's office. At this time, however, scientists are well aware that heart disease can no longer be viewed as a multifactorial disease. We now need to see and understand heart disease as well as obesity, high blood pressure, risk-related blood fats, and adult-onset diabetes as the changing faces of insulin's powerful and far-reaching impact.

With the discovery of the insulin connection, risk factors that had appeared separate and unconnected reveal themselves as reinforcing disorders linked by insulin's influence. Many of these formerly separate risk factors make up what scientists now refer to as Insulin Resistance Syndrome (or as it is also known, Syndrome X or Metabolic Syndrome).

For research scientists and physicians alike, the dream is to discover a single factor, a *profactor,* that links and is responsible for several different important illnesses. Ideally, the correction or removal of the underlying factor would result in the prevention or elimination of the related illnesses as well.

For carbohydrate addicts hyperinsulinemia appears to be their "profactor," and what had been their curse in the past now becomes a blessing for today and tomorrow.

> Along with the discovery of hyperinsulinemia's powerful connection to heart disease came an understanding of how to prevent or correct it.

DISABLING INSULIN'S POWER

The Carbohydrate Addict's Healthy Heart Program has been designed to help lower your risk of coronary artery disease and coronary heart disease by eliminating the *cause* of all three critical changes. If you have already had a heart attack, the Program is designed to remove the cause of your problem and allow your heart, insofar as possible, to repair itself and reverse any damage done. Thwarting hyperinsulinemia's powerful and dangerous "triple play" of artery narrowing depends on eliminating or greatly reducing excess levels of insulin. The need for a program that would do just that led Professor M. W. Stolar of Northwestern University Medical School to make a clear and open call for a heart disease treatment program that would minimize insulin levels.

We are grateful that along with the discovery of hyperinsulinemia and its connection to heart disease came an understanding of how to prevent or correct it. As high levels of insulin and insulin resistance decline, signs of atherosclerosis often decline or disappear; cholesterol and triglyceride levels drop; lower-density lipids (LDL—the "bad" fats in the blood) drop; and higher-density lipids (HDL—the "good" cholesterol) rise.

Our clinical practice and scientific research have shown that within three months after an individual starts following The Carbohydrate Addict's Healthy Heart Program, many indicators of heart disease can drop dramatically and in some cases begin to disappear. As patients and research participants alike continue on the Program, many find that their total cholesterol may drop by as much as 20 percent. Blood pressure levels greatly improve as well. It is not unusual to see triglycerides drop by half, with the greatest decrease found in those with the highest blood fat levels. In some rarer cases, total triglycerides have been shown to decrease by as much as 150 points. In addition, cravings disappear, and in their stead a significant, steady, and easy weight loss is more the rule than the exception.

The Carbohydrate Addict's Healthy Heart Program is easy and simple. It requires little time and will not require you to give up the foods you love. You will never have to weigh, measure, or make exchanges. Real people can't live by numbers. Most important, The Carbohydrate Addict's Healthy Heart Program may be crucial in reducing your insulin-related link to heart disease. If you or someone you love carries the burden of an insulin-related risk for heart disease, this can be the greatest gift of all.

> The Carbohydrate Addict's Healthy Heart Program can be crucial in breaking hyperinsulinemia's link to heart disease. For those of us who carry the heart disease risk factor burden, this can be the greatest gift of all.

4

ARE YOU A CARBOHYDRATE ADDICT AT RISK?

ADDICT: from the Latin *addicene*, to surrender or to be captured into slavery. —*Webster's Dictionary*, second edition

- How do you know whether you are a carbohydrate addict?
- How do you know whether you have Insulin Resistance Syndrome?
- How do you know whether you are at risk for a heart attack or heart disease?
- If you have already had a heart attack, how do you know whether you are at risk for another?
- How do you know whether you have Syndrome X (Metabolic Syndrome)?

These are some of the questions that people ask as they learn more about the powerful impact of carbohydrate addiction and the importance of insulin and insulin resistance to heart health. Three key questions must be answered: (1) What is the best way to test for carbohydrate addiction? (2) How can a carbohydrate addict determine the stage of Insulin Resistance Syndrome to which he or she has progressed? (3) What can be done to stop and reverse a carbohydrate addict's progression through the stages of Insulin Resistance Syndrome?

In the many letters we receive, as well as in our lectures and patient consultations, we are asked to recommend reliable laboratory procedures that will test for carbohydrate addiction, excess insulin release, and insulin resistance. We explain that a blood test that evaluates a patient's fasting insulin levels is *not* necessarily an accurate indicator of any of these problems. A blood test that measures fasting insulin levels can, in fact, be quite misleading if the result falls in the normal range.

> **Blood tests that measure insulin levels after fasting can be quite misleading.**

Remember that if you are a carbohydrate addict, you release excess levels of insulin, which can remain high for a prolonged period of time. Your insulin levels rise after you eat or drink high-carbohydrate foods or beverages as well as in response to stress. You may never realize you are overreleasing this powerful hormone, but the signs will be evident in blood tests— *if the right tests are given at the right time.*

Here is a vital error that many physicians and scientists make: the most commonly ordered blood test for determining your insulin level measures your blood insulin levels after fasting. Only a single reading is taken, and it is taken after you have had no food or drink for a period of eight to twelve hours. In addition, you are usually told to come for testing early in the morning, when your stress levels tend to be the lowest.

Since insulin levels normally rise in response to eating or drinking high-carbohydrate foods or beverages or experiencing stress, if insulin levels are calculated after you have had *no* food or drink and when you have been stress-free for a good period of time, insulin levels may *appear* normal. They may rise to risk-related levels when, upon leaving the physician's office, you eat some breakfast or you return home or go to the office and face your daily routine.

A second problem with this testing occurs because, after you drink a mixture of glucose (sugar) and water after fasting, your body can release insulin at a different rate than it does after you have had a mixed meal (which includes a balance of protein and high-carbohydrate foods). Since many tests use the glucose mixture (called a "challenge") for testing after fasting, the results can be somewhat misleading.

Even if the test had been performed after you had something to eat or drink or while you were under stress, a single sample reveals nothing about how high your insulin levels will remain over a period of hours. The fasting insulin test can be irrelevant in determining your post-eating insulin levels.

> Unfortunately, a fasting insulin test
> is often the only insulin test given—
> if it's given at all.

Unfortunately, a fasting insulin test is often the only insulin test given—if it's given at all. Although the test itself is problematic, perhaps the most significant error occurs in the evaluation of your test results.

Many physicians assume that if your fasting insulin test indicates a normal level of insulin, you cannot have an insulin imbalance. There is an abundance of research to show that they are wrong. Physicians who make this false assumption fail to realize that an overrelease of insulin usually takes place only when something stimulates it, such as stress or high-carbohydrate food or drink. Since in clinical practice many physicians assume that a diagnosis of insulin resistance and Insulin Resistance Syndrome depends on finding high levels of insulin, when fasting insulin tests are used, these diagnoses are often missed.

Relying on a fasting insulin test to determine whether you release too much insulin when you eat high-carbohydrate foods is like being tested for a strawberry allergy when you have been instructed to avoid strawberries for several days before the test. Chances are, after you stay away from strawberries, your skin will show no rash and you will report neither congestion, itching, nor headache. It is likely you will have no signs or symptoms of strawberry allergy whatsoever, and in all likelihood you will be found to be allergy-free. You might protest that the test was invalid because the instructions you were given eliminated any chance of your having the very allergic response for which the test was performed.

Attempting to determine a patient's typical insulin response to the consumption of high-carbohydrate foods (often referred to by physicians as *postprandial reactive hyperinsulinemia*) by using a fasting insulin test is totally illogical. It simply makes no sense. Unfortunately, this is the way many people are currently tested—if they are tested at all.

To make matters worse, patients given fasting insulin tests are often told that since their insulin levels are normal, they need not be tested again. For the carbohydrate-addicted patient, these conclusions can be very wrong and potentially dangerous.

Most of us do not think twice about fasting before a blood test; it is done all the time. In the case of an insulin test, however, the information you get after fasting may fail to show evidence of the problem for which the physician should be looking.

Some patients, often those in the later stages of Insulin Resistance Syndrome, do show high levels of insulin while fasting, but in the earlier stages abnormally high levels of insulin are evident only after the consumption of high-carbohydrate foods and beverages or during stressful situations. For those in the early stages of Insulin Resistance Syndrome, a fasting blood insulin test is *not* the appropriate test to confirm a diagnosis of carbohydrate addiction or document its progression through the stages of Insulin Resistance Syndrome.

Some laboratories offer postprandial insulin tests that measure insulin levels after you have had something to eat or drink, but they have no standard basis for comparison, so there is nothing against which to compare the results. This means that once you get the lab results, most likely neither you nor your physician will be able to make sense out of the numbers in the report. In addition, these tests often measure your insulin levels after you have drunk a mixture of very sweet sugar (glucose) and water. Although such a test may indicate what happens after you have ingested only pure sugar, it tells you nothing about your normal response to "real food."

> **If an insulin test were to be accurate,
> it would have to measure your insulin response to food, drink,
> and all the daily changes you encounter.**

If an insulin test were to give an accurate reading, it would have to measure how much insulin is released as your body responds to food, drink, changes in the environment, stress, and daily and hourly fluctuations, as well as medication and menstrual-cycle changes.

At the very least, an accurate test would have to have been administered to a variety of people so that a standard range of normal limits could be established comparable to the limits you see on medical laboratory test reports in relation to cholesterol, triglyceride, and blood sugar (glucose) levels.

Scientists are aware of the lack of, and the need for, good insulin testing, but they are still debating the positives and negatives of a whole battery of tests that are generally used for these purposes in research situations only. At this time each of the tests under consideration has been shown to have major drawbacks, and it appears that none can reasonably be relied on for an accurate clinical diagnosis.

With that said, if laboratory testing is necessary, the one test that appears to be the best choice is the three-hour oral glucose tolerance test with insulin sampling. This test measures blood sugar (glucose) and insulin levels after fasting and again at regular intervals after the consumption of an intense sugar mixture (the glucose challenge). Although this test fails to take into account the differences between a sugar drink and a typical meal that contains protein and fat as well as carbohydrates, it can be used to help diagnose an overrelease of insulin.

If the three-hour oral glucose tolerance test with insulin sampling is done, of particular interest should be the comparison of blood sugar readings at fasting versus two to three hours after the glucose challenge. We have found that in the most severely addicted, at two to three hours after the high-sugar drink is consumed, blood sugar readings fall to a lower level than they were after the eight- or ten-hour fast. This hypoglycemic response is, in our opinion, one of the most powerful indicators of abnormally high insulin surges. (Incidentally, these findings also confirm the blood sugar swings that so many carbohydrate addicts report.) In full-blown adult-onset diabetes, blood sugar levels no longer fall due to severe insulin resistance and/or the body's inability to produce or use insulin.

Although oral glucose tolerance tests with insulin sampling can be done if necessary, the time, expense, and discomfort of taking and testing multiple blood samples can make it less than an ideal choice, and with your physician's approval, the three-hour oral glucose tolerance test with insulin sampling may not be necessary.

Through our scientific studies and clinical practice, we have developed a reliable pen-and-paper quiz that samples a wide variety of insulin and insulin resistance risk factors. Your responses to this quiz will help to determine whether you are a carbohydrate addict at risk for insulin-related heart disease.

> There is a reliable pen-and-paper quiz that can help determine whether you are a carbohydrate addict at risk for insulin-related heart disease—without the need for extensive blood testing.

This quiz has been refined, researched, reevaluated, and revised for ten years. We have incorporated risk-factor evaluations from *The Surgeon General's Report on Nutrition and Health* along with data from the finest medical research available. Each year, as results of new research become available, new findings are incorporated.

We have found that when compared with scientific research protocols and traditional blood-testing methods, The Carbohydrate Addict's Heart Health Quiz can be quite reliable in determining the level of carbohydrate addiction, hyperinsulinemia, and insulin resistance, which can greatly influence your risk for heart disease. The heart disease risk profiles following the scoring subsection can also help you ascertain your heart disease risk and determine the stage of Insulin Resistance Syndrome to which you may have progressed. With this information in hand, you will be ready to begin your program and with each passing day reduce your risk for insulin-related heart disease and make positive changes to restore your heart health.

THE CARBOHYDRATE ADDICT'S HEART HEALTH QUIZ

BEFORE YOU BEGIN

The Carbohydrate Addict's Heart Health Quiz requires only a few minutes to complete. This test takes into account the contributions of your environment, your genetics (from your family's medical history), your personal medical history, and your lifestyle.

At the end of the evaluation, you will be given a subscore in each of the four areas of insulin-related heart disease risk factors:

1. Your Family and Personal Medical History
2. Your Nutritional Profile
3. Your Activity Level
4. Your Stress Level

Your Combined Heart Disease Risk Score is the number that will indicate your overall risk for heart disease in relation to insulin's powerful influence.

A JOURNEY OF DISCOVERY

You are about to begin an enlightening and exciting journey. You have already begun to discover the ways in which your health, well-being, and happiness may be influenced by the hormone insulin and its impact on your body.

As you complete The Carbohydrate Addict's Heart Health Quiz, you will begin to understand why each of your four subscores along with your Combined Heart Disease Risk Score are essential in helping you lower your insulin-related risk for heart disease or reverse insulin-related heart problems that you may already have encountered. Best of all, as you begin the Carbohydrate Addict's Healthy Heart Program, your quiz results will help you keep track of your own progress and success.

THE CARBOHYDRATE ADDICT'S HEART HEALTH QUIZ

Part 1: Your Family and Personal Medical History

Check all of the following that apply.

ONE OR MORE OF MY GRANDPARENTS HAVE OR HAD:

_____	high blood pressure.	(1 point)
_____	adult-onset diabetes.	(1 point)
_____	heart disease or atherosclerosis.	(1 point)
_____	difficulty controlling weight.	(1 point)
_____	risk-related fat levels in the blood.	(1 point)

ONE OR MORE OF MY PARENTS HAVE OR HAD:

_____	high blood pressure.	(2 points)
_____	adult-onset diabetes.	(2 points)
_____	heart disease or atherosclerosis.	(2 points)
_____	difficulty controlling weight.	(2 points)
_____	risk-related fat levels in the blood.	(2 points)

I HAVE:

_____	high blood pressure.	(4 points)
_____	adult-onset diabetes.	(4 points)
_____	heart disease or atherosclerosis.	(4 points)
_____	risk-related fat levels in the blood.	(4 points)

Check the *one* sentence that applies to you.

I AM:

_____	not overweight, and I don't struggle to control my weight.	(0 point)
_____	not overweight, but I do struggle to control my weight.	(1 point)

(continued)

_____	less than 20 pounds overweight.	(2 points)
_____	20–50 pounds overweight.	(3 points)
_____	51–100 pounds overweight.	(4 points)
_____	more than 100 pounds overweight.	(6 points)

Check the *one* sentence that applies to you.

I AM:

_____	under 35 years of age.	(0 point)
_____	between 35 and 49 years of age.	(1 point)
_____	between 50 and 64 years of age.	(2 points)
_____	over 65 years of age.	(3 points)

Check if the following applies to you.

_____	I hold quite a bit of weight in my tummy or belly.	(3 points)

Family and Personal Medical History Subscore: _____

Part 2: Your Nutritional Profile

Check all of the following that apply.

_____	During the day I snack between meals.	(2 points)
_____	When I feel like snacking, I often eat either a piece of fruit or some snack food (chips, cookies, crackers, or candy).	(4 points)
_____	Between meals I drink coffee or tea that contains milk, creamer, sugar, or sugar substitutes.	(2 points)
_____	I often chew gum or eat mints or hard candies (regular or "diet").	(2 points)
_____	I often eat when I am not really hungry.	(2 points)
_____	I usually include at least one of the following in every meal: bread, pasta or some other starch, fruits, or sweets.	(2 points)
_____	Between meals I drink soda or other beverages (regular or "diet").	(2 points)
_____	I eat foods high in saturated fats almost every day.	(2 points)
_____	At least one meal a day usually lasts for	

(continued)

	more than an hour.	(2 points)
_____	I often snack at night.	(2 points)

Nutritional Profile Subscore: _____

Part 3: Your Activity Level

Check the *one* sentence that describes you *in general*.

I AM:

_____	a very active person *and* participate in a regular exercise regimen.	(0 point)
_____	a very active person *or* participate in a regular exercise regimen.	(1 point)
_____	a moderately active person.	(3 points)
_____	not active.	(8 points)

Activity Level Subscore: _____

Part 4: Your Stress Level

Check the *one* sentence that applies to you.

I EXPERIENCE A GREAT DEAL OF STRESS:

_____	rarely or never.	(0 point)
_____	at my job but not at home.	(2 points)
_____	at home but not at work.	(3 points)
_____	at home *and* at work.	(6 points)

Check the *one* sentence that applies to you.

I SMOKE:

_____	never.	(0 point)
_____	less than one pack of cigarettes a day.	(2 points)
_____	between one and two packs of cigarettes a day.	(6 points)
_____	more than two packs of cigarettes a day.	(8 points)
_____	cigars or a pipe.	(3 points)

Check the *one* sentence that applies to you.

I DRINK BEER OR WINE:

_____	very rarely.	(0 point)
_____	on occasion, but then in pretty large amounts.	(2 points)

(continued)

_____ once or twice a week.	(1 point)
_____ once a day only, no more than two glasses.	(0 point*)
_____ twice a day or more.	(5 points)

Check the *one* sentence that applies to you.

I DRINK MIXED DRINKS:

_____ very rarely.	(0 point)
_____ on occasion, but then in pretty large amounts.	(1 point)
_____ once or twice a week.	(1 point)
_____ once a day.	(2 points)
_____ twice a day or more.	(6 points)

Check if the following applies to you.

_____ I regularly take birth control pills or female hormone replacement medication.	(2 points)

Stress Level Subscore: _____

*Research studies have indicated that consuming up to no more than two glasses of beer or wine each day, in a single sitting, can reduce the risk for heart disease. We believe this may be to the chromium content of wine and beer. Consumption of greater amounts appear to negate such benefits.

SCORING

To the right of each of the items on The Carbohydrate Addict's Heart Health Quiz, you will find the point value for that item.

Total the points separately for Parts 1, 2, 3, and 4. When adding up your scores, be certain to include points for each item you checked. Each of the four parts of the quiz will provide you with subscores for your insulin-related heart disease risk in relation to your Family and Personal Medical History, Nutritional Profile, Activity Level, and Stress Level. At the end of each part, write in your subscore (the total points for that part).

Then write all four subscores on the following summary list and add them up to get your Combined Heart Disease Risk Score. Now notice where each subscore places you in relation to the total number of possible points. Did you place near the low end, middle, or high end? Your relative placement as well as the actual score will help you understand your risk for insulin-related heart disease and make choices that can greatly improve your heart health now and for many, many years to come.

	Your Subscores	Total Possible Points
Part 1: Family and Personal Medical History	_____	0–43
Part 2: Nutritional Profile	_____	0–22
Part 3: Activity Level	_____	0–8
Part 4: Stress Level	_____	0–27
Combined Heart Disease Risk Score	_____	0–100 (total)

WHAT YOUR HEART DISEASE RISK SCORES MEAN

If you are a carbohydrate addict, by definition, your body releases too much insulin in response to eating high-carbohydrate foods on a frequent basis. Chances are, you also release high levels of insulin after you eat or drink foods that are *not* high-carbohydrate but that your body perceives as sweet. It does not matter whether the food or drink you are consuming contains a sugar substitute (artificial sweetener) rather than "real sugar"; if your body "thinks" a food or drink contains carbohydrates, your body can and will release insulin. Chances are, you also release insulin in response to foods that contain free glutamates (including, but not limited to, monosodium glutamate) as well as during or after periods of intense stress.

In time, unless you take some action to halt or reverse insulin's influence, cells in your body will become insulin resistant, and over time you will progress through the four stages of Insulin Resistance Syndrome. At each stage of the syndrome, new heart disease risk factors emerge, and in the final stage heart attack and heart disease become a clear and present danger.

The higher your Combined Heart Disease Risk Score, the greater your risk for high blood pressure, risk-related blood fat levels, obesity, adult-onset diabetes, atherosclerosis, and, over time, insulin-related heart disease. Your Combined Heart Disease Risk Score indicates your current probability of insulin-related heart disease *if you take no risk-reducing action.*

Your Combined Heart Disease Risk Score will place your risk in one of four ranges: doubtful, mild, moderate, or high.

Your Combined Heart Disease Risk Score will place you in one of four ranges: doubtful risk (indicating that your insulin levels do not appear to influence your heart health) or one of the heart disease risk levels (mild risk, moderate risk, and high risk), in which insulin and insulin resistance have a major impact. These Heart Disease Risk levels include: mild risk, moderate risk, or high risk. A score that places you in the high-risk range suggests that you are at greater immediate risk for insulin-related heart problems than someone whose score indicates a moderate or mild risk. In general, a higher score also indicates that you are at a more advanced stage of Insulin Resistance Syndrome, though depending on changes in lifestyle or stress, unexpected illness or trauma, someone at a lower risk level can progress quickly to a higher risk level and a more advanced stage of Insulin Resistance Syndrome.

> As you grow older, your Combined Heart Disease Risk Score will naturally rise.

As you grow older, your Combined Heart Disease Risk Score will naturally rise, so if your score places you in the mild or moderate range now, use this program and this time wisely, so that you may avoid progressing "naturally" into the high-risk range. If, on the other hand, your Combined Heart Disease Risk Score is already high, we are very happy that you have found this program now and can benefit from the work and experience of all those who have come before you.

YOUR COMBINED HEART DISEASE RISK LEVEL

The sum of your subscores (that is, your combined score) provides you with your combined heart disease risk level. Find the risk level that corresponds to your combined score, then read the heart disease risk profile for that risk level.

Risk	Combined Score:
Doubtful	0 – 11
Mild	12 – 18
Moderate	19 – 36
High	37 or higher

YOUR HEART DISEASE RISK PROFILE
DOUBTFUL RISK PROFILE

A Combined Heart Disease Risk Score of 0–11 suggests that most likely you are not at significant risk for insulin-related heart disease and its risk factors. It's important to remember, however, that being at doubtful risk for insulin-related heart problems does *not* mean that you are somehow immune to heart disease and other diseases that might stem from factors other than excess insulin and insulin resistance.

> Being at doubtful risk does *not* mean that you are immune to heart disease.

Although some people who scored in the doubtful risk range have improved their general health and risk-factor indicators while on The Carbohydrate Addict's Healthy Heart Program, it should be noted that the Program was not specifically designed for those who fall into the doubtful risk range. If you are in this range, however, it would certainly be advisable to continue your sensible and balanced lifestyle.

MILD RISK PROFILE

A Combined Heart Disease Risk Score of 12–18 suggests that you have a small but notable risk for all of the following insulin-related health problems: high blood pressure, risk-related blood fats, obesity, adult-onset diabetes, and heart disease. Many carbohydrate addicts at mild risk are in stage 1 of Insulin Resistance Syndrome (see page 57).

A score that indicates a mild risk for insulin-related heart disease may be the result of a scattered family history of insulin-related problems along with nutritional factors and activity- and stress-related lifestyle factors that have already begun to intensify your inherited tendency toward hyperinsulinemia. Although your health is probably not suffering significantly at the moment, there are many things you can do now to prevent or reduce your risk for insulin-related heart disease in the years to come.

A mild risk for insulin-related heart disease may also be the result of a moderate to strong family risk for an insulin imbalance combined with your own healthy lifestyle choices. If so, you may have been working very hard to counteract your family's tendency toward hyperinsulinemia and insulin resistance through the strength of your own commitment to your health and well-being. You may literally be holding insulin-related problems at bay—at least for the time being.

> A mild risk score means that you are still in an early stage of Insulin Resistance Syndrome. There are many things you can do to help stop the progression now.

In order to keep your risk in the mild range without fight or sacrifice, or even move yourself back down into the doubtful risk range, you need a program that has been designed to correct the cause of your insulin overload, a program that will allow you to make health-promoting choices while enjoying your well-earned peace of mind and the pleasures that make life so worthwhile. If you are at mild risk for insulin-related heart disease, The Carbohydrate Addict's Healthy Heart Program will offer you simple, effective ways to reduce your risk even further, while enjoying a life filled with freedom and pleasure.

MODERATE RISK PROFILE

A Combined Heart Disease Risk Score in the 19–36 range suggests that you have a moderate but significant risk for all of the following insulin-related health problems: high blood pressure, risk-related blood fats, obesity, adult-onset diabetes, and heart disease. Many carbohydrate addicts at moderate risk are in stage 2 of Insulin Resistance Syndrome (see page 57), in some cases a precursor to Syndrome X (Metabolic Syndrome).

If you are still relatively young, a moderate risk level may reflect the fact that your youth is compensating for a strong insulin imbalance that comes from genetic and/or lifestyle factors. If your age is holding your insulin imbalance at bay, you can almost surely expect your combined heart disease risk level to rise dramatically in the years to come. Starting your insulin-balancing program now may very well help you avoid debilitating and life-threatening insulin-related health problems as you grow older.

A moderate risk level can also be the result of a mild genetic predisposition toward insulin-related health problems in combination with nutritional, activity, and stress factors that increase your basic risk level. In some cases you may inadvertently have increased your insulin imbalance while

> If you are at moderate risk,
> you will be happy to discover how easy it can be
> to halt, then reverse, your
> insulin-related heart risk—for life.

trying to get healthy by following traditional one-size-fits-all recommendations. In other instances you may have given up on trying to achieve a healthier lifestyle due to the self-denial and sacrifice associated with conventional programs. You may have come to the conclusion that, though you wanted to follow a health-promoting program, most programs did not offer you practical, livable, and satisfying choices and, as you may have found out later, never corrected the underlying cause of your insulin imbalance.

A moderate risk for insulin-related heart disease may also be the result of a strong family history of insulin-related disorders that you are keeping in check by your own healthy lifestyle choices. Compensating for a strong genetic predisposition toward hyperinsulinemia and insulin resistance can be difficult at best, especially when you do not know the key guidelines for correcting the imbalance. You will probably find The Carbohydrate Addict's Healthy Heart Program a delight since it gives you the health benefits you have been working for without the deprivation you may have thought inevitable.

If your score places you in the moderate risk range for insulin-related heart disease, the Program can provide an easy way to lower your insulin-related risk while you enjoy the simplicity and pleasures that make a healthy life worth living. And after all, isn't that what it's all about?

HIGH RISK PROFILE

A Combined Heart Disease Risk Score of 37 or more suggests that you have a strong risk for all of the following insulin-related health problems: high blood pressure, risk-related blood fats, obesity, adult-onset diabetes, and heart disease. Depending on how long you have been in the high-risk range, chances are you are in either stage 3 or stage 4 of Insulin Resistance Syndrome (see pages 57–58). You may be suffering from Syndrome X (Metabolic Syndrome). The higher your Combined Heart Disease Risk Score, the more likely you are to progress rapidly through the stages of Insulin Resistance Syndrome *if you take no risk-reducing action.*

If you are in your twenties or thirties, a high risk level indicates that as you grow older your genetic and/or lifestyle factors appear to make you a strong candidate for insulin-related heart disease. The Carbohydrate Addict's Healthy Heart Program may be a very important discovery for you, in particular, and following the program may well make the difference between a life plagued and shortened by insulin-related problems and one filled with pleasure, enjoyment, health, and peace of mind.

If you are middle-aged or older, a high risk level indicates that you have a very strong genetic predisposition for insulin-related heart disease and/or that you have begun to show some of the signs of insulin-related heart problems. The good news is, we know what causes your excess levels of insulin and insulin resistance, and best of all, we know how to correct it. Your biology is not your destiny, and any damage that you may have done through unwise or misinformed choices can, in many cases, be stopped and, in some cases, reversed.

> If you are at high risk for insulin-related heart disease, the guidelines in this book may well make the critical difference between a life dominated by limitations and cut short by illness and a life of freedom, health, and vitality.

WHAT DO YOUR SUBSCORES TELL YOU?

As you begin your program, your subscores along with your Combined Heart Disease Risk Score will help guide you in making the easiest and most beneficial choices that are appropriate *for you*. Your subscores will show you the ways in which your genetics, nutrition, activity, and stress work in combination to affect your personal overall risk for insulin-related heart disease. Your subscores will give you an understanding of the relative power of each of the forces that is raising your risk for insulin-related heart disease.

> Your subscores will show you the ways in which your genetics, nutrition, activity, and stress work in combination.

To the right of each of your four subscores (Family and Personal Medical History, Nutrition, Activity Level, and Stress Level), you will find the number of points—the highest and lowest scores—that is possible in each of the areas.

The position of your subscores in relation to the total range that is possible tells you how much influence each area is having on your risk for insulin-related heart disease. For instance, if any of your subscores fall in the lower end of a range, this category of risk factors may be helping you keep your overall heart disease risk low. A low score in one area may also help to counteract the risks associated with higher subscores in other areas.

A subscore in the lower Family and Personal Medical History range, for instance, may help offset a high Stress Level subscore. You may have witnessed this "helping-hand" phenomenon if you have ever seen a person who has a family history free of insulin-related heart disease and can handle high levels of stress without suffering any heart health–related repercussions.

If your subscore is very high in a particular area, however, it may cancel out some of the benefit that you might normally gain from a low subscore in a different area. If, for example, your Stress Level subscore is somewhat low, the heart health benefit it might otherwise provide may be offset by a very high subscore in your Family and Personal Medical History. In that case you might find that although you have no noticeable physical problems in low-stress conditions, you may start to have difficulties when you find yourself facing stressful situations. Your high subscore in Family and Personal Medical History may make your heart health vulnerable to prolonged stress.

The impact of two or more high subscores is equal to far more than the sum of their parts. Risk factors do not stand alone but are compounded and influenced by other risk factors. So if you have several high subscores, the combined impact will probably increase your risk for insulin-related heart problems more than you'd suspect by considering each one separately.

This same process works in your favor, however, for as you reduce your subscore levels, the effect is also multiplied. As you lower two or more subscores, for instance, you are likely to find a greater reduction in your combined heart disease risk level than you might normally expect.

The Carbohydrate Addict's Healthy Heart Program will guide you in reducing your insulin-related risk by incorporating the changes *you* prefer to make. If you are a sports lover, for instance, you will find that you can choose bonus activity options to help reduce your hyperinsulinemia and insulin resistance through movement or exercise alternatives. On the other hand, if you hate to exercise but are willing to make additional nutritional changes, you will find you can further reduce your insulin-related risk factors without involving yourself in long or complicated exercise regimens.

> **For a program to keep working, it must be compatible with your needs, your preferences, and your time limitations.**

For a program to work and keep working, it must be compatible with your needs and be adaptable to your preferences and time limitations. Any program that says that everyone must make the same choices simply cannot work in the long run.

In the pages to come, you will discover a wide variety of options that can help you to prevent and reverse your insulin-related heart disease risk and to restore your heart health as well. We will show you how to use The Carbohydrate Addict's Healthy Heart Program to help correct what has been called the "pathological link" to atherosclerosis, high blood pressure, excess weight, coronary artery disease, adult-onset diabetes, and heart disease. Your personalized program will take into account your individual preferences while offering you peace of mind and helping you to improve your chances for a long and healthy life—all without deprivation or sacrifice.

PART TWO

TAKING IT TO HEART:

THE BASIC PLAN—

A PROGRAM OF BALANCE

5

THE CARBOHYDRATE ADDICT'S HEALTHY HEART PROGRAM

STEP 1: BALANCED NUTRITION

The first step is one which makes the rest of our days.—*Voltaire*

Most of us would never accept an eyeglass prescription from an eye doctor who had failed to test our vision. If we did try the prescription, we would most certainly not blame ourselves if we found that the glasses failed to help us see well. Yet, when it comes to heart health, carbohydrate addicts fall into exactly this type of bind.

The majority of carbohydrate addicts find it difficult, if not virtually impossible, to stay on one-size-fits-all heart health programs because these plans are not designed to correct the underlying insulin imbalance that causes them to crave high-carbohydrate foods and at the same time puts them at great risk for insulin-related heart disease and its associated risk factors. When they do manage to struggle with the near-impossible demands of most other programs, many find that these plans simply don't produce the heart health results they had been led to expect.

You are about to discover a health-promoting plan unlike any you have ever encountered. The Carbohydrate Addict's Healthy Heart Program is tailored to fit the needs of carbohydrate addicts: to reduce and balance high levels of insulin and insulin resistance that put them at risk for high blood pressure, easy gain of excess weight, risk-related blood fat levels, adult-onset diabetes, and in the end, for heart disease as well.

> You are about to discover a health-promoting plan unlike any you have ever encountered.

The Carbohydrate Addict's Healthy Heart Program is divided into two stages: (1) The BASIC Plan and (2) Heart Health–Enhancing Options.

The first stage, The BASIC Plan, is composed of three steps that work together; each step adds power to the other two, helping to balance excess levels of insulin and reduce or eliminate insulin resistance. These three steps, when combined, will bring you:

Balance through
Activity,
Supplementation, and
Insulin-regulating
Carbohydrate intake

The second stage of the program includes Heart Health–Enhancing Options (called Enhancing Options for short) and is composed of five choices. Added to The BASIC Plan, each option will strengthen and enhance the insulin-balancing effects of the first part of the program. The more Enhancing Options you choose, the more powerful your program.

Both stages, in combination, can reduce or eliminate your insulin connection to heart disease for life. The more Heart Health–Enhancing Options you choose to combine with The BASIC Plan, the better your ability to greatly reduce your risk for insulin-related heart disease.

AN IMPORTANT NOTE BEFORE YOU BEGIN

As with any change in diet, activity, or dietary supplementation, it is important that you check with your physician. Please do so before beginning this program and throughout its duration. Your own unique needs, medical concerns, and limitations may negate or alter some of the guidelines that follow. Your physician may recommend alternatives or may prefer that you follow a different plan. Your physician's recommendations should always take priority. Never stop, reduce, or change diet, medications, supplements, activity, or anything else recommended by your physician without his or her express approval.

THE PROGRAM IN A NUTSHELL
THE BASIC PLAN: AN OVERVIEW

In Step 1 you will find four simple, clear, and livable nutritional guidelines to help you balance your insulin levels and reduce your insulin resistance without struggle or deprivation. The four guidelines that make up Step 1 will help you reduce the number of times each day that you eat high-carbohydrate foods while helping you to increase the quality of the high-carbohydrate foods you do eat. Each day you will enjoy the high-carbohydrate foods you need and love without ever having to measure, count, or weigh your food.

You will discover that on this program there are no exchanges to track, and as long as your physician has not said otherwise, no foods are "off-limits." High-fiber and unsaturated fat recommendations will help enhance the insulin-regulating effect of the easy carbohydrate-related changes you will be making. As your insulin levels drop, often within three to four days, you will feel your cravings for high-carbohydrate foods drop away as well.

In Step 2 you will be offered selections of optional supplemental nutrients useful in balancing insulin levels, reducing insulin resistance, and lowering your risk for insulin-related heart disease. Based on your own requirements and preferences, you will be able to choose from a variety of supplements, many with proven insulin-regulating heart-enhancing properties, including any of the following: glucose tolerance factor chromium, foods high in fiber, vitamins C and E, folic acid, and magnesium.

In Step 3 you will choose from a wide variety of insulin-regulating physical activity and exercise options. You will find easy, fun-filled choices for almost every level of ability and inclination, including many especially designed for the time-challenged. The frequency, duration, and intensity of your activity or exercise choices will vary depending on your ability and preferences.

HEART HEALTH–ENHANCING OPTIONS

In addition to The BASIC Plan, the broad range of Enhancing Options that make up the second part of the program can bring essential balance to your mind, body, and spirit, along with health enhancement to your heart.

In the Enhancing Options (see Chapter 8), you will be able to choose from a broad selection of additional nutritional measures, alternative activities, explorations, and exercises that ease your mind, strengthen your body, and nurture your spirit while enhancing the insulin-regulating benefits of The BASIC Plan.

ESSENTIAL POINTS

On The Carbohydrate Addict's Healthy Heart Program, you will add one step at a time, building your success on each of the previous steps.

When you are ready to begin, read over the Step 1 guidelines that follow. Make certain that you understand all four nutritional guidelines before you begin. Apply all four guidelines from Step 1 at the same time. Do not move on to Step 2 until you feel you have mastered Step 1.

Once you feel comfortable incorporating the four nutritional guidelines of Step 1, you are then free to add Step 2. Wait until you have incorporated each step into your regular routine before adding the next step.

Continue to follow the guidelines detailed in each previous step while adding the next step. If you find that you have moved too quickly, discontinue the new step, but make certain that you continue all previous steps.

GETTING STARTED ON
THE BASIC PROGRAM: STEP 1

Before you begin the Program, make certain that you have read the "Essential Points" subsection. These instructions will help you understand the best ways for you to move through the program. As with any program, you should be aware of what to expect.

> Within a matter of days, you should notice a dramatic decrease or an elimination of your cravings for high-carbohydrate foods.

Within a matter of a few days after you begin Step 1, you should notice a dramatic decrease or an elimination of your cravings for high-carbohydrate foods. A drop in cravings is often the first sign that the insulin-balancing guidelines of Step 1 are reducing or eliminating your hyperinsulinemia as well as your insulin resistance.

Many people also report a rise in energy and a renewed sense of well-being. (If your cravings for high-carbohydrate foods are not greatly reduced or

STEP 1: BALANCED NUTRITION

> ## Good News about
> ## Low-Fat, Low-Salt, and Other Health Agency Dietary Recommendations
>
> The Carbohydrate Addict's Healthy Heart Program is compatible with the *Dietary Guidelines for Americans* as recommended by the Department of Health and Human Services (U.S. Department of Agriculture) as well as the guidelines of the American Heart Association and the American Cancer Society.
>
> These well-respected agencies have offered their guidelines as an aid in the prevention of obesity, high blood pressure, adult-onset diabetes, and heart disease. Recommendations contained in these reports* are easy to include in The Carbohydrate Addict's Healthy Heart Program.
>
> You will find simple suggestions for incorporating these dietary guidelines into your program in the appendix to this book, "Incorporating Low-Fat, Low-Saturated Fat, Low-Salt, and Other Health Agency Dietary Recommendations into Your Program."
>
> Before including any recommendation in your eating plan, be certain to consult with your doctor to make sure that all health agency dietary guidelines are appropriate for you.
>
> *The U.S. Department of Health and Human Services' *Dietary Guidelines for Americans,* 4th ed. (U.S. Department of Agriculture); the American Heart Association's guidelines, *Eating Plan for Healthy Americans;* and the American Cancer Society's *1996 Guidelines on Diet, Nutrition, and Cancer Prevention.*

eliminated by your fourth day on the program, see Chapter 11 for information and help.)

GUIDELINE 1: EAT A BALANCED REWARD MEAL® EVERY DAY

Once each day eat one well-balanced Reward Meal. Your other daily meals and snacks will be detailed in the guidelines that follow, but for now it is important to know that your Reward Meal should contain a salad, followed by a well-balanced meal of protein (meat, fowl, fish, low-carbohydrate dairy and textured vegetable protein, and tofu—that is, soybean curd); low-carbohydrate, nonstarchy vegetables; and high-carbohydrate foods (including starchy vegetables, breads, snack foods, fruits, juices, and sweets). If appropriate and desired, at this meal you may also have a modest amount of alcohol,* unless—as in the case of those with adult-onset diabetes and other conditions—your doctor advises otherwise.

You may choose any time of day for your Reward Meal, but generally, make your choice ahead of time. The majority of our readers, patients, and research participants choose their evening meal as their Reward Meal, although some enjoy their Reward Meal at lunch or breakfast. The choice is up to you. Most people find that they look forward to the same meal each day as their Reward Meal. Now and then they may enjoy the freedom of changing the timing of their Reward Meal, depending on social engagements, vacations, holidays, and celebrations.

Balance, Balance, Balance
On the Program, you never need to weigh or measure your food; you never need to be concerned about percentages, exchanges, or counting. Naturally slim people don't live by the numbers, and neither will you. You must be certain, however, to include a good balance of low- and high-carbohydrate foods in your Reward Meals. This balance will give you the nutrition you need while helping your body to regulate your insulin release and reduce your insulin resistance.

To balance your Reward Meal, start the meal with at least two cups of fresh salad† made from lots of leafy green vegetables and, if you like, some dressing. The rest of your Reward Meal should consist of equal portions:

- $1/3$ low-carbohydrate protein (including meat, fish, fowl, low-carbohydrate dairy and textured vegetable protein, and tofu)
- $1/3$ low-carbohydrate (nonstarchy) vegetables
- $1/3$ high-carbohydrate foods (including bread and other grains, starchy vegetables, fruit, and dessert)

*Diabetes and other disorders may preclude your being able to consume alcoholic beverages. Be certain to check with your physician, and if you are able to include an alcoholic beverage as part of your Reward Meal, always be certain to drink in moderation.

† If you cannot or do not wish to eat salad, you can choose to include at least one cup of cooked low-carbohydrate vegetables instead. These vegetables take the place of salad only; continue to include additional low-carbohydrate vegetables in your main meal as well. You may choose different low-carbohydrate vegetables for your meal or more of the same as those eaten in place of salad. If, due to a medical concern, salads and vegetables are not permitted, consult your physician for alternative suggestions.

STEP 1: BALANCED NUTRITION

Simply estimate your portions so that each represents about one-third of the total amount of food you anticipate eating at that meal. A good guide is to imagine a plate divided into thirds. Now, in your mind's eye, place the vegetables, the protein, and the carbohydrates (including dessert) into each of the thirds on the plate. They should look just about equal.

Start by taking average-sized portions first. You can always go back for seconds, but once again include one-third portion from each group—protein, low-carbohydrate vegetables, and high-carbohydrate foods.

Although they are generally not regarded as carbohydrates, alcoholic drinks can cause your body to release insulin, so when balancing your Reward Meal, consider all alcoholic drinks to be part of the high-carbohydrate portion of the meal.

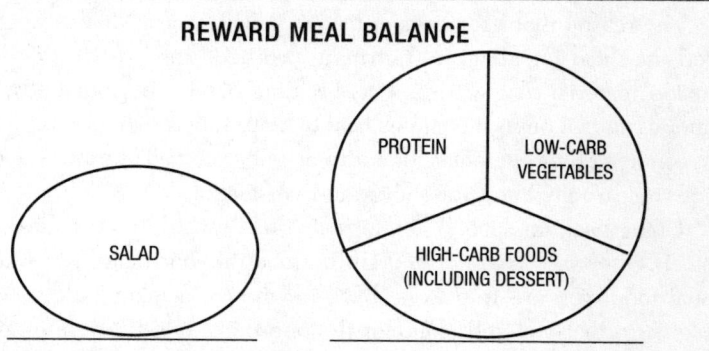

Salad: All greens and a wide variety of low-carbohydrate vegetables. (See pages 133–134.)

One-third low-carbohydrate protein (regular or low-fat varieties): Includes meat, poultry, fish, cheese, eggs, egg substitutes, low-carbohydrate textured vegetable protein, and tofu—that is, soybean curd. (See complete list of low-carbohydrate foods on pages 132–134.)

One-third low-carbohydrate vegetables: Includes all nonstarchy vegetables. (See complete list of low-carbohydrate foods on pages 133–134.)

One-third high-carbohydrate foods (including dessert): Includes all starches (breads, pasta, rice, and so forth), starchy vegetables (potatoes, peas, corn, carrots, and so forth), snack foods, fruits, juices, sweets, and any alcoholic beverages, as appropriate. (See partial list of high-carbohydrate foods on pages 135–137 and the special information about alcoholic beverages on page 142.)

Remember, your Reward Meal must be balanced. Your Reward Meal should be a healthful combination of food, not a binge. Your Reward Meal cannot consist only of high-carbohydrate foods. A meal comprised of pizza, potato chips, cookies, cake, and ice cream is *not* a balanced Reward Meal; that kind of unbalanced meal has no place in this Program. If you do not balance your Reward Meal on a regular basis, you may not get the important health benefits of this Program. Unbalanced Reward Meals will not help you reduce your insulin levels or your insulin resistance, nor will they help lower your risk for insulin-related heart disease.

So don't use the Reward Meal as an excuse to eat only carbo-rich foods; keep it balanced. (If you are having difficulty getting yourself to eat a balanced Reward Meal, or if you are eating too many carbohydrates at your Reward Meal [that is, carbo drifting], see Chapter 11, "Helping Hands.")

The reason that balance is crucial in your Reward Meal is simple. You need the salad for fiber and nutrition; you need the protein-rich foods to provide material that will serve as building blocks for your body, for the minerals and vitamins it contains, and to help stabilize your blood sugar levels; you need the vegetables for additional fiber as well as nutrition; and you need the carbohydrates for energy and satisfaction.

Going back for second helpings at your Reward Meal is always an option. If, after you have finished all the food on your plate, you want additional food, you are free to go back for more. In taking additional food, make sure that you still maintain the one-third, one-third, one-third portions. Be certain that you *do not go back just for more high-carbohydrate foods.*

Remember, if you go back for seconds, you *must* have equal portions of seconds of everything (except for the salad). These seconds can be large (if you are very hungry) or small (if you just want a bit more), but the amount you eat of all three portions must be equal. (Don't take equal portions and eat only the carbs—we know that trick!) In the same way, if you are not hungry enough to eat all of your first plateful, eat less of *all* of the three portions; do not eat most of the high-carbohydrate foods and leave most of the vegetables.

Keep in mind that your cravings, weight, blood pressure, blood fats, blood sugar, and the very health of your heart depend on the amount of insulin your body releases. The more *often* you eat high-carbohydrate foods or the more carbohydrate-heavy your meals, the higher your insulin levels and the greater your insulin resistance. The higher your insulin levels and the greater your insulin resistance, the greater your risk for heart disease.

On the other hand, one balanced Reward Meal each day, in combination with low-carbohydrate meals (which we will discuss later), provide a carbohydrate frequency and balance that lead to balanced insulin levels and reduced insulin resistance. In this way, balance of diet brings balance of body. You can have the satisfaction of eating the foods you love while reducing your cravings, your tendency to gain weight, and your risk for insulin-related heart disease and its associated risk factors—all at the same time.

> **Regardless of whether you want to lose weight, balanced insulin levels and lowered insulin resistance can make your Reward Meal a double reward for heart health.**

Within a few days, as cravings disappear, you will find it easier to balance your Reward Meal, but remember, balance really is essential. In addition, as you continue to follow the program, chances are your body will become better able to handle the high-carbohydrate foods that you do eat at your Reward Meal. As you become less insulin resistant, your insulin levels will be less likely to peak as high.

If you are overweight, chances are you will find that you are less prone to quickly convert the food you eat into fat, which means you will be able to use more of the food energy you take in rather than storing it as fat. In any case, regardless of whether you want to lose weight, the benefits of balanced insulin levels and lowered insulin resistance can make your Reward Meal a double reward for heart health.

If you choose breakfast as your Reward Meal, remember that you must still follow the recommendations for balancing Reward Meals, as discussed in this subsection.

GUIDELINE 2: COMPLETE YOUR REWARD MEAL® WITHIN ONE HOUR

From start to finish it's important to complete your Reward Meal within sixty minutes. This might seem like an odd recommendation. Most heart health–enhancing programs put limits on what you can eat and on how much you can eat, but you have probably never been given a maximum limit on how long you can eat.

The reason for a time limit is simple but important. Every time you eat high-carbohydrate foods, your body releases insulin in two waves. Scientists call this the *biphasic* (two-phase) release of insulin. The first wave, or phase, which is basically an on-off mechanism, starts within a few minutes of tasting or just seeing, smelling, or thinking about food. This release of insulin depends on how often you have eaten high-carbohydrate foods in the previous twelve to twenty hours and how much of them you ate.

> Consuming great quantities of high-carbo foods,
> or eating or drinking them throughout the day,
> signals your body to release extra insulin
> in preparation for the next carbohydrate onslaught.

If you have been snacking on high-carbohydrate foods or beverages often throughout the day and/or if you have been eating great quantities of them, your body assumes that each new meal or snack will also contain more high-carbohydrate foods. In order to handle this anticipated high-carbo intake, your body releases high levels of insulin.

You have probably experienced the effects of this first wave of insulin release after taking a bite or two of food and suddenly finding that you were hungrier than you thought you were before eating. This quick jump in hunger as well as the intense pleasure that the food gave you is often evidence of your body's first wave of insulin.

For a moment, think back to Guideline 1. The purpose of one Reward Meal each day is to give you the carbohydrates that you need for good nutrition while making sure that the first phase of insulin release is kept as low as possible. Your body wants to conserve as much energy as it can while getting you the nutrition you need. The hormone insulin is designed to help you save. Just as a nursing mother's body will produce more milk the more her baby suckles, your body will produce more insulin the more often you eat high-carbohydrate foods.

> When the thought, taste, or smell of food
> makes you feel hungrier than you thought you were,
> you are feeling the effects of your first release of insulin.

If, as per Guideline 1, you have high-carbohydrate foods only once each day, then, when you begin to eat high-carbohydrate foods at your Re-

STEP 1: BALANCED NUTRITION

ward Meal, your body will no longer expect a high-carbohydrate meal and will have far less insulin in reserve to release. Guideline 1 helps you keep the first phase of insulin release low. Lower insulin levels usually means both lower insulin resistance and lower insulin-related heart disease risk.

The second phase of insulin release, however, is *not* a preset amount. The amount of insulin that is released in the second phase does not depend on how much high-carbohydrate food you have had at previous meals but rather on how long you continue eating high-carbohydrate food at this particular meal.

> **When you eat over a long period of time and begin to feel less satisfied, that's the result of your second release of insulin.**

The second phase of insulin release is your body's fail-safe mechanism. If you lived in prehistoric times, it would have helped you if you had suddenly come across high-carbohydrate foods (a patch of ripe berries, for instance). You would have needed insulin in order to handle the high sugar content of the fruit. At that time, as now, your body assumes that the longer it takes you to eat, the more you must be eating. So as a backup, your body has the ability to release extra insulin on the spot should you need it. This second phase of insulin kicks in if your high-carbohydrate meal lasts for an extended time.

Chances are you have experienced the effects of this second phase of insulin release at times when meals have continued for extended periods—at leisurely restaurant meals, family celebrations, or holidays, for example. At these times you may have eaten until you were satisfied only to find that as you continued to eat, you became *less* satisfied than you had been before. You may have felt that the more you ate, the less satisfied you were. You might have eaten to the point of being uncomfortable and felt less satisfied or "finished" than you had felt earlier in the meal.

This is usually evidence of insulin's second wave. It reaches its peak at about sixty-five or seventy minutes after you start eating, and it is the very reason that Guideline 2 is needed.

> **Each of the four guidelines of Step 1 can help reduce insulin release as well as your insulin resistance.**

If you finish your Reward Meal within sixty minutes, your insulin levels will most likely remain far lower than if you had continued eating past the one-hour limit. Guideline 2 helps ensure that you finish your meal *before* the second wave of insulin has reached its peak. As you finish your meal, your body is then able to sense that no more insulin is needed, and with insulin levels remaining lower, you will feel far more satisfied, both at the meal and afterward. Once again, less insulin means less insulin resistance and lower risk for insulin-related heart disease.

Although both phases of insulin release may have made a great deal of sense in prehistoric times, today, with high-carbohydrate foods available twenty-four hours a day, every day of the year, we can no longer afford to continuously tell our bodies that it is time to eat.

Guidelines 1 and 2, in combination with Guidelines 3 and 4, will help turn off the "keep-eating" signal that directs your body to continue releasing high levels of insulin.

You can be sure that all the high-carbohydrate foods that you love and need are available to you every day in your Reward Meal (your other meals and snacks are addressed in Guideline 3). Just be certain to keep your well-balanced Reward Meal confined to one hour—from start to finish.

GUIDELINE 3: EAT ONLY LOW-CARBOHYDRATE FOODS AT ALL OTHER MEALS AND SNACKS

At all meals and snacks other than your Reward Meal, eat low-carbohydrate foods *only*. You will find a complete list of low-carbo foods on pages 132–135. At these meals eat or drink only foods that are on the "Low-Carbohydrate Foods List."

In general, low-carbohydrate foods include high-fiber vegetables (such as salad and cooked vegetables) and protein-rich foods (including meat, fowl, fish, low-carbohydrate dairy and textured vegetable protein, and tofu). Low-carbohydrate meals and snacks should be well balanced and should include both high-fiber and protein-rich choices.

The quantity of food you consume during low-carbohydrate meals is not limited, as long as you include both high-fiber vegetables (raw or cooked) and protein in equal portions. We will address special breakfast balances in a moment, but for now, as a starting point, assume your meals will be half protein and half vegetables.

Never weigh or measure your portions. As with Reward Meal servings, there is no need to do so. Just judge with your eye to estimate that you are taking equal-sized portions (approximately equal by the size of the portions, that is, not by weight).

You are free at any time to lean a bit more heavily toward the vegetable side of your low-carbohydrate meal (up to two-thirds vegetables and one-third protein), but always include *some* protein. You may find it more pleasurable and appealing to include two kinds of vegetables—a salad of raw vegetables and a cooked vegetable, for instance—along with some protein. Be certain to include only low-carbohydrate vegetables at these meals and snacks. We generally recommend that you take average-sized portions and go back for more if you like. You may be surprised at how satisfying these meals and snacks can be.

> Since this program has been designed
> to correct the cause of your cravings,
> **sticking with it becomes easier with each passing day.**

Remember, on this program, you don't have to worry about limiting yourself to tiny portions. As insulin levels normalize, your cravings will decrease dramatically, and most people find that at times they may literally "forget to eat." Since this program has been designed to correct the cause of your cravings, sticking with it becomes easier with each passing day, and working toward ideal heart health can be struggle-free forever. We know that seems impossible to believe right now, but you are almost sure to see things quite differently after a short time on the Program.

You can skip a low-carbohydrate meal if you simply are not hungry, but don't skip meals because you think that less food will make you lose weight and that losing weight by skipping meals is good for your heart. That kind of crash dieting never does any good for you or your health. On the other hand, if you don't want to eat because you just aren't hungry, which happens a great deal on this program, then skip that meal as long as it does not present a health problem (get your doctor's okay) and you continue to feel well. If you are considering skipping most or all of your low-carbohydrate meals, be certain to read "The Food Frequency–Reducing Option" in Chapter 8.

Although you may skip low-carbohydrate meals, do not, under any circumstances, skip Reward Meals on a regular basis. You need carbohydrates for your good health. On the other hand, if you want a snack, you are free to enjoy a low-carbohydrate snack at any time. (The desire for between-meals snacks is unusual on this program. If you find that you want snacks or

Low-Carbohydrate Foods List

Note: This list does not constitute a list of recommended foods but, rather, all foods that are low in carbohydrates and less likely to cause an insulin release. Depending on fat/saturated fat/cholesterol levels, some foods may not be appropriate for all readers. Any food that does *not* appear on this list should be considered to be a high-carbohydrate food and must be saved for your daily Reward Meal. Portions at your low-carbohydrate meals and snacks depend on your individual needs. Unless your physician advises otherwise, choose average-sized portions. Go back for more if you like. There is no need to measure or weigh food. If in doubt about the carbohydrate level of a particular food, save it for your Reward Meal.

MEATS—all regular and lean meats, including:

Beef, lean	Pork, lean	Veal
Hamburger, lean	Rabbit	Venison
Hot dogs (all lean meat, no added sugar)	Sausages (all lean meat, no added sugar)	
Lamb		

Most luncheon meats now contain added sugars, fillers, monosodium glutamate, and other carbohydrates and carbohydrate act-alikes. In addition, these prepared meats are high in saturated fats (another source of insulin release). It is strongly recommended that you do not include luncheon meats in your program.

FOWL—light or dark varieties, with or without skin, including:

Capon	Duck	Quail
Chicken	Goose	Squab
Cornish hen	Pheasant	Turkey (ground or whole)

FISH AND SHELLFISH—all varieties, canned, jarred (no sugar), or cooked (no bread crumbs), including:

Bass	Crabmeat	Monk
Bluefish	Flounder	Oysters
Calamari	Haddock	Salmon
Clams	Halibut	Sardines
Cod	Lobster	Scallops

(continued)

STEP 1: BALANCED NUTRITION

Low-Carbohydrate Foods List (continued)

Scrod
Shrimp
Smelt
Sole
Sturgeon
Swordfish
Trout
Tuna (not packed in broth, which often contains carbohydrate act-alikes. Check ingredients)

DAIRY AND NONMEAT ALTERNATIVES — regular or low-fat varieties of:

Cheese (regular and low-fat, all varieties except low-fat ricotta)
Cream cheese (regular only)
Eggs
Egg substitutes°
Egg whites
Sour cream (regular and low-fat)
Textured vegetable protein (TVP)°
Tofu (soybean curd)°

Vegetarian meat alternatives and TVPs that contain 4 grams of carbohydrates or less per average serving can be eaten at low-carbohydrate and Reward Meals.

It appears that many brands of cottage cheese may now contain glutamates. We think it best for carbohydrate addicts to avoid these entirely. See page 139 for more information on glutamates.

Milk, cream, or half and half can be consumed at all Reward Meals and, in addition, once a day at non–Reward Meal times (that is, at low-carbohydrate meals or in between). Limit the one non–Reward Meal portion to no more than 2 ounces daily and include it in no more than one cup of coffee or tea or in cooking. Do not use non-dairy creamers. Finish the coffee or tea within fifteen minutes.

VEGETABLES — fresh or cooked (no breading), steamed, or boiled nonstarchy vegetables, including:

Alfalfa sprouts
Arugula
Asparagus
Bamboo shoots
Bean sprouts
Broccoli°
Brussels sprouts°
Cabbage (all)
Cauliflower
Celery
Chives
Cucumbers
Endive
Green beans
Greens (all)
Kale
Lettuce
Mushrooms
Okra
Parsley
Peppers (green)
Radishes

(continued)

Low-Carbohydrate Foods List (continued)

Scallions
Snap beans

Sorrel
Sour grass

Spinach
Wax beans

Onions (at low-carbohydrate meals use as seasoning only, 2 teaspoons or less)

Tomatoes, raw (at low-carbohydrate meals include no more than 1/4 per meal)

OILS, FATS, AND DRESSINGS:

Saturated fats have been shown to release high levels of insulin. Use unsaturated fats (U) whenever possible. Fats and oils that are liquid at room temperature should be considered unsaturated and are better choices than solid, saturated fats. Avoid hydrogenated fats whenever possible.

Butter or margarine, regular or low-fat substitutes: Avoid or use very sparingly.

Mayonnaise: Include regular mayonnaise only (not low-fat) in low-carbohydrate meals (use sparingly or thin with water for lower-fat alternative). Avoid brands that contain glutamates (see the "Carbohydrate Act-Alikes" list, page 142). Avoid low-fat mayonnaise, which can contain a great deal of added sugar.

Oils: All varieties, including olive oil (U), corn oil (U), safflower oil (U), sesame oil (U), sunflower oil (U), and liquid vegetable oil (U).

Salad dressings: All regular and low-fat varieties in which sugar is not among the first four ingredients. Avoid brands that contain glutamates. (See page 143.)

EXTRAS:

Capers (for garnish only)
Dill pickles
Garlic (fresh or powdered)
Herbs
Horseradish
Hot sauce
Mustard
Olives (green or black; no pimentos)
Onion powder
Pepper, ground
Salt
Spices
Vinegar (white, all other varieties)*

*If you are particularly sensitive to carbohydrates or naturally occurring glutamates, you may find that these foods can cause excess insulin release, as evidenced by rebound cravings, reduced weight loss, or increases in insulin-related heart disease risk factors. If so, or if you are concerned about these foods, save them for Reward Meals or avoid them entirely.

(continued)

Low-Carbohydrate Foods List (continued)

BEVERAGES:
Carbonated water   Seltzer (nonflavored)   Tea (hot or cold)
Coffee (unflavored only)
Herbal teas vary in carbohydrate content and insulin impact. Use nonfruity, non-grain-based teas at low-carbohydrate meals.

High-Carbohydrate Foods List

(To be balanced with low-carbohydrate foods at Reward Meals)
Note: This list contains *examples* of some of the many high-carbohydrate foods you can balance with low-carbohydrate foods at your daily Reward Meal. This list does not constitute recommendations but rather a partial listing of foods according to their carbohydrate count. All foods that are not specifically listed on the companion low-carbohydrate foods chart should be considered high-carbohydrate foods and reserved for Reward Meals. As always, follow physician recommendations.

Portions depend on your individual needs. Unless your physician advises otherwise, choose average-sized portions. You can go back for more if you like. There is no need to measure or weigh food. See page 125 for a guide to balancing foods at Reward Meals.

BREADS, GRAINS, CEREALS—all varieties (regular, low-fat, low-sugar, whole-grain, and so forth), including:

Bagels	Couscous	Stuffing
Biscuits	Croissants	Tabuli
Breads	French toast	Tahini
Breakfast bars	Granola	Tempura coating
Cereals (hot or cold)	Grits	Waffles
Corn meal	Pancakes	

DAIRY—regular, frozen, and low-fat varieties of:

Breakfast drinks	Ice cream	Milk
Cream	Ice milk	Yogurt (regular or
Creamers (nondairy)	Low-fat	low-fat, creamy
Half and half	ricotta cheese	or frozen)

(continued)

High-Carbohydrate Foods List (continued)

FRUIT AND JUICES—all fruits (cooked, dried, fresh), fruit juices, or vegetable juices, including:

Apples	Grapefruit	Papaya
Bananas	Grapes	Peaches
Cantaloupe	Kiwi fruit	Pears
Carrot juice	Lemons	Pineapple
Cherries	Limes	Plums
Dates	Mangoes	V-8 juices
Figs	Oranges	

LEGUMES, SEEDS, NUTS, AND NUT BUTTERS—all varieties, including:

Baked beans	Hummus	Pumpkin seeds
Black beans	Kidney beans	Sesame seeds
Cashews	Lentils	Soybeans°
Chestnuts	Peanut butter	Split peas
Chickpeas	Peanuts	Walnuts
Flaxseed	Pistachios	Water chestnuts
Garbanzos		

"HIGH-PROTEIN" POWER BARS, POWER DRINKS, PROTEIN POWDERS, SOY PROTEIN POWDER:
Those sweetened with sugar or to which you add fruit juice are usually high in carbohydrates and should be reserved for Reward Meals, if they are consumed at all. Those sweetened with sugar substitutes should be avoided entirely.

Important note: "Unsweetened" often means that the product is sweetened with a sugar substitute and, for the carbohydrate addict, should be avoided entirely.

PASTA, NOODLES AND RICE—all fresh and dry varieties, including:

Chinese noodles	Rice (all varieties)	Spaghetti
Egg noodles	Rigatoni	Spinach noodles
Macaroni	Shells	Tabbouleh
Pasta (all varieties)		

SNACK FOODS, SWEETS, AND EXTRAS: All varieties of snacks sweetened with sugar should be kept in balance at Reward Meals.

Cakes	Chips	Cookies
Candies	Chocolate	Crackers

(continued)

STEP 1: BALANCED NUTRITION

High-Carbohydrate Foods List (continued)

Fructose
Gelatin desserts
Honey
Mints
Popcorn
Pretzels
Puddings
Rice cakes
Snack bars and mixes
Sugar

SUGAR SUBSTITUTES should be avoided in all foods and beverages, including snack foods and desserts. For details see Guideline 4 (page 139).

VEGETABLES: All vegetables *not* listed as low-carbohydrate should be considered high-carbohydrate, including fresh, stir-fried, sautéed, with or without breading, steamed, or boiled varieties.

Artichokes
Beets
Carrots
Corn
Leeks
Onions
Pea pods
Peas
Peppers (red)
Potatoes
Squash
Tomatoes (when more than 1/4 per meal)
Zucchini

EXTRAS: Reserve all of the following for Reward Meals. Check ingredients. If glutamates are added, avoid entirely. (See page 143 for information on carbohydrate act-alikes.)

Ketchup (catsup)
Salsa
Soy sauce°
Steak sauce
Teriyaki sauce°

BEVERAGES—NONALCOHOLIC:
All fruit juices and drinks
All sugar-sweetened drinks and sodas
All flavored seltzers and club sodas
All herbal teas (Although not high in carbohydrates, they may stimulate insulin release.)

BEVERAGES—ALCOHOLIC
Beer, wine, mixed drinks, liqueurs, and so forth should be treated as if they were high-carbohydrate foods. Save alcoholic drinks for your Reward Meal and, for ideal meal balance, consider them to be part of your one-third portion of carbohydrates.

°Some individuals are particularly sensitive to glutamates, even glutamates that are naturally occurring and eaten at Reward Meals. In these cases glutamates may cause excess insulin release, as evidenced by rebound cravings, reduced weight loss, or increases in insulin-related heart disease risk factors. If you find this to be the case, or if you are concerned about these foods, avoid them entirely.

(continued)

High-Carbohydrate Foods List (continued)

SUGAR SUBSTITUTES should be avoided in all foods and beverages, including diet drinks. For details see Guideline 4 (page 139) and the subsection on sugar substitutes (page 142).

CHEWING GUM AND MINTS:
Sweetened with SUGAR: Reserve for Reward Meals. Count as high-carbohydrate in balance and finish within the meal's one-hour time limit.

Sweetened with SUGAR SUBSTITUTES: Avoid entirely. For details see Guideline 4 (page 139).

---

mini-meals on a regular basis, make certain that you are not eating any high-carbohydrate foods at your low-carbohydrate meals or snacks and that you are avoiding all carbohydrate act-alikes. These errors can cause your carbohydrate cravings to return. If you need some assistance, see Chapter 11, "Helping Hands.")

By definition, a low-carbohydrate breakfast does not include the usual cereals, fruits, breads, or pastries that you may be used to having in the morning. The reason is quite clear. These high-carbohydrate foods set in motion the carbohydrate-craving cycles, hyperinsulinemia, and insulin resistance that brought you to this program.

Your choices for breakfast are many. You can decide to skip breakfast (you may find you really don't want it!) or have only a cup of coffee or tea (with milk or cream).* If you prefer to eat a small breakfast or a full meal in the morning, you can choose from any of the low-carbohydrate foods on pages 132–135. In addition, Chapter 12 contains a variety of low-carbohydrate recipe suggestions. A low-carbohydrate breakfast at home or at your favorite restaurant might include a mushroom omelette (made of eggs or real egg whites) and some cucumber slices. You may want to add some cheese (regular or low-fat) to the omelette as well. Some of our readers, patients, and research participants ask for a bowl of lettuce and cucumbers with oil and vinegar as a substitute for the potatoes that usually accompany omelettes. Others ask for a special plate of sautéed green peppers on the side. Some of our more adventurous carbohydrate addicts en-

---

*We have found that including milk or cream in one cup of coffee or tea outside Reward Meal times can be allowed. Be sure to finish the beverage within fifteen minutes. Do not use nondairy creamer. Coffee or tea without lightener can be enjoyed at any time.

STEP 1: BALANCED NUTRITION

joy lunch or dinner foods at breakfast, including chicken salad, strips of chicken wrapped in lettuce leaves, or poached or smoked salmon.

Although low-carbohydrate lunches and snacks are easy to balance, many people find that their low-carbohydrate breakfasts contain few vegetables or none at all. We recommend that you include a portion of vegetables and/or salad with breakfast if you can, but if a breakfast with sliced cucumber, fresh mushrooms, or celery is decidedly unappealing, don't worry. Just be sure to include a good portion of low-carbohydrate vegetables with your other low-carbohydrate meals on days when you have not included vegetables at breakfast. If you are not having salad and veggies at breakfast, don't make breakfast your Reward Meal more than once or twice a week.

Low-carbohydrate lunches are easy to make and delicious, whether you are eating at home or in a restaurant. A typical example of a low-carbohydrate lunch might include a broiled chicken breast, sautéed mushrooms and green peppers, along with a salad with a low-carbo dressing. A Greek salad is often a nice choice (you should have some extra protein on the side). If you want tuna, ask for it straight from the can, often called "individual tuna plate." Restaurants usually serve tuna fish salad, chicken salad, egg salad, and shrimp salad that is packed with bread, monosodium glutamate, and other fillers—not good for carbohydrate addicts or their hearts. A burger (turkey or lean beef) can be enjoyed as a delicious low-carbohydrate lunch, but omit the bun, though you can top the burger off with some cheese (regular or low-fat) and enjoy a salad and dill pickle with it as well.

GUIDELINE 4: AVOID CARBOHYDRATE ACT-ALIKES THAT CAN RAISE INSULIN LEVELS: GLUTAMATES AND SUGAR SUBSTITUTES

Glutamates
Monosodium glutamate (MSG) and other glutamates (called free glutamates) can appear naturally in foods or may be included as additives by manufacturers in order, among other reasons, to increase the popularity of their products. Some carbohydrate addicts experience an addictive response to foods that contain glutamates and return to glutamate-added foods that they might not otherwise choose or enjoy if these foods did not contain this additive. In some cases, without realizing why they are doing so, carbohydrate addicts may find themselves selecting brands that contain high levels of added glutamates over other brands that do not.

> **Glutamates are hidden in our foods
> under a wide variety of names.
> They can release high levels of insulin.**

Scientists are just learning what food manufacturers have apparently known for years: we have glutamate receptors in our taste buds that drive us to seek out foods that contain glutamates. We are driven to eat foods containing glutamates even when we cannot taste the glutamates. Glutamates appear to enhance other tastes and perhaps the sensation of taste as well. The problem is that there is a high price to pay for the pleasure that glutamates provide.

> **Even as you read these pages,
> glutamates are being added to our foods.
> Foods that you always thought were glutamate-free suddenly
> have glutamates added, though their labeling has not changed.**

When glutamates are added to foods, they can release high levels of insulin, which cause changes in our metabolism. As Drs. N. A. Togiyama and A. Adachi reported in the medical journal *Physiological Behavior*, even applying monosodium glutamate to the tongues of animals will cause them to release high levels of insulin within three minutes. The hunger that follows such an insulin response could increase cravings, cause weight gain, and if repeated over time, increase the likelihood of adult-onset diabetes. The body's response to this *excitotoxin* may elevate blood pressure, increase blood fats, and increase the overall risk of insulin-related heart disease.

Still, there is a great deal more to learn about the effects of monosodium glutamate; research exploring the full impact of glutamates is still under way. Unfortunately, food manufacturers seem to have a jump on the research. Even as you read these pages, glutamates are being added to our foods. Foods that you always thought were glutamate-free may suddenly appear with glutamates added, though there has been no noticeable change in package labeling.

The latest of these "quick switches" has taken place in the canned fish industry. Most food manufacturers have started adding glutamates to canned tuna. They have cleverly added free glutamates under one of the dozen or more names used to hide its presence. Two of those names are *broth* and *hydrolyzed protein*. Only a few of the low-fat, low-calorie brands of canned tuna have no glutamates. You can spot the glutamate-free brands because their ingredients list reads "tuna, water" (and nothing else).

> Check out the ingredients in a recently purchased can of tuna.
> If it now contains broth or hydrolyzed protein,
> it may very well contain glutamates.

Although manufacturers may not lie, they don't always tell the whole truth. When we called the two top canned tuna fish manufacturers, we were told that no monosodium glutamate had been added. When we asked specifically whether *free* glutamates had been added to their products, both companies confirmed our suspicion. Though they knew that, for our purposes, there was little difference between free glutamates and monosodium glutamate, both companies refused to admit the presence of this additive until forced to do so.

Their secrecy is not surprising.

Glutamate is powerful stuff. It breaks down the muscle fiber of animals and causes brain damage in laboratory animals. Did you know that scientists who want obese lab animals with which to do experiments call the supply house and ask for MSG-fattened rats? The rats are made obese simply by adding monosodium glutamate to their feed! Yet glutamate manufacturers apparently hire spokespersons to polish their image and lobby for their position in political circles, and their advocates seem to be doing their job.

So although others may say there is nothing wrong with glutamates, we say, if you are a carbohydrate addict, stay away from MSG and added glutamates. They can greatly increase your insulin levels and, from everything we can see, your risk for insulin-related heart disease as well.

One woman who came to see us had stroke-level blood pressure. She had taken every medication available, and none of them helped. She exercised, adhered to a rigid and stringent diet, never drank, and cut out salt. Nothing helped. Her food diary revealed that she was eating the same canned foods day after day. She told us that she loved dips, canned vegetables, and soups. Every one of the foods that she was eating was filled with glutamates. Within three weeks of following our program and being careful to avoid glutamates, her blood pressure was that of a healthy young woman. She felt better than she had in years, and happy and healthy to this day; she swears the change saved her life.

Added glutamates appear to be more of a problem for carbohydrate addicts than are naturally occurring glutamates. You probably will not be able to avoid glutamates altogether. At least one-third of all the food you eat in restaurants contains added glutamates. You are almost forced to put up with glutamates in order to live a normal life, but when you have a choice, when you buy foods in stores, read the label and avoid foods that have added glutamates.

On the ingredients listing, added glutamates can be hidden under a variety of names, many of which are shown in the "Carbohydrate Act-Alikes" chart (below).

So whenever you can, for your heart's sake, avoid foods that contain *added* glutamates. A rose by any other name may smell as sweet, but glutamates by any other name do not.

> At least one-third of all the food you eat in restaurants contains added glutamates.

Carbohydrate Act-Alikes

Although these foods and beverages are not necessarily high in carbohydrates, many carbohydrate addicts respond to them as if they indeed were high in carbohydrates. Carefully read the recommendations for each category.

SUGAR SUBSTITUTES: These can release insulin as if they were high-carbohydrate foods and should generally be avoided. For details see Guideline 4 (page 139).

ALCOHOLIC BEVERAGES: Though alcohol in itself is not a carbohydrate, it can be metabolized along some of the same metabolic pathways as carbohydrates. Your body may respond to alcoholic beverages as if they were high in carbohydrates. Alcoholic drinks should be confined to Reward Meals and counted as a carbohydrate when balancing that meal.

(continued)

STEP 1: BALANCED NUTRITION

> ## Carbohydrate Act-Alikes (continued)
>
> **MONOSODIUM GLUTAMATE AND FREE GLUTAMATES AS ADDITIVES**: When glutamates appear naturally in foods, in many cases their level of concentration does not seem to present an insulin-related problem. When they are added to foods, however, they seem to release far higher levels of insulin, acting as if they were intensely sweet high-carbohydrate foods. Natural glutamates can be included in meals as per the preceding lists, but added glutamates should be avoided whenever possible. For details see Guideline 4 (page 139).
>
> Check your ingredient listing. Glutamates can go under a variety of names, including:
>
> | | | |
> |---|---|---|
> | Anything enzyme-modified | Calcium caseinate | Malt extract |
> | Anything fermented | Carrageenan | Maltodextrin |
> | Anything protein fortified | Flavoring | Natural flavors (or natural flavoring) |
> | Anything ultra-pasteurized | Gelatin | Pectin |
> | Autolyzed yeast | Hydrolyzed oat flour | Plant protein extract |
> | Barley malt | Hydrolyzed plant protein | Potassium glutamate |
> | Broth | Hydrolyzed soy protein | Sodium caseinate |
> | Bouillon | Hydrolyzed vegetable protein | Soy protein |
> | | | Soy sauce |
> | | | Stock |
> | | | Textured protein |
> | | | Whey protein |
> | | | Yeast extract |
> | | | Yeast food |
>
> Note: Cottage cheese and canned tuna, once free of glutamates, now usually contain glutamates and should be avoided by carbohydrate addicts. Canned tuna manufacturers may include the glutamates under the ingredient "broth." Read ingredients labels.

Sugar Substitutes

One of the most powerful triggers for insulin release is the one that most carbohydrate addicts never think about: sugar substitutes. Whether in the form of a natural or an artificial sweetener, either type of sugar substitute can signal the body to release high levels of insulin. For purposes of simplicity, we will refer to all artificial and natural nonsugar sweeteners as sugar substitutes. Whether they are marketed as artificial sweeteners, little blue packs, pink packs, sweeteners, or referred to by their brand name, it really doesn't matter. We have found that if you are a carbohydrate addict, sugar substitutes can raise your insulin levels, increase your insulin resistance, and cause greater blood sugar swings than almost any other food or beverage.

> **If you are a carbohydrate addict, sugar substitutes can raise your insulin levels, increase your insulin resistance, and cause blood sugar swings.**

The reason is simple. As you have already learned, when you consume foods or drinks that are naturally sweet, the carbohydrates in those foods or drinks are turned into simple sugar. The insulin that is released ushers the sugar into any cells that will allow it to enter. Insulin then signals the liver to turn any unused blood sugar (what remains in the bloodstream) into blood fat so that it can be channeled into the fat cells. Over time, if no other high-carbohydrate foods are eaten, insulin levels drop and glucagon levels rise. The fat cells open, and some of the energy they have held within is released into the bloodstream to keep blood sugar levels stable and to feed cells throughout the body. In time your body will use up the energy available in your blood supply, and when you eat once again, the cycle begins anew.

When carbohydrate addicts eat foods that are sweetened with sugar substitutes, however, the cycle can be thrown out of balance. Sugar substitutes did not exist when our bodies evolved a few million years ago. Your body was made to handle "real" sugar, and to this day it will treat anything that tastes sweet as if it contained real sugar. Therefore, when you consume foods or beverages that contain sugar substitutes, your body releases insulin just as it would if you were eating or drinking the real thing.

The problem occurs because there is no incoming sugar for the insulin to work on—no incoming sugar for it to usher into cells. So insulin rounds up the only sugar available—the sugar in your blood. If you are insulin resistant at all, chances are the energy will end up in your fat cells. You may experience blood sugar swings. You may feel hungry and irritable and out of sorts and most likely will reach for more food or drink sweetened with sugar substitutes, keeping the insulin-releasing cycle going. Since insulin levels remain high, glucagon never gets a chance to allow the fat to leave the fat cells. The result? You are caught on a merry-go-round of insulin peaks, blood sugar swings, craving, weight gain, and insulin resistance—all of which are precursors for heart disease.

STEP 1: BALANCED NUTRITION

In time, as you progress through the stages of Insulin Resistance Syndrome, your body will become more and more insulin resistant until even your fat cells shut down to the incoming blood sugar and insulin. Blood sugar, trapped in your bloodstream, leads to a cascade of problems we call adult-onset diabetes, and in the end your pancreas may become incapable of producing insulin.

> **Are you, or is someone you know, addicted to diet drinks?**

Look to your own experience:

- Do you find that an hour or two after having a diet drink, you crave more of the same?
- Do you then want a snack or sandwich or something sweet to eat with your diet drink?
- Do you rationalize, telling yourself that it's a good thing that you drink diet sodas because they help you cut down on calories, yet know that you seem to eat as much with or without the diet drinks?
- Do you get a special feeling of satisfaction when you take your first sip?
- Did you dislike the taste of diet drinks at first, only to find that you no longer noticed the unpleasant taste as much?
- Do you ever think you might be addicted to diet drinks? Or to gums or mints sweetened with sugar substitutes?
- Do you find it hard even to consider the idea of giving sugar substitutes up altogether?

"Yes" answers to any of these questions indicate that you may be experiencing an addictive response to sugar substitutes. The greater the number of yes answers, the greater the probable addiction.

We have found that for the carbohydrate addict, avoiding sugar substitutes is very important. The high levels of insulin that can result from eating or drinking sugar substitutes are the same insulin responses as you would experience with "real" sugar consumption; in fact, we have found that they are often higher. And the insulin that is released can lead to the same high risk for elevated blood pressure, blood fats, weight gain, adult-onset diabetes, and heart disease.

So for your heart's sake eliminate the sugar substitutes that may have become a part of your daily routine. If, on the other hand, the thought of doing without sugar substitutes sends fear and anxiety to the core of your being, we can offer some help by way of a four-day challenge.

An Exciting Four-Day Challenge
If you would like to follow the program but are unsure how to bring yourself to give up diet sodas and other foods sweetened with sugar substitutes, we may have a solution. Rather than asking you to give up your diet drinks and artificially sweetened desserts for life, we suggest that you simply do without them for four days. Remember that you can still enjoy the sugar-sweetened foods, drinks, and desserts you love as part of your balanced Reward Meal; we just don't want you to have sugar substitutes. Be certain to follow the program at the same time.

> Rather than giving up your diet drinks for life, we suggest that you do without them for four days. As your cravings disappear, so will your desire for diet drinks.

Here's why. As you follow all three steps of the program (even if you are just following the guidelines for Step 1 at the time), your addictive connection to sweets—real and artificial—will be broken, and you will be able to feel the difference between a body overloaded with insulin and one in fine balance. With your insulin levels in better balance, you will most likely find that the addictive hold that sugar substitutes had on you has disappeared.

If you do not eliminate sugar substitutes, even for only a limited time, you may never know the freedom from cravings and the wonderful promise of health that a life without hyperinsulinemia can offer. So while following the Program, give up sugar substitutes for a just a little while—four days. We feel sure that when you experience the freedom from cravings that comes with breaking free of your addiction to carbohydrates, you will continue to be sugar substitute–free and to reach out and claim all the fine health and promise that await you.

A VITAL LIQUID ASSET

You may have heard it before, but rest assured, you will hear it again here. As part of any health-promoting program, unless your physician indicates otherwise, be sure to drink six to eight glasses of water every day.

Taking in enough water may sound simple at first, but as your intake of soda is cut and your cravings and general desire to eat decrease, it is easy to forget to take in enough liquid. So make your daily water quota available (get a large insulated mug, if you like) and desirable (we love cool springwater), but most of all, drink it!

How Sweet It Isn't: Valerie's Story

DRS. RICHARD AND RACHAEL HELLER REMEMBER

For more than two years, Valerie had been waiting to be part of our ongoing research project at Mt. Sinai School of Medicine in New York. Now, just when an opening appeared, it looked as if her elevated blood pressure levels were going to put her participation on hold.

"There are different studies opening up," we explained. "The study you signed up for is for those with no apparent heart-related problems, and given your high blood pressure, you will need to wait for a different study." We felt terrible. We knew how much Valerie had been looking forward to working with us. We had called her personally to tell her that the Normative Study had an opening. Now, because of her blood pressure, she would be put back on the waiting list.

"But I never had high blood pressure before," Val went on. "And I've waited to be part of the program for so long."

At first we were at a loss as to what to do. Valerie appeared to be someone who would be a highly motivated research participant. She was serious and committed, and we knew that once she was part of the research group, she would do everything she could to help reduce her risk factors for heart disease. These were the same risk factors that had taken her mother, father, and older twin brothers, all before the end of their fifth decade. Surprisingly, though heart disease was rampant in her family, Valerie had shown none of the expected signs of oncoming heart disease—until now.

Suddenly, when Valerie was only fifty-three years old, her blood pressure had jumped from a reading well within the normal range to a level of great concern. Her cholesterol and triglyceride levels had been rising slowly over the years, and her levels of HDL, the good cholesterol, had been steadily falling—all signs of progressive Insulin Resistance Syndrome and the ongoing hyperinsulinemia that fueled it. It was at her most recent visit to her physician, however, in preparation for joining our study, that she discovered this sudden change in blood pressure.

"I don't know what's causing the problem," Valerie explained. "I'm not doing anything different and," she added, tears filling her wonderfully expressive eyes, "I would hate to lose the chance I have been waiting for for so long. I would do anything to be part of the group. My friend Ally has already been accepted, and I was the one who told her to put her name on the waiting list."

Without a word to each other, the two of us knew that we, too, would do whatever we could to make it possible to work with Val. Our schedule was impossible. We were working eighteen hours a day, and our four-and-a-half-year waiting list to join the program was growing steadily. Seeing anyone privately was out of the question. Valerie's high blood pressure bumped her onto a different waiting list, which might put off her participation by another two years or more. The only solution was to help her bring her high blood pressure down—and fast. We racked our brains for solutions. Drugs were not an option. They would also put her into a different category of study. Her personal physician had already indicated that if Valerie was unable to bring down her blood pressure within a short period of time, she would have to start taking medication, which, in turn, would also preclude her participating in the original study.

In the end the solution came easily and naturally, from Valerie. Although we had tried to understand what changes might account for her sudden rise in blood pressure, at first Valerie was unable to offer any possible explanations. We reviewed all the typical changes that often lead to elevations in blood pressure: changes in medications, diet, activity, stress. In Valerie's case nothing appeared to have changed. But she was not about to give up.

"There must be something I'm missing," she mused, then offered to write down everything she did and ate for several days in hopes that when we reviewed her log, we would be able to identify the culprit.

One week later she returned, her daily inventory in hand. Her spirits were not high. "Well, I brought it," she said, handing us the sheets. "I wrote down everything I did for the whole week, and I don't see anything different. Maybe you can find something, but I don't think there's anyplace to go."

We read through the carefully detailed pages she handed us and then compared them to the food inventory Valerie had completed two years earlier, when she had first asked to join our research program. The difference was clear and evident to us. Valerie was drinking diet soda several times a day. On two occasions she had consumed five diet sodas in one day.

"That couldn't be the answer, could it?" she asked with a mixture of hope and disbelief. Yet she had to admit, it was the only change that might account for her jump in blood pressure.

We explained the impact that sugar substitutes could have on insulin levels, and Valerie listened intently. One part of her was relieved to find the potential cause of her problems; another part was unwilling to give it up. "It's the only treat I let myself have," she explained, then added, "but I really want to bring my blood pressure levels down, and if I don't have to take medications . . ." Her voice trailed off.

We offered Val our four-day challenge. Just four days without diet soda and we bet she would no longer mind doing without it. Valerie, with her usual willingness, took up the challenge.

Seventy-two hours later, almost to the minute, Valerie was on the phone. "I don't know if my blood pressure has dropped," she said excitedly, "but something has changed already.

"I feel better than I have in months. My cravings are so much less, I can hardly believe it, and I'm not holding water in my ankles and fingers like I was. I just feel better, you know?" We knew, but we wanted to hear it from her.

"I woke up this morning full of energy. That just isn't me. I am not a morning person, but this morning I felt great. And I haven't had a headache in two days. I really didn't want to talk about it, but I've been pretty much living with these headaches, and I was wondering if they were related to my high blood pressure. I feel so good. I can't believe it was just the diet soda!"

We slowed Valerie down a bit to make certain that the only changes that she had made were with regard to her diet soda

> consumption and, when we were assured that this was indeed the case, arranged to follow her progress and consult with her physician.
>
> One month later a bright, happy Valerie took her place with our new research group. Her blood pressure was now well within normal levels, and she was more than ready to learn about the other changes that she could make to lower her insulin levels and maximize her heart health.
>
> "One request," Valerie had said, when we called to tell her that we had saved her a place in the group. She clearly was excited to be part of our group but asked a favor. "When it comes to talking about why they should eliminate diet sodas, let me tell my story."
>
> Our answer? Better than that, Valerie, with your permission, we've included it here for the whole world to see.

ON TO THE NEXT STEP

When you feel you have mastered the four guidelines of Step 1, you are ready to move on to Step 2 (supplementation) and Step 3 (Activity).

Many people stay at Step 1 for quite a while, experiencing the wonderful lack of cravings and enjoying their newfound health benefits. You are welcome to linger at Step 1 for as long as you like.

This is a plan of choice. If you are going to stick with a program for life, it must be flexible and meet your needs. When, and only when, you are ready to continue on your health-promoting adventure, continue to the next chapter to learn more about Step 2. If you prefer to skip Step 2 and move on to Step 3, that is fine, too. Step 3 begins on page 187. Either Step 2 or Step 3 can help you to further balance your insulin levels and reduce your insulin-related heart risks, as will the Heart Health–Enhancing Options in Chapter 8. For the best results, follow all three steps, supplemented later by the Heart Health–Enhancing Options.

Although we encourage you to move in order through the steps as we have outlined them, it is more important for you to choose changes that are livable and that you are ready to make. If you bypass Step 2, you are welcome either to return to Step 2 at a future date or to continue on to the Heart Health–Enhancing Options. Each of the steps and Enhancing Options you find within the Program will provide a special focus that can, in

STEP 1: BALANCED NUTRITION

its own way, help you to balance your insulin levels and reduce your insulin resistance.

Best of all, as you move from step to step and through the options, with each new change you make, your success brings with it a greater and greater chance for a future filled with joy, freedom, and health.

> Your success brings with it
> a greater and greater chance for
> a future filled with joy, freedom, and health.

6

THE CARBOHYDRATE ADDICT'S HEALTHY HEART PROGRAM

STEP 2: BALANCED SUPPLEMENTATION

*The first step begins the journey,
the second ensures its success.*—Ben Franklin

THE RIGHT LITTLE ANECDOTE

A young court clerk at his first case took his place beside the judge. The clerk listened carefully as both sides presented their cases, then anxiously awaited the judge's ruling.

"Well," said the judge, turning to the defendant, "I think you're right." The clerk held his breath, for he had not expected so direct and instantaneous a judgment, especially one that did not agree with his own unspoken opinion.

"And," the judge continued, turning to the plaintiff, "I think you're right."

Beside himself and unable to contain his thoughts, the clerk spoke out. "But judge," he cried, "you turned to the defendant and said he was right, then you turned to the plaintiff and said he was right." The clerk stopped short, surprised by his own passion, and waited for a ruling that would put his anxiety to rest.

"Hmmm," remarked the judge, stroking his chin a moment. Then, turning to the clerk, he responded, "I think you're right."

Our little story describes perfectly the state of affairs when it comes to dietary supplementation: there is rarely one right answer, and many considerations must be weighed in determining which supplements, if any, are best for you.

THE WAR BETWEEN THE STATES

The preceding story represents the divided court of scientific and public opinion with regard to the use of nutritional supplementation.

By definition nutritional supplementation is the addition of nutrients with the intent of bringing about a specific, positive health-related result. Nutritional supplementation can be accomplished by eating or drinking the nutrient in its natural form or by means of extracted or synthesized forms in specially prepared tablets, capsules, or other formulations.

> Opposing views on nutritional supplementation make for The War between the States.

The nutritional supplementations that are offered as options in this chapter have been chosen because they have repeatedly been shown through extensive scientific research to promote and enhance heart health and in many cases to greatly reduce your risk for heart disease.

When it comes to nutritional supplementation in general, you will probably hear opposing arguments that support two schools of thought—both sides having very well-documented points of view, both having powerful arguments and even more powerful advocates. And both are right, in their own way. Yet they remain so diametrically opposed that we have sometimes referred to their disagreement as The War between the States.

The first side in this battle represents The State of Deficiency. These well-respected scientists and physicians contend that supplementation should be employed only when there is a clear deficiency of a specific vitamin, mineral, or trace element that leads to a nutrition-related disease or disorder. They would agree, for example, that it is necessary and appropriate to give vitamin B_{12} supplementation to an elderly person who is no longer capable of absorbing the vitamin from his or her food and is showing signs of memory-related problems as a result of this vitamin deficiency. In order for them to recommend supplementation, a patient's blood test would have to reveal a lower-than-normal level of B_{12}, and supplementation would be given until a normal level was reached. In all likelihood, however, these scientists and physicians would not recommend B_{12} supplementation as a means of preventing this problem.

The problem with The State of Deficiency school of thought is twofold. First, those who support this approach assume that (1) they know the appropriate levels of nutrients, and (2) the appropriate levels of nutrients are the same for all individuals, with some leeway allowed for age and gender differences. This one-size-fits-all approach to nutritional supplementation has some major shortcomings. Just as there are individual differences in the need for food or water, some people need more of one nutritional supplement than do others. In addition, although some people can tolerate extremes of nutritional deficiency with seemingly little impact, others may be so sensitive as to be unable to continue functioning well.

> Just as there are individual differences
> in the need for food or water,
> some people need more of
> one nutritional supplement than do others.

The second problem with the deficiency approach to supplementation is its reliance on laboratory tests. Although some testing procedures may produce good, reliable, verifiable results, others may offer less reliable results that may fail to account for individual differences or may give a false sense of normality. In the case of B_{12} testing, for instance, a standard test is given to reveal how much of the vitamin a person is able to absorb.

The fault with standard testing lies in the fact that the form in which the vitamin is given during testing is not the same as the form in which the vitamin appears in "real" food. The test results, then, may show no problem even though a deficiency does exist. The inability to determine and meet the needs of a given individual may lead to severe, even life-threatening, deficiencies. If the deficiency approach to nutritional supplementation is based on the assumption that one cannot make the human body healthier than it can be at its best state, the question remains as to who and what determines the best state for an individual's body. So although The State of Deficiency approach to supplementation is logical, this philosophy of "less is more" may not be an approach by which you can achieve ideal heart health.

In the fight for your heart health, the side opposing The State of Deficiency might best be referred to as The State of Therapeutics. Those who

STEP 2: BALANCED SUPPLEMENTATION

support this side of the nutrition argument say that some vitamins, minerals, and trace elements can offer heart-related health benefits to those who may not necessarily show signs of deficiency. Providing nutritional supplementation to these individuals is, then, therapeutic.

Some of the advocates for the therapeutic approach are well-respected scientists and physicians who use strict scientific methods to evaluate the benefits of a wide variety of nutrient supplements. Unfortunately there also exist, within the confines of this approach, those of questionable backgrounds, those who would make nutritional recommendations without sufficient proof of their value or who would overgeneralize and exaggerate the potential benefits.

> For the individual who seeks ideal heart health, nutritional deficiencies must be eradicated.

From the finest minds to the most suspect frauds, The State of Therapeutics contains some of the best and worst in the area of nutritional advice. In addition, some advocates recommend megadoses of nutrients that, in time, may lead to severe, even life-threatening, overdoses. To make matters worse, concentrated doses of some nutrients can either interfere with the absorption of other nutrients or cause an increased excretion of those nutrients. So, again, although this approach is logical and is correct in many respects, it, too, cannot be assumed to ensure your attainment of ideal heart health.

It appears that, as in the court scene described at the beginning of this chapter, both sides are right. For the individual who seeks ideal heart health, nutritional deficiencies must be eradicated. At the same time, appropriate therapeutic doses of supplements may also be beneficial for many.

STEP 2: SUPPLEMENT YOUR NUTRITION AS PER YOUR INDIVIDUAL NEEDS

In this step you will learn about six simple nutrients, available at your local supermarket or health food store, that may be very important to your heart health. As always, consult with your physician before beginning your nutritional supplementation and continue under his or her guidance.

Although everyone has been taught the value of good nutrition (over and over again), few people are aware of the importance of ideal individualized nutrition. Ideal individualized nutrition is that food balance which best meets the needs of your body and your lifestyle. When food alone cannot supply the right vitamin, mineral, and trace element or nutrient combination to meet your needs, supplementation of the right kind may prove to be vital in restoring and maintaining ideal heart health.

> Each supplement we have included in this chapter
> has been selected for its
> importance to insulin-related heart health.

Each of the vitamins, minerals, or trace elements that we have included in this chapter has been selected for its importance to heart health in relation to insulin balance. This is an essential consideration for carbohydrate addicts. Some of the supplementation choices that follow have been shown to reduce hyperinsulinemia, some to improve your body's ability to handle carbohydrates, some to restore the imbalance that hyperinsulinemia can bring; some do all three.

In consultation with your physician, choose those supplementation options which appear to best meet your needs and, if you like, add them as your way of completing Step 2 in your heart health promotion program. We recommend that you start with the first option, chromium (in the form of glucose tolerance factor) and, as you wish, add other supplementation options one at a time. Wait at least one week before adding each new supplement. You may move on to Step 3 while you continue to add supplementation options, or if you like or if your doctor prefers, you may move directly to Step 3 of the program, bypassing all supplementation options.

If you choose to supplement your nutrition, read over the descriptions of the preferred supplementation options that follow. As you make your selections, keep in mind your family's medical history, your own personal history, and your lifestyle. The choices presented here have been compiled in order to provide you with options for your ideal individualized nutrition; choose those that are right for *you*. Under no circumstances should you change the dosages of any medications your physician has prescribed, nor should you stop taking them, unless your doctor recommends such a change.

> Studies by scientists at the U.S. Department of Agriculture have found that nine out of ten diets do *not* supply enough chromium.

SUPPLEMENTATION OPTION 1: CHROMIUM BALANCING INSULIN LEVELS NATURALLY

Of all the nutritional supplementation options that we have researched, by far the most powerful and important to the carbohydrate addict is chromium.* Chromium occurs naturally in our foods but can be lost when foods are processed or refined. Dr. R. A. Anderson and his research team at the United States Department of Agriculture now report that the diets of as many as nine out of ten Americans do *not* supply them with adequate amounts of chromium.

> Many of the foods and beverages we consume— including soda, snack foods, and junk foods— literally rob our bodies of chromium.

In addition, many of the foods and beverages that we consume regularly—including soda, snack foods, and junk foods—can literally rob us of our vital chromium stores. Even foods and beverages that are often considered "healthy"—like milk, fruits, and juices—can drain our body's dwindling chromium supply. To add to this chromium piracy, emotional and physical stress as well as extremes in activity can further deplete our bodies of this precious nutrient. So given today's challenges, keeping our bodies supplied with adequate chromium by eating chromium-rich foods may no longer be possible.

Chromium has been called the "essential cofactor" of insulin. We often describe it as insulin's partner, helping insulin to do its jobs. And like partners working together, when one is unable to do his or her part, the second may be forced to compensate. So it is with insulin and chromium. When your body does not have enough chromium, it needs more insulin to do its work and releases extra insulin whenever high-carbohydrate foods or drinks are consumed.

---

*Throughout this book, unless otherwise indicated, the term *chromium* can be assumed to mean the trivalent, nutritional form of chromium.

> **Chromium is a vital cofactor for insulin.
> Too little chromium in our diet
> can mean higher insulin levels in our blood.**

A simple deficiency in chromium can begin a powerful cycle of excess insulin release followed by insulin-related cravings and weight gain as well as blood sugar and heart-related problems. An insulin resistance cycle can be initiated in which the muscles, brain, and other organs shut down to insulin and blood sugar. First, insulin and blood sugar are channeled into the fat cells (leading to weight gain and low blood sugar swings). Later, the fat cells resist the onslaught of insulin, trapping insulin and blood sugar in the bloodstream (leading to adult-onset diabetes and high blood pressure, and laying the foundation for heart disease).

For years scientists have confirmed the important role that chromium deficiency plays in the development of heart disease. More than twenty years ago, Dr. K. N. Jeejeebhoy and his colleagues reported in the *American Journal of Clinical Nutrition* that chromium deficiency resulted in abnormal blood sugar levels, risk-related blood fat levels, and slower metabolic rates.

> **The very process of aging and its relationship to heart disease
> may be tied to the chromium-insulin connection.**

Repeatedly, over the past two decades, scientists such as Dr. A. S. Kozlovsky and his colleagues, reporting in the scientific journal *Metabolism*, have confirmed that chromium deficiency is common to heart disease and adult-onset diabetes, and as researcher and author Dr. Richard A. Passwater reported, chromium deficiency "results in arterial plaque formation, which in turn can induce blood clotting, which causes a heart attack."

The very process of aging and its relationship to heart disease may be tied to the chromium-insulin connection as well. The older we get, the more our bodies appear to need chromium but the more likely it is that (1) we are not taking in the chromium we need and (2) stress and other factors are robbing us of our vital chromium stores. When we look at both facts together, we realize that as we grow older, our bodies have less chromium available just when we need it the most. And with each passing decade, lower levels of chromium can lead to higher levels of insulin and, through insulin's actions, an increased risk for heart disease.

The good news is that correcting a silent chromium deficiency is both easy and inexpensive. Supplementing your diet with chromium can have a powerful effect on preventing or reversing many of the heart-related health problems and heart disease risk factors that have long been associated with the "natural process of aging."

> Correcting a silent chromium deficiency
> is both easy and inexpensive.

NATURAL VERSUS SUPPLEMENTAL CHROMIUM

Natural food sources of chromium include brewer's yeast, black pepper, mushrooms, wine, and beer, among others. It is, however, almost impossible to avoid or correct a chromium deficiency by consuming these foods and beverages. The ways in which these foods are prepared, the quantities needed, and the stress to which we are exposed make it virtually impossible for Americans to keep chromium stores high by natural means.

After all, you can eat only so much brewer's yeast and black pepper, and there is only so much beer or wine you should consume. In addition, although we can limit how many times each day we take in high-carbohydrate foods, the chromium depletion that follows the consumption of processed or refined foods, as well as the stresses we encounter daily, are virtually unavoidable.

Though it is generally preferable to get the nutrients you need from the food you eat, supplementing your chromium intake with a daily dose of the right kind of chromium may prove to be the easiest ways for the carbohydrate addict to help keep insulin levels in balance.

GLUCOSE TOLERANCE FACTOR:
CHROMIUM BY ANY OTHER NAME

A special form of the inexpensive and common nutrient chromium is available from virtually all health food stores. This form of chromium has been found to have significant effects on insulin levels and on the weight- and heart-related health problems that can often result from an insulin imbalance.

The specific form of chromium that has been shown to be so effective and that we give our research participants and private patients is called *glucose tolerance factor chromium,* or GTF chromium for short.

You may have heard a great deal about other forms of chromium, including chromium picolinate, chromium polynicotinate, and others. We cannot recommend other forms of chromium. Chromium picolinate is still somewhat new, and for a while there was some concern about the safety of the picolinate portion of the product. Chromium polynicotinate is a special form of chromium that has been combined with niacin. In our opinion this coupling can be problematic. Because niacin has a critical level of intake that is very low, it is easy to overdose on the niacin. Although combining niacin and chromium may be a good idea profitwise (it allows manufacturers to come up with new patents), for your ideal individualized nutrition balance, we think it is far better to keep these supplements separate. In that way you are far less likely to take too much niacin while trying to get enough chromium. In addition, this combination has not been tried and tested over the years in the same way as GTF chromium has.

> Not all chromium supplements are the same.
> We think biologically active GTF (glucose tolerance factor) chromium is the best choice.

GTF chromium seems far and away the best choice. In our opinion it is the safe and effective way to take in this essential nutrient. In the future you may hear about a whole host of other chromium combinations. Each new type of chromium-nutrition cocktail offers two benefits to the manufacturers that may not be in your best interests. First, these gourmet chromium-nutrient combinations can usually be made more cheaply than GTF chromium, yet they can be sold for the same price as GTF chromium or more. Lower production cost with the same selling price equals greater profit.

Second, chromium-nutrient combinations can be patented, whereas GTF chromium is a simple nutrient that no single company or person can own. When a chromium-nutrient combination can be patented, a company can charge a higher price for it and, in turn, will often sink big advertising bucks into promoting its sales. Plain old GTF chromium cannot be hyped or sold at high prices, so manufacturers often prefer to "jazz it up" in order to patent it and then make it more attractive to the public. Like aspirin, GTF chromium is a good old standby that does its job quietly and dependably.

WHAT TYPE OF CHROMIUM IS BEST?

There are many types of chromium that you can buy at your local health food store but only one that we would suggest at this time:[*] GTF chromium. When buying GTF chromium, make certain that the label clearly states that it is "certified biologically active." Several brands meet these guidelines; we ourselves use Solgar's GTF chromium, which is certified biologically active.

A word of caution: be certain that you read the label carefully. The tablets should contain *only* glucose tolerance factor chromium; no niacin, polynicotinate, or other "added nutrients." We strongly suggest that you choose GTF chromium and GTF chromium alone.

> Solgar and other companies
> produce more than one kind of chromium,
> so read the label carefully.

If your health food store does not have Solgar's GTF chromium or you do not want the brand it carries, do not let the store clerk talk you into something else. Stick with GTF chromium. You might ask the store to order the GTF chromium you want. In general, it should cost about $9 to $11 for one hundred tablets, each containing 200 micrograms (200 µg) of GTF chromium.

The National Research Council says that 50 to 200 micrograms of trivalent chromium each day is the "safe and adequate" intake for adults. *Most* pills contain 200 micrograms, so one pill each day fulfills the "safe and adequate" daily intake recommendation. Not all brands contain 200 micrograms, so it is important to read the label.

> Do *not* take your GTF chromium with
> food, vitamins, or medications.

Take your GTF chromium at the same time every day, but do *not* take it with food or medications. Zinc—found in so many of your foods, in your

[*]Individual health needs and concerns should be considered. Therefore, check with your physician before adding GTF chromium supplementation to your diet. Since GTF chromium may reduce the need for insulin, diabetics who take GTF chromium should be closely monitored by their physicians.

multivitamins, or as supplement tablets themselves—can interfere with the absorption of the chromium, so take your GTF chromium with water and nothing else.

The benefits of GTF chromium may begin to show within one to two months. However, long before you notice the difference, your body will already be responding to this often much-needed nutrient.

SUPPLEMENTATION OPTION 2: FIBER
FIRST AND FOREMOST, FAVOR FIBER

When it comes to choosing a food source that could literally save your life, you can probably do no better than selecting foods high in fiber. We know you've heard it before, but this time we'll make it palatable and fun. First, the facts. Some researchers have concluded that omitting fiber from your diet puts you at as much risk for heart disease as does cigarette smoking, high cholesterol, or high blood pressure. Every gram of fiber that you eat widens the distance between you and a heart attack, yet most people eat less than half the amount they need.

> The fact that fiber is not "sexy" may have helped claim thousands of lives.

The reason for the lack of interest in fiber is threefold. First, fiber is not "sexy." After all, most people would rather say that they are on a high-protein diet (which sounds young and vibrant, as if you were preparing for some athletic challenge) than admit they are on a "high-fiber" diet (which sounds as if you needed some sort of laxative). Say "low-fat" and you think of a slim woman admiring herself in a mirror; say "high-fiber" and you imagine a frail, old person hunched over a cereal bowl. Albeit inaccurate, fiber's image persists—and no doubt about it, the image gets in the way.

Second, the whole fiber issue seems confusing, although it doesn't have to be. In the following paragraphs we'll explain it in a few sentences, and you'll feel like an instant expert.

Third, ensuring a high-fiber diet sounds neither easy nor appetizing. Most people would rather just take a pill. Surprise! Simply following Step 1 of this program helps ensure that you'll get a good portion of your recommended daily intake of fiber. By making a few additional high-fiber choices

STEP 2: BALANCED SUPPLEMENTATION

when selecting your high-carbohydrate foods, you can supplement your program with additional heart healthy fiber.

Fiber is the textured portion of fruits, vegetables, and grains. It passes through your body without being digested. It has no caloric value and provides the body with no important vitamins or minerals, yet it is absolutely essential for a heart healthy program.

Although most people refer to fiber as if it were a single entity, there are many foods that supply different kinds of fiber. Fiber is divided into two main groups, soluble and insoluble. *Insoluble fiber* does not dissolve in water and cannot be broken down by stomach acid, so it moves quickly through the gastrointestinal tract and promotes the swift elimination of fecal matter. Although insoluble fiber has been shown to relieve constipation and prevent hemorrhoids and many researchers have reported its importance in the reduction of the risk for colon cancer, it does not necessarily balance insulin levels. As your physician recommends, insoluble fiber may be an important adjunct to your eating program. Insoluble fiber-rich foods include fruits, vegetables, and whole-wheat products that include the wheat bran.

Soluble fiber, on the other hand, dissolves in water (even though it remains intact while inside the body). In the intestines, soluble fiber forms a jelly-like mass that binds with cholesterol and promotes its excretion from the body. Due to its binding effect, soluble fiber has a powerful cholesterol-lowering effect, reducing both total cholesterol and low-density blood fats—actions that are important in reducing your risk for heart disease.

> **Soluble and insoluble fiber have different properties.**
> **Soluble fiber helps balance insulin levels**
> **and improve sugar metabolism.**

Of greatest importance, soluble fiber has been shown to balance insulin levels and improve sugar metabolism as well. For the carbohydrate addict in particular, a diet rich in soluble fiber along with other insulin-balancing changes can greatly reduce heart disease risk and improve and help restore heart health.

Soluble fiber can be found in grains, beans, oats, barley, soybeans, fruits, and vegetables. It is always best to get your fiber from your food. Although soluble fiber can also be found in psyllium seed, pectin, and guar gum, the use of concentrated fiber supplementation from these high-fiber sources is *not* recommended unless your physician thinks it necessary. If a fiber supplement has been prescribed, take it at Reward Meal times only.

Adding high-fiber foods to your eating program is easy! Low-carbohydrate, high-fiber vegetables can be included in all meals, whereas high-carbohydrate, high-fiber grains, beans, fruits, and so on should be reserved for your Reward Meals. If your present diet is low in fiber, a gradual approach to increasing fiber is recommended. If, for instance, your diet now provides very little fiber and you suddenly and greatly increase your fiber intake, you may well experience unpleasant bloating, gassiness, and other symptoms.

Some high-fiber foods are more likely to produce gassiness than others. Beans and other legumes are quite well known for their gas-producing abilities. If you find that a particular food creates a gas problem, cut back on the portion or substitute another choice that contains a similar fiber. A person who cannot tolerate beans, for instance, may have no problem with celery, apples, or oatmeal. It is generally agreed that your intake of fiber should come from a variety of foods and that the intake should be spread throughout the day to avoid a sudden overload to your digestive system.

Most dietary recommendations indicate that your daily intake of fiber should be between 20 and 35 grams. Most people take in about 10 to 12 grams, a decidedly inadequate amount of this heart-important substance. On page 165 you will find a list of high-fiber foods that are delicious and easy to include in your meals. You can raise your fiber intake at all meals by including higher-fiber vegetables such as green beans, asparagus, spinach, cabbage, and Brussels sprouts. Salads rich in celery, lettuce, spinach, mushrooms, bean sprouts, and green peppers are another high-fiber, low-carbohydrate choice that can be included in all meals.

> **You can raise your fiber intake easily and naturally.**

At Reward Meals, you can raise your fiber intake easily and naturally by including, as part of your one-third high-carbohydrate portion, high-fiber complex carbohydrates (such as whole-grain bread and pretzels, popcorn, and fiber-rich whole fruits) rather than low-fiber high-sugar foods (such as candy or soda). At Reward Meals eat the whole fruit rather than drink fiber-depleted juices. Your heart will thank you. If your doctor agrees, as you increase your fiber intake you may do as many nutrition experts advise and increase your water intake by two glasses more than the generally recommended six to eight glasses per day.

STEP 2: BALANCED SUPPLEMENTATION

Heart-Healthy High-Fiber Foods

Food	Serving	Fiber (grams)	Include in Low-Carbo Meals	Include in Reward Only
Vegetables (Raw)				
Carrots, sliced	½ cup	1.9		√
Celery	1 stalk	1.0	√	√
Green pepper	1 cup	1.0	√	√
Lettuce, chopped	1 cup	0.9	√	√
Mushrooms	½ cup	0.9	√	√
Spinach	1 cup	1.2	√	√
Sprouts, bean	½ cup	1.5	√	√
Vegetables (Cooked)				
Asparagus	½ cup	1.0	√	√
Broccoli	½ cup	2.2		√
Brussels sprouts	½ cup	2.3	√	√
Cabbage	½ cup	1.7	√	√
Carrots	½ cup	2.6		√
Green beans	½ cup	1.6	√	√
Okra	½ cup	1.5*	√	√
Onions	½ cup	1.1*		√
Parsnips	½ cup	2.7		√
Peas	½ cup	3.6		√
Potatoes, with skins	1 medium	2.5		√
Spinach	½ cup	2.5	√	√
Squash, summer	½ cup	1.4		√
Turnips	½ cup	1.7*		√
Zucchini	½ cup	1.8		√
Breads, etc.				
Bran muffin	1 small	2.5		√
Bread, French	1 slice	0.7		√
Bread, pumpernickel	1 slice	1.0		√
Bread, whole-wheat	1 slice	1.4		√
Rye wafers	3 wafers	2.3		√

Heart-Healthy High-Fiber Foods (continued)

Food	Serving	Fiber (grams)	Include in Low-Carbo Meals	Include in Reward Only
Cereal				
100% bran cereal, cold	1/3 cup	8.5		√
Oat bran, cooked	3/4 cup	2.2 °		√
Oat bran cereal, cold	3/4 cup	1.5 °		√
Oatmeal, uncooked	1/3 cup	1.4 °		√
Oats, whole, cooked	3/4 cup	1.6		√
Shredded wheat, cold	2/3 cup	2.6		√
Wheat flakes, cereal	1 cup	2.0		√
Wheat germ	1/4 cup	3.4		√
Fruit				
Apple, with skin	1 medium	3.5		√
Apricots, dried	5 halves	1.4		√
Apricots, fresh	3 medium	1.8		√
Banana	1 medium	2.4		√
Blueberries	1/2 cup	2.6		√
Cherries	10	1.2		√
Grapefruit	1/2 large	3.1		√
Mango	1/2 small	1.7 °		√
Peach	1 medium	1.9		√
Pear	1 medium	3.2		√
Pineapple	1/2 cup	1.1		√
Prunes	3 medium	3.0		√
Strawberries	1/2 cup	1.5		√
Legumes (Cooked)				
Baked beans, canned	1/2 cup	2.6 °		√
Black beans	1/2 cup	2.4 °		√
Butter beans	1/2 cup	2.7 °		√

Heart-Healthy High-Fiber Foods (continued)

Food	Serving	Fiber (grams)	Include in Low-Carbo Meals	Include in Reward Only
Chickpeas	½ cup	1.3*		√
Kidney beans, canned	½ cup	2.0*		√
Navy beans	½ cup	2.2*		√
White beans, canned	½ cup	2.2*		√
Pasta/Rice (Cooked)				
Macaroni	1 cup	1.6		√
Rice, brown	½ cup	1.0**		√
Spaghetti, regular	1 cup	1.1		√
Spaghetti, whole-wheat	1 cup	3.9		√
Snacks				
Popcorn	1 cup	1.6		√
Popcorn cakes	4	1.1		√
Pretzel, hard	1	0.8		√
Pretzel, whole-wheat, hard	1	2.2		√

*Soluble fiber.
**White rice contains only one-fifth the fiber of brown rice. Brown rice makes a far better high-fiber choice when appropriate.

SUPPLEMENTATION OPTION 3: VITAMINS C AND E: ANTIOXIDANTS TO HELP KEEP YOU YOUNG AT HEART

To understand why antioxidants are so important to your heart health, you need to know a little about oxygen. Everyone knows that we need oxygen for life, but few people think about the fact that with each breath you take, as every cell in your body is drenched with life-giving oxygen, your body gets one breath older. This aging process is the result of *oxidation*.

Oxidation is a chemical reaction that occurs when the oxygen you breathe combines with the fats that are present in your cells. It is similar to the process that turns a shiny metal tool into an ugly, rusted one. Although our bodies don't rust, oxidative damage within our bodies brings about much of the wear and tear that we call aging and that can lead to heart disease. Oxidative reactions within our body form *free radicals*, compounds that can attach themselves to cells and interfere with normal functioning. Fortunately, antioxidants provide a simple way of blocking the potential damage that can be done by free radicals.

When you think of antioxidants, imagine millions of little trash cans traveling around your body "scooping up" any harmful debris or leftover material they find along the way. Antioxidants help extend the life of our cells. Oxidants are a natural part of chemical reactions in our bodies, but they can be greatly stimulated by air pollution, tobacco smoke, radiation, rancid foods, and herbicides as well as the unavoidable physical effects of aging. Because of this unexpected onslaught of oxidants from many sources, our natural antioxidants are not enough to keep the body from being damaged. Therefore, it becomes important to extend our body's antioxidant supplies by taking in foods and supplements that contain antioxidants.

> Each of the antioxidant vitamins, E and C,
> helps to promote heart health in its own unique way;
> combined, they can bring added benefits.

Today the powerful effects of antioxidants are being explored by scientists in record numbers, but at this time the two antioxidants that appear to be most important are vitamins C and E. Each of these antioxidants helps to promote heart health in its own unique way, and each should be considered as an important potential supplement to your program. As always, consult with your physician.

VITAMIN E: THE AGE FIGHTER

Vitamin E has been compared to a nutritional Swiss Army Knife, a most handy item that is capable of performing a wide variety of functions. The list of the health benefits that have been traced to vitamin E goes on and on: it modifies blood fats so that they protect against heart disease, improves circulation by helping to prevent the formation of blood clots that can block the flow of blood to the heart (and helping to dissolve those blood clots that do form), protects red blood cells from oxygen damage, boosts our "good" cholesterol, and improves our immune system so that we are better protected from bacterial infections (a newly discovered cause of heart disease).

A high concentration of vitamin E can be found in a wide variety of seeds, nuts, and oils, including olive oil, wheat germ and wheat germ oil, sunflower seeds and oil, almonds, pecans, hazelnuts, safflower oil, corn oil, soybean oil, peanut butter, and peanut oil. Whole grains, leafy green vegetables, desiccated liver, organ meats, soybeans, and eggs are rich in vitamin E as well.

Processing, refining, freezing, heating, and the presence of chlorine and iron can strip foods of much of their natural vitamin E. For that reason processed and refined cereals that state that they contain added vitamin E (especially those with added ferric iron and other vitamins) may not deliver adequate and usable amounts of vitamin E to your body. Just because the vitamin was added during "manufacture" does not mean it is available *in a usable form* when you eat the food. The processing itself or the addition of competing vitamins or minerals may remove vitamin E or render it useless. Oils that are cold-pressed (such as olive oil) and whole grains are far more likely to retain their vitamin E content than those that have been heated, processed, or refined.

Even if your diet is rich in vitamin E, many drugs—such as cholesterol-lowering medications, oral contraceptives, and some antibiotics—can impair the absorption or utilization of the vitamin.

> **Cholesterol-lowering medications, oral contraceptives, and antibiotics can make it difficult for your body to use the vitamin E it gets.**

Hyperinsulinemia's reduction of vitamin E stores had been suspected for many years, but the link and its connection to heart disease were confirmed only in the last few years. Recent reports, such as the groundbreaking work by Dr. A. G. Galvan and his research team, published in 1996 in the medical journal *Metabolism*, have provided vital information regarding insulin's link to vitamin E. Studying four groups of subjects—those who were overweight, diabetic, hypertensive, or free from any physical problems—Dr. Galvan found that in all groups vitamin E levels dropped significantly when subjects were made hyperinsulinemic. The team concluded that high levels of insulin drastically deplete the body of vitamin E. This vitamin depletion would leave the body unprotected, open to oxidant injury, cell aging, and an increased risk for heart disease.

> **High levels of insulin can deplete your body of vitamin E.**

An understanding of vitamin E's powerful and widespread health benefits is just emerging. Although the population at large has come to accept that vitamin E is good for you, scientists are rushing to document its amazing benefits. From dissolving blood clots at Duke University Medical Center's Department of Surgery to lowering blood sugar levels of adult-onset diabetics (as reported at meetings of the American Heart Association), vitamin E's potentially lifesaving abilities make good heart sense.

Vitamin E supplementation has been shown to significantly reduce angina (heart pain), and researchers are now speculating that vitamin E may play a special role for those with adult-onset diabetes, lowering the insulin resistance that traps sugar in the bloodstream. Reducing insulin resistance would result in lower blood sugar levels, a primary goal for adult-onset diabetics. It is likely that future research will confirm vitamin E's powerful potential to reduce insulin resistance as well as diabetics' risk for heart disease.

> **Vitamin E supplementation has been shown to dissolve blood clots and reduce angina and may help balance blood sugar levels.**

Whenever possible, foods rich in vitamin E should be included among your daily choices (see page 169). Supplementation is encouraged only after consultation with your physician. If you smoke or have high blood pressure, diabetes, or rheumatic or ischemic heart disease, vitamin E supplementation may not be appropriate for you or your intake may have to be modified. Discuss these and all other medical concerns with your doctor.

Vitamin E supplementation may not be advisable if you are taking blood-thinning medications or have any medical condition that can contribute to vitamin K deficiency, such as malabsorption syndrome or liver disease. These and all other concerns should be discussed with your physician before you start vitamin E supplementation.

Vitamin E can be found in eight supplemental forms. The most common and active supplemental form is called *alpha-tocopherol*. The recom-

STEP 2: BALANCED SUPPLEMENTATION 171

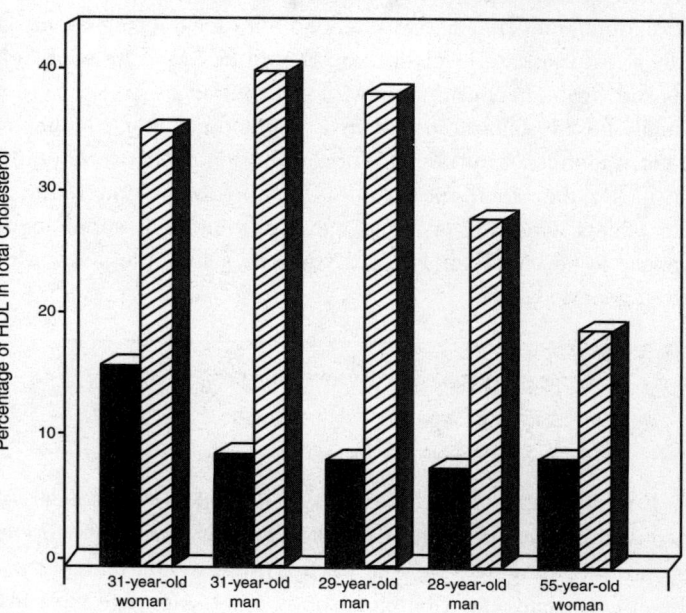

■ Before Vitamin E
▨ After Vitamin E

In his study published in the *American Journal of Clinical Pathology*, Dr. William Hermann gave 600 to 800 I.U. of vitamin E per day* to five people with very low levels of the good cholesterol, HDL. After one month or more of taking the nutrient, HDL-cholesterol levels rose to normal, indicating a far lower risk for heart attack.

*Chart adapted from data provided by study. Individual readers' dosages may vary. Check with your physician before beginning your own regime of vitamin E therapy.

mended daily allowances (RDAs) for tocopherol are 8 international units (I.U.) per day for nonpregnant women and 10 international units per day for men. Dr. L. A. Simons, in his 1996 research report "What Dose of Vitamin E Is Required to Reduce Susceptibility of LDL to Oxidation?," found that 500 international units per day brought about desired change, whereas Dr. H. M. Princen and other researchers reported that although greater amounts of vitamin E brought about greater LDL reduction, a dosage of only 25 international units per day was needed in order to bring about significant change. Appropriate levels for you should be based on your individual needs and, again, in consultation with your physician.

It is usually best to choose a vitamin E supplement that contains no other vitamins, minerals, or nutrients. When appropriate, choose vitamin E soft-gel capsules rather than the vitamin E supplementation found in multivitamin tablets. Choosing a brand name of vitamin E supplements does not appear to add any benefit, so if you like, select a less-expensive though trusted generic label.

> Some iron supplements destroy vitamin E;
> don't take both supplements at the same time.

Vitamin E is oil-soluble and is better absorbed if taken with a meal. Inorganic (ferric) iron destroys vitamin E. Therefore, if ferric iron supplement tablets are recommended by your doctor, these should be taken at a different time of day than your vitamin E supplement. Although most iron supplements contain the organic (ferrous) form of iron, which does not interfere with vitamin E uptake, unless you are certain, take them at different times. Do not take vitamin E with oral contraceptives, antibiotics, or other medications that can interfere with its absorption, and if you take more than one capsule, take them at different times to increase their power to enhance your heart health.

VITAMIN C: IT'S NOT JUST FOR COLDS ANYMORE

When most people think of vitamin C supplementation, their thoughts turn either to Linus Pauling's research or to the plethora of cold remedies that include vitamin C in one form or another. Few people are aware of vitamin C's connection to heart health.

Like other antioxidants, vitamin C (also known as ascorbic acid) has the

STEP 2: BALANCED SUPPLEMENTATION

ability to neutralize many of the potentially harmful effects of oxidation; in particular, it can help disarm free radicals before they attack artery walls. You may have witnessed vitamin C's antioxidant abilities yourself, in your kitchen, if you have ever used the juice of a lemon to keep the cut surfaces of apples, peaches, or avocados from turning brown.

> Vitamin C appears to have a protective effect to help keep your arteries and heart healthy. In those who have experienced heart failure, vitamin C improves the flow of blood to and through the heart.

In addition, vitamin C has been shown to boost immunity, speed healing, and slow aging, three indirect but very important links in the heart disease chain. Scientists have witnessed vitamin C's positive effects on both men and women and across all age groups and found that not only does vitamin C appear to have a protective effect to help keep your arteries and heart healthy, but in those who have experienced heart failure, vitamin C also improves the flow of blood to and through the heart.

Not only has a deficiency in vitamin C been connected to the initiation and progression of heart disease as well as associated chest pain (angina), but vitamin C can also enhance the positive effects of other nutrients—in particular, other antioxidants—in the battle for heart health. Because it is such a good partner to other antioxidants, we often refer to vitamin C as the complementary vitamin.

The complementary nature of vitamin C may be especially important for the carbohydrate addict. Although the exact mechanism is still not clear, it appears that vitamin C may have difficulty entering cells where it is needed; as cells close down in response to high insulin levels, vitamin C may be shut out as well. Supplementing your diet with vitamin C and vitamin E may be a simple approach to the maintenance or improvement of heart health. As vitamin E reduces insulin resistance, opening the "doors" for vitamin C to enter, it is quite reasonable to expect that vitamin C will find it far easier to bring its benefits to the very cells that need it most.

Researchers are still discovering some of vitamin C's other beneficial and complementary actions. Dr. K. G. Losonczy and his team at the National Institutes of Health reported their findings in the *American Journal of Clinical Nutrition*. Studying more than 11,000 people, these scientists found that among those studied, research participants who supplemented their diet with both vitamins E and C showed a reduction of more than 50 percent in coronary heart disease mortality. Vitamin C has been shown to protect other fat-soluble vitamins—for example, vitamins A and E—keeping them capable of activity until your body calls them into action.

Your body cannot produce vitamin C, so all the vitamin C you need must be supplied by your diet or supplementation. A high concentration of vitamin C can be found in fruits, vegetables, nuts, wine, and beer. Red and green peppers, broccoli, orange and cranberry juices, papaya, strawberries, and citrus fruits are particularly rich in vitamin C. Because vitamin C is both water-soluble and heat-sensitive, it is important to understand that cooking destroys vitamin C, so if you are eating foods rich in vitamin C, remember that only fresh, uncooked forms of a food will contain optimal levels of vitamin C. As always, use caution in preparing foods so that uncooked fruits and vegetables contain no harmful bacteria.

> Your body cannot produce vitamin C, so all you need must be supplied by your diet or supplementation. Birth control pills and aspirin can destroy your body's reserves.

In addition to the difficulty of getting enough vitamin C from our diets, many of us lose the vitamin C our bodies have in storage. The anti–vitamin C action of birth control pills and heavy doses of aspirin can reduce vitamin C stores. Certainly it is always best to get your vitamin C from your food, but since that is sometimes impossible, with your physician's approval you may find it beneficial to supplement your intake with over-the-counter vitamin C tablets, available at your local supermarket, drugstore, or health food store. Although vitamin C supplements are inexpensive and easy to obtain, they are not all created equal.

Before you purchase any vitamin C supplement, you should know just a bit about vitamin C as it appears in food. Vitamin C in citrus fruit comes in the perfect package. The thick skin that surrounds oranges, grapefruits, lemons, and limes is lightproof, thereby protecting its precious contents. Inside the fruit the vitamin C gets a boost from the citrus bioflavonoids that are naturally found in the peel of these fruits. These vitaminlike molecules can improve your ability to hold and use vitamin C by up to 35 percent. The good news is that you can now purchase vitamin C supplements that are produced with helper bioflavonoids packed into each tablet.

If at all possible, choose a vitamin C supplement that contains no

STEP 2: BALANCED SUPPLEMENTATION

other vitamins, minerals, or nutrients. Brand names of vitamin C supplements do not appear to be any better than generic, so if you like, choose a less-expensive though trusted generic label.

In consulting your physician, discuss vitamin C interaction with any medications that you may be taking, including (but not limited to) aspirin, oral contraceptives, or other drugs that can interfere with vitamin C absorption. In addition, it should be pointed out that vitamin C may increase the absorption of aluminum, which is found in some antacids as well as other medications. Since aluminum can be toxic, never take vitamin C with any medications (over-the-counter or prescription) that contain aluminum. High doses of vitamin C (1 gram or more per day) can interfere with your ability to absorb vitamin B_{12} from your food or other supplements you may be taking. Vitamin C intakes of more than 200 milligrams per day may reduce the effectiveness of many antidepressants. Although vitamin C supplementation has become commonplace because it can provide many valuable benefits, as with any nutrient, it should be taken with caution and medical monitoring.

The RDA for vitamin C is 60 milligrams per day for adult men and nonpregnant women. Many scientists and physicians alike are speaking out, saying that optimal levels (for more than just the prevention of deficiency diseases) should be much higher. Researchers such as Dr. L. Mosca of the University of Michigan's Preventative Cardiology Program, publishing in the *Journal of the American College of Cardiology*, have reported that for research participants with coronary artery disease, 1,000 milligrams per day of vitamin C, in combination with vitamin E and beta-carotene supplementation, helped reduce the oxidation of low-density lipids (LDL, or "bad," cholesterol).

Individual needs and appropriate doses vary depending on the source of the vitamin C as well as dietary and lifestyle choices. Smoking, for instance, has been shown to reduce levels of vitamin C by 25 to 40 percent. Pain relievers, antidepressants, anticoagulants, and steroids have all been shown to deplete the body's store of vitamin C as well. In general, it may be best to avoid the chewable varieties of vitamin C, which can damage tooth enamel. High doses can result in false-negative readings in tests for blood in the stool, and some people experience stomach irritation with any vitamin C supplementation. So although vitamin C can be a helpful part of a heart health–enhancing program, do not megadose and always let your doctor be your guide.

SUPPLEMENTATION OPTION 4: FOLIC ACID: THE HOMOCYSTEINE CONNECTION TO HEART DISEASE

Until recently a lack of folic acid (also called *folate* and one of the family of B vitamins) was not considered to be central to the development of heart disease. It had been shown, many years ago, that children with a rare genetic defect that resulted in abnormally high blood levels of a substance called homocysteine developed arterial disease at a very early age. Yet the connection of low folic acid and high homocysteine levels to adult-onset heart disease remained under investigation and poorly understood. It is only recently that the work of so many researchers over so many years has confirmed the powerful folic acid–homocysteine connection to heart disease.

> Folic acid helps break down homocysteine, an emerging risk factor for heart disease.

One of the actions of folic acid is to promote the breakdown of homocysteine, an amino acid (a building block for protein) that is normally present in the blood. Adults with moderately high levels of homocysteine have been found to be significantly more likely to suffer from severe arterial disease than people with normal levels of homocysteine. Future research may offer new understandings, but at this time it is thought that homocysteine damages arteries and that folic acid converts it into a substance that does not. Although scientists are aware that there is a relationship between homocysteine levels, folic acid, B_{12}, and B_6, investigations continue, exploring this vital connection.

Perhaps the most important research finding for the carbohydrate addict was the discovery that folic acid can reduce insulin levels. Again, the research is so new that how folic acid lowers insulin levels remains unknown, but this potentially powerful connection may make folic acid an even more important supplement for heart disease risk reduction than ever before.

"We think that there is good enough evidence that the whole population would benefit from increasing folic acid intake," says Shirley Beresford, associate professor of epidemiology at the University of Washington, School of Public Health, Seattle, as quoted in *USA Today* (November 10, 1995).

STEP 2: BALANCED SUPPLEMENTATION

Her team analyzed the findings of thirty-eight studies and discovered "very strong evidence" that folic acid can reduce heart disease risk caused by increased levels of homocysteine.

> Researchers have estimated that taking folic acid supplements daily could prevent up to 27,000 deaths each year.

Research indicates that 400 micrograms of folic acid daily could prevent up to 27,000 deaths in this country each year. Unfortunately, although 400 micrograms of folic acid had been the recommended daily allowance in the past, that RDA was reduced by half in 1989. Clinical trials are continuing to validate the importance of folic acid in reducing heart disease risk, and although recommendations may soon change to include folic acid as a vital tool in the fight for heart health, it appears that most scientists and physicians would now agree with a report that appeared in the *Journal of the American Medical Association* in September 1997 that called for clinical trials but added, "In the meantime, policies for increasing folic acid intake could have a considerable effect."

Dr. Meir Stampfer, of Brigham and Women's Hospital, Boston, has noted that research suggests that moderate elevations of homocysteine are linked to a three times higher risk of heart disease and that high levels of homocysteine generally can be reduced "with modest levels of folic acid." Further studies led by Harvard's Mu-En Lee show that homocysteine turns on genes that activate the growth of cells in blood vessel walls. These cells become atherosclerotic plaques. When exposed to folic acid, the genes shut off. So for the carbohydrate addict, who might well be among the estimated 21 percent of the population with high homocysteine levels, folic acid supplementation would seem to be a very good idea.

The matter of folic acid supplementation for heart health is still in a state of flux. Originally the American Heart Association issued a statement that it "does not recommend widespread use of folic acid and B vitamins to reduce the risk of heart disease and stroke." The statement recommended a healthy, balanced diet that includes five servings of fruits and vegetables a day. For folic acid the AHA's recommended daily value was 400 micrograms. (The RDA is 200 micrograms for men and 180 micrograms for women.) The recommendation listed several good sources of folic acid—including "citrus fruits, tomatoes, vegetables, and grain products"—and added that "[i]n January 1998, wheat flour became fortified with folic acid to add an estimated

100 micrograms per day to the average diet" and that "[s]upplements should only be used when diet is not adequate to achieve these intakes."

> **The risk for heart disease was more than double in those with high homocysteine levels.**

Recently, in their *Recommendations: Homocysteine; Folic Acid and Cardiovascular Disease* (1999), the American Heart Association announced that: "[t]wo recent reports have strengthened the evidence for this [heart disease–high homocysteine] relationship.

1. A large multicenter European trial, published in the *Journal of the American Medical Association*, found that among men and women younger than age 60, the overall risk of coronary and other vascular diseases was 2.2 times higher in those with plasma total homocysteine levels in the top fifth of the normal range compared with those in the bottom four-fifths. This risk was independent of other risk factors, but was notably higher in smokers and persons with high blood pressure.

2. A Norwegian study, published in [the] *New England Journal of Medicine*, found that among 587 patients with coronary heart disease, the risk of death after four to five years was proportional to plasma total homocysteine levels. The risk rose from 3.8 percent in those with the lowest levels (below 9 μmol per liter) to 24.7 percent [in those] with the highest levels (greater than 15 μmol per liter)."

The AHA added that "other evidence suggests that homocysteine may have an effect on atherosclerosis by damaging the inner lining of arteries, and promoting thrombosis [blood-clot formation]."

The AHA went on to make the crucial homocysteine–folic acid connection:

Plasma homocysteine levels are strongly influenced by diet, as well as genetic factors. The dietary components with the greatest effects are folic acid and vitamins B_6 and B_{12}. Folic acid and other B vitamins help to break down homocysteine in the body. Several studies, including the recent multicenter European trial, have found that higher blood levels of B vitamins (including folic acid) are related, at least in part, to lower concentrations of homocysteine. Other recent evidence shows that low blood levels of folic acid are linked with an increased risk of fatal coronary heart disease and stroke.

The AHA report continued by observing that as yet

there has been no controlled treatment study showing that folic acid supplements reduce the risk of atherosclerosis, or that taking these vitamins has an effect on the development or recurrence of cardiovascular disease. Researchers have studied varying amounts of folic acid to lower homocysteine levels, but it is still not clear what an optimal dose might be and to what extent a dietary supplement might be required to lower homocysteine levels.

The AHA added, "Although evidence for the benefit of lowering homocysteine levels is lacking, patients at high risk should be strongly advised to follow an overall diet that ensures adequate intake of folic acid and vitamins B_6 and B_{12}."

Many researchers believe that the evidence is compelling and clear that folic acid reduces homocysteine levels. Dr. Manuel R. Malinow, of the Oregon Health Services University in Portland, theorized that fortifying cereal-grain products with folic acid, which the United States Food and Drug Administration has recommended as a way to prevent congenital (birth) defects, might lower plasma homocysteine levels as well.

In a study involving seventy-five patients with coronary heart disease, ranging in age from forty-five to eighty-five, Dr. Malinow and his colleagues measured the effects of folic acid–fortified breakfast cereals on subjects' plasma homocysteine levels. The cereals contained one of three levels of folic acid.

Plasma homocysteine levels did not decrease significantly among patients who consumed 127 micrograms of folate daily, "approximating the increased daily intake that may result from FDA's enrichment policy," Dr. Malinow and his colleagues reported in the *New England Journal of Medicine*. According to the study, folic acid levels of 449 micrograms and 665 micrograms, however, decreased homocysteine levels by 11 percent and 14 percent, respectively. Dr. Malinow's study shows that even a well-balanced diet may not contain enough folate or folic acid to lower homocysteine levels and prevent heart attacks.

Other prominent researchers support the need for folic acid supplementation in addition to a folate-rich diet. "The evidence linking heart attacks with homocysteine levels and folate intake is very strong," commented Godfrey Oakley Jr., M.D., director of the division of birth defects and developmental disorders at the Centers for Disease Control and Prevention in Atlanta.

> Obtaining the folic acid you need from your food may not be possible.

Obtaining the folic acid you need from your food may not be possible. Helenbeth Reiss Reynolds, a nutritionist in Plymouth, Minnesota, and a spokesperson for the Chicago-based American Dietetic Association, has noted that "[n]aturally occurring folate is not as bioavailable as folic acid, so fortification is very important." She also noted that the average American eats only 200 to 250 micrograms of folic acid each day, enough to prevent folate deficiency but not enough to reduce homocysteine levels.

So what is the bottom line for the person who wants to reduce heart disease risk? We believe that in consultation with your physician, you might want to strongly consider a diet rich in folic acid along with additional vitamin supplementation. Brewer's yeast, citrus fruits, tomatoes, green leafy vegetables, and grain products are particularly rich in folic acid. The jury is still out in relation to B_6 supplementation; some concerns and questions remain unanswered. In addition to other recommendations, some scientists are advising that, when folic acid intake levels are increased, it is important to keep B_{12} intakes high so that folic acid's powerful benefits do not mask a hidden B_{12} problem. Certainly foods rich in B_{12} and vitamin supplementation of B_{12} might be a good adjunct to added folic acid. In addition to the need for other nutrient balance, folic acid supplementation may require the addition of magnesium (see Supplementation Option 5). As in all dietary matters, check with your doctor, and for your heart's sake, talk folic!

SUPPLEMENTATION OPTION 5: AMAZING MAGNESIUM

We are not quite sure why magnesium has not yet received the media attention we think it deserves. It is odd that given the strength of the compelling research that documents magnesium's contribution to heart health, so few people are aware of this amazing mineral.

> **Magnesium deficiencies show up consistently
> in patients with atherosclerosis, angina,
> congestive heart failure, hypertension,
> heart attack, arrhythmias, and more.**

Magnesium is essential to heart function, and magnesium deficiencies show up consistently in patients suffering from atherosclerosis, angina, congestive heart failure, hypertension, heart attack, arrhythmias, and more. Magnesium helps regulate the balance of sodium and calcium in cells, particularly in the blood vessels and the heart. This electrolyte balance may not sound important, but infinitesimal quantities can mean the difference between life and death. Adequate amounts of magnesium help to keep blood vessels relaxed and elastic and ensure that the heart continues to beat regularly and smoothly.

Magnesium's importance does not stop with its direct heart-related function; it takes part in more than three hundred biochemical reactions within the body, including glucose metabolism, the manufacture of proteins, muscle contraction, regulation of vascular tone, and the conversion into energy of all the food you eat.

A magnesium deficiency can interfere with the regulation of calcium in and out of your cells, leaving them more susceptible to muscle spasm. In the case of your heart, the result can be inadequate oxygen due to involuntary contractions of the smooth muscles of artery walls, which in turn can lead to a heart attack. Recent studies have revealed that people who are given intravenous magnesium supplementation immediately after an acute heart attack have a much better chance for survival. For some, magnesium has literally saved their lives.

> **As many as 50 percent of Americans
> may be deficient in magnesium, and
> blood tests don't always reveal magnesium deficiencies.**

Yet as many as half the people in the United States may be deficient in magnesium. Blood tests don't always reveal magnesium deficiencies. Researchers administered magnesium to research participants who had heart dysrhythmias (nonrhythmic heartbeats). Although their blood magnesium levels appeared within normal limits, the addition of magnesium reduced or eliminated the dysrhythmias, indicating that regardless of whether the blood tests showed a lack of magnesium, a deficiency apparently existed. Whereas a below-normal blood magnesium level indicates that you are deficient in this mineral, a normal blood test does not necessarily mean that you are not deficient.

In addition to other causes, low magnesium levels are more common in those who are taking some diuretics (water pills) or digitalis; the absorption of magnesium may be reduced when calcium supplementation is taken (either by pill or in the form of antacids) or if you are eating foods high in either fiber, protein, sugar, iron, or fat. Supplements of folic acid and vitamin D can increase the need for magnesium. Alcohol, caffeine, and potassium all drain the body of its magnesium stores as well.

> Chances are, the higher your insulin levels,
> the lower your magnesium levels.

Of particular interest to the carbohydrate addict is the fact that magnesium stores are dependent upon insulin action, and the higher your insulin levels and insulin resistance, the lower your natural stores of magnesium are likely to be. For some time scientists were divided as to which came first, hyperinsulinemia or low magnesium levels; opposing evidence was available to support both views.

The one vital observation appeared to be that where scientists found hyperinsulinemia, they found low levels of magnesium (and vice versa). Then in 1995 Dr. M. S. Djurhuus and her research team, reporting in the medical journal *Diabetes Medicine*, finally revealed the process by which hyperinsulinemia significantly increased the amount of magnesium excreted in the urine. Observing the loss of this vital mineral, these researchers concluded that excess levels of insulin might well be responsible for the "magnesium depletion observed in various hyperinsulinaemic states, diabetes mellitus, atherosclerosis, hypertension, and obesity."

Research in this area is ongoing, and although taking magnesium supplements cannot ensure balanced insulin levels, the research does indicate that magnesium may prove to be an important adjunct in the prevention and elimination of many magnesium deficiency–related disorders, including diabetes, atherosclerosis, hypertension, and obesity. Certainly consult with your doctor to determine whether magnesium supplementation should be part of your overall insulin-reducing plan.

Magnesium is a component of plant chlorophyll and, although the

> ## Do You Have Signs of Magnesium Deficiency?
>
> A magnesium deficiency can produce any of the following symptoms:
>
> - Agitation or anxiety
> - Anemia
> - Cold hands and feet
> - Confusion or disorientation
> - Depression
> - Exaggerated startle response
> - Hallucinations
> - Heart rhythm disturbances (including rapid heartbeat)
> - High or low blood pressure
> - Hyperactivity
> - Irritability
> - Loss of balance while walking
> - Loss of hair
> - Muscle weakness
> - Nausea
> - Nervousness
> - Numbness and tingling
> - Restless leg syndrome
> - Restlessness
> - Seizures
> - Spasm
> - Stomach upset
> - Subnormal body temperature
> - Tremors or twitching
> - Vertigo
> - Weakness
>
> If you have any of these symptoms and the cause remains unexplained, it would certainly seem wise to discuss magnesium supplementation with your physician. In addition, in view of magnesium's relationship to insulin and insulin resistance, the use of magnesium supplementation as part of a heart healthy program would seem an important issue to explore.

amount varies widely, is found in all unprocessed foods. You will find that the richest sources of magnesium are nuts, legumes, wheat germ and other unprocessed grains, and whole seeds. The removal of the husk and germ layers of grain (milling) removes up to 80 percent of the magnesium, but unless you intend to use the whole grain, unmilled, you will probably be happy to hear that other good food sources of magnesium include soybeans, cornmeal, shrimp, crab, clams, oysters, and green vegetables.

The RDA for magnesium for adult men and women is 4.5 milligrams per kilogram of body weight. This recommendation calculates out to an average intake of about 350 milligrams per day for most men and 280 milligrams per day for most women (more or less, depending on individual weight levels). Physicians can prescribe sustained-release forms of magnesium. Although there are over-the-counter preparations, we must caution you that they can be mixed with other ingredients that may make it inadvisable for you to take them. For now it is best to be aware of magnesium's powerful potential, discuss it with your physician as appropriate, and look for it to become the new "hot" helper in heart health.

THINGS TO COME

Many new supplementation alternatives are about to break through and become part of conventional heart health promotion. They await additional scientific confirmation or in some cases a bit more media attention. For a peek at our picks for the up-and-coming supplement choices, see Chapter 9, "On the Horizon: Emerging Warriors in the Battle for Heart Health."

Young at Heart: Beth's Story
DR. FREDERIC VAGNINI REMEMBERS:

The intake sheet indicated that Beth was only forty-nine years old, but as I entered the examination room, the woman I saw could easily have been a dozen years her senior. Beth's hair was gray, her skin pasty, her back hunched. She look tired and beaten, and my heart went out to her.

Her blood reports told part of the story: high triglycerides, almost three times normal; low levels of "good cholesterol," high levels of "bad cholesterol." Her blood pressure was a bit high, and she was significantly overweight; even more worrisome was the fact that she carried the excess weight in her abdominal area, often a sign of impending insulin-related heart disease.

Still, I felt that there was more to consider than the results of laboratory tests, and my hunch was right. We spoke for a bit, and within a short time Beth opened up and shared her worry and frustration. She was suffering from extremes in mood and cravings, something she related to low sugar. Although many causes may be responsible for changes in thinking and motivation, Beth felt that her inability to concentrate or think clearly often occurred about

STEP 2: BALANCED SUPPLEMENTATION

two hours after eating, a sign that, indeed, blood sugar problems might be contributory.

Although a fasting blood sugar test did not indicate any abnormality, given the incidence of adult-onset diabetes in Beth's family, I asked her to consent to an oral glucose tolerance test. A three-hour testing of her blood following a high-glucose drink provided the information we needed. Not yet "officially" diabetic, she was well on her way, and her test results clearly indicated that her body was unable to handle sugar in a normal manner. Her insulin response to the glucose was more than three times normal, and within two hours after consuming the glucose drink, her blood sugar level was lower than it had been after she had been fasting for more than eight hours.

I explained that although low blood sugar levels seemed as if they might be the opposite of the high blood sugar levels so often associated with adult-onset diabetes, they were often very closely related.

Beth's mother and father had both been diabetic; her father had succumbed to heart disease in his fifties, her mother in her early sixties. Beth needed help, and she needed it now.

We discussed a low-frequency-of-carbohydrates diet in which high-carbohydrate foods were to be eaten once each day, with other daily meals consisting of low carbos. Beth was also told to begin taking glucose tolerance factor chromium each day.

"Take it between meals," I explained, "and without any other supplement. Zinc competes with chromium, and if you take them together or if you take your chromium with any food containing zinc, it could keep your body from absorbing this precious mineral."

Beth wanted to know more about chromium, and I was happy to help her understand its importance. "Nine out of ten American diets are deficient in chromium. You don't get enough in your diet. When you eat processed foods that have lots of sugar, or drink milk, you lose even more of the chromium you have already stored away. Chromium is an important helper to insulin, and when you don't have enough chromium, your body tries to make up for it by releasing extra insulin. That's the last thing we want your body to do!" I added with emphasis.

I recommended glucose tolerance factor chromium, a well-researched form of chromium that has been shown to be highly effective. Beth agreed to check back in about three months.

The woman I saw a few short months later looked many years younger and a great deal happier. "I feel like a whole new woman," she exclaimed. "My mood swings are gone. I can't tell you how wonderful that is. And, well, I feel so . . . young."

Tests confirmed what Beth already knew. Her blood pressure was down, triglycerides were within normal levels—a great improvement—and the rest of her blood work showed important improvements. A repeat three-hour glucose tolerance test showed remarkable changes; had I not seen her only three months earlier, I would never have considered her to be prediabetic now.

"I know that chromium's important," Beth told me as I shared the test results. "The diet took away the cravings, and I know it helps keep my blood sugar in line, but—I can't explain it—I feel better after I take the chromium. Something just feels right."

Her eyes were bright, her cheeks were warm with the natural glow of health, and her manner was confident. She had a new energy, and she smiled as she excitedly shared her experiences and feelings.

"Yes," I thought. "Something is very right." And I smiled in response as I thought how young at heart my patient had become.

7

THE CARBOHYDRATE ADDICT'S HEALTHY HEART PROGRAM

STEP 3: BALANCED ACTIVITY OPTIONS

Active minds and active bodies never grow old.—*Lee Salk*

MOVERS AND SHAKERS

Some people are movers: they simply love to be active. Some people are shakers: they shake their heads in wonder and disbelief as they sit and watch the movers.

You will hear us say it again and again: one size does not fit all—and when it comes to an activity program, that truth still holds. Although hundreds of scientists have documented the ways in which activity reduces high insulin levels as well as insulin resistance, and although we will encourage you to be as active *as is appropriate for you and your individual needs and preferences*, if you are unable or unwilling to add an activity component to your program (either for the time being or indefinitely), that is clearly your prerogative.*

Regular and appropriate activity reduces both insulin levels and insulin resistance. These changes can help lower high blood pressure, improve your total blood fat levels, elevate HDL ("good" cholesterol) and lower LDL ("bad" cholesterol), reduce your risk for adult-onset diabetes, and decrease your weight and risk for insulin-related heart disease.

---

*All decisions regarding activity choices should be made in consultation with your physician.

In all likelihood an active lifestyle will have a synergistic effect, multiplying the benefits gained from following the first two steps of this program, to put you at even less risk for insulin-related heart disease. Still, if you cannot or do not wish to be part of an ongoing activity program (even one that is very mild and nondemanding), you can still reap the heart health benefits that come from balanced insulin levels afforded by the other steps in this program.

> **Activity reduces insulin levels and insulin resistance.**

If you choose to skip this step, do so with the thought that you are passing on it "for now." In time the impact of Steps 1 and 2 may make you more willing and motivated, and perhaps more able, to enjoy the pleasures and benefits of an active lifestyle. At that time you can return to this step.

We hope, then, that you can join us in this "moving" step to heart health, but if you cannot, feel free to proceed to the Heart Health–Enhancing Options, in the next chapter.

STEP 3: ADD AN ACTIVITY THAT FITS YOUR INDIVIDUAL NEEDS

Step 3 consists of three levels of activity, which will allow you to select the degree of intensity of activity. In addition, you will be able to choose how often you would like to take part in an activity.

Before you decide on an activity, there are two people with whom we would like you to speak. First and foremost, of course, you must check with your physician. You should always consult your doctor before making any changes to your activity/exercise routine.

Second, we would like you to take the time to consult with yourself. Have a real "heart-to-heart" talk. Really, we want you to take careful stock of the time and energy you are willing to put into the activity portion of your program. No wishful thinking here, just down-to-earth reality.

> **Be realistic in your choices.**
> **Select an activity that's fun and easy**
> **and that fits into your schedule.**

STEP 3: BALANCED ACTIVITY OPTIONS

Consistency is the key to this step, as it is to all the steps of the Program, but the good news is that you will have a wider latitude of choice than you have probably ever encountered before. We encourage you to select an activity that is so easy and/or so much fun that consistency will not be a problem. Choose a level of activity that will make you feel good and will be easy to maintain.

Consistency need not involve a daily commitment. It is far better to pick a mild activity and stick with a three-times-a-week schedule than to select a vigorous daily activity and skip it several times each week. Your body may not know the difference at first, but your mind will. And as you know, if you don't feel good about breaking a promise, even (or especially) to yourself, you will avoid the source of your guilt.

Select an activity that's fun and easy to fit into your schedule. Start slowly and increase activity as appropriate. You may find that as you continue incorporating Steps 1 and 2 into your life, your energy levels

> **Don't force yourself to do something you don't want to do. You will come to resent it.**

will rise. You may be more inclined to be active, less easily tired, and more motivated. Again, with your physician's okay, step up your activity as you desire. If, at any time, you feel that you would prefer to return to your former level of activity or change to another activity, do so *immediately*. Don't force yourself to do something you don't want to do. You will come to resent it and avoid the activity altogether.

We cannot tell you how many people talk themselves out of their own feelings and push themselves past their own endurance until they come to hate what they used to enjoy. Finally they rebel against the very things they wished to accomplish. So right here, right now, please try to be loving, understanding, firm, and compassionate with yourself. In the end it makes good heart sense, on all levels.

IF YOU ARE ALREADY ACTIVE OR EXERCISE REGULARLY

If you are already leading a very active lifestyle or take part in sports or exercise regularly, you may consider your current activity level your starting point. As appropriate—with regard to your physical abilities, time

Setting Yourself Up for Success
WHEN IT COMES TO CHOOSING AN ACTIVITY, USE YOUR HEAD

When you select your activity within this step, take time to consider your own needs and limitations. Be realistic. Think about the following:
- How much time can you commit on a *regular* basis?
- Do you prefer a single activity, or are you willing to take part in a changing variety of activities that will keep up your interest?
- When the weather is bad, can you continue performing your selected activity?
- When time and work demands become difficult, will you be able to keep your commitment?
- Is there something you can do to make your choice more rewarding?

Consider physical limitations carefully. Try to avoid making promises that you will later break and for which you could later blame yourself. If you do change your mind, be forgiving. Learn from your experience and make a more informed choice the second time.

It is far better to select an activity that takes less time and effort but is one that you can comfortably continue doing than to select a much more rigorous activity that you are forced to abandon because it is simply not right for you.

Start off with an "easier" commitment; as your insulin levels and weight decrease, and as your energy levels increase, you can always move to something more difficult. Being consistent with an easier alternative will yield much greater rewards than being on-again, off-again with a more demanding choice. Always check with your physician before beginning any new activity program.

---

constraints, motivation, and physician's recommendations—you may choose to continue your current activities or increase them.

Sometimes simply becoming consistent with an activity is enough to make you feel that you are making positive changes; in other cases you may be quite happy with the changes you have already made. Remember that you can always increase your activity level, frequency, or duration, whenever you like, as long as you are already keeping your current commitments to yourself. With no pun intended, in activity as well as nutritional change, it does not pay to bite off more than you can chew. So when deciding whether or not you wish to increase your activity level (intensity, duration, or frequency), allow your head—not your hopes—to lead the way.

ACTIVITY CHOICES

Choose one activity level (light, moderate, or vigorous) and a frequency level (how often you will take part in the activity).* Within your activity level, you can either select one specific activity or, if you prefer, vary your choices.

For example, let's suppose you decide to begin with a light activity level and choose a moderate frequency level. You might select walking (at a brisk but easy pace) as your regular activity, to be done for half an hour three times a week. As an alternative within that same activity level, you could choose to walk for half an hour one day a week, and do pool exercises for half an hour on each of the other two days.

Write down your selection and plan your activities and times in advance. For best results mark your goal on your calendar and schedule the time of day that you will keep open for this very important heart healthy choice.

Frequency Levels

    Low Frequency. Fifteen minutes, three times a week
    Moderate Frequency. Fifteen minutes every day or half an hour three times a week
    High Frequency. Thirty minutes every day or one hour three times a week

Activity Levels

LIGHT ACTIVITIES
    Biking (regular or stationary): easy, even pace
    Bowling
    Dancing: bouncy but easy pace
    Golf

*Please select only activities that do not conflict with your personal physician's recommendations.

Pool exercises: a wide variety of light, easy activities
StepMaster, NordicTrack, treadmills, and the like: very easy, even pace
Stretching exercises
Tai chi
Walking: brisk but easy pace
Yoga

MODERATE ACTIVITIES
Aerobics: light pace
Biking (regular or stationary): moderate pace
Dancing: moderate pace
Free weights: moderate pace with some rest time included
Jogging: light, brisk running
Pool exercises: moderate, fun activities
Roller skating: easy, even pace
Rope jumping: light, even pace
Skiing (cross-country or downhill): light pace
StepMaster, NordicTrack, treadmills, and the like: moderate, even pace
Swimming: moderate, even pace
Tennis, racquetball, volleyball: light, easy pace
Walking: moderate pace

VIGOROUS ACTIVITIES
Aerobics: moderate or fast pace
Biking (regular or stationary): fast pace
Dancing: fast pace without interruption
Free weights: intense workout
Jogging: moderate or intense running
Pool exercises: brisk exercises without interruption
Roller skating: moderate or fast pace
Rope jumping: moderate pace
Skiing (cross-country or downhill): moderate or fast pace
StepMaster, NordicTrack, treadmill, and the like: fast pace
Swimming: fast pace
Tennis, racquetball, volleyball: moderate or fast pace
Walking: fast pace without interruption

IN THE WEEKS TO COME

As you start to feel comfortable with your activity, and after getting your physician's okay, you can begin to increase your duration (how long) and frequency (how often). Or you may prefer to move to more challenging activities (from mild to moderate, or from moderate to vigorous). Choose to increase your activity in the way that seems most appealing to you. If you really enjoy your walking routine, for instance, you might find that it is easy to extend the length of time you spend walking. If, on the other hand, you don't have the time or desire to prolong your walking but prefer to pick up speed and walk at a faster pace or walk more often, that, too, is your prerogative. Just remember to move on only when you are consistent with your current activity commitment.

KEEPING YOUR PRIORITIES STRAIGHT

Some people have been told that the more demanding an activity and the more you "work up a sweat," the better for your heart. For the carbohydrate addict, this is not always so. Your body is bent on saving energy. An important way to pull it out of its "saving" mode is to maintain an active lifestyle—rather than a demanding exercise regimen that you cannot keep up.

When you are active, your risk for hyperinsulinemia decreases. By adding a regular activity to your carbohydrate-balancing and supplementation steps, you can begin to make a real change in your insulin levels and in your risk for insulin-related heart disease factors.

> Gentle, regular activity can pull your body out of a "saving" mode, lower insulin levels, and reduce your risk for heart disease.

Fast-paced aerobics or other formal exercise regimens can have their place, though your ability to participate in a rigorous exercise regimen cannot be determined here. For the purpose of balancing insulin levels and reducing insulin resistance, however, gentle and regular activity can bring about results similar to those of more rigorous workouts. Furthermore, an enjoyable, easy walking, movement, or dancing routine may be the type of activity that you will be most likely to maintain, and that, in the end, will bring about the best insulin-reducing results possible. In addition, strenuous workouts are more likely to deplete your body of chromium and other nutrients that are vital to balanced insulin and blood sugar levels.

> Be realistic. Don't place impossible demands on yourself. Give yourself credit for all the good work you do. Be gentle.

Increase your activity level, length of time, and/or frequency as you desire, and in keeping with your current health status. This is your program. Don't impose unnecessary rules and demands on yourself. Be gentle and appreciative of your own hard work. If you begin to skip your activity times, see whether something might be done to make your choices more fun or rewarding. As always, give yourself credit for all the good work you do, and if you aren't keeping up with some activities, don't fix blame. Instead, find out why—then fix the problem.

PART THREE

HEART HEALTH ENHANCERS

FOR TODAY AND TOMORROW

8

HEART HEALTH–ENHANCING OPTIONS—FOR LIFE

The greatest power that a person possesses is the power to choose.
—*J. Martin Kohe*

SIMPLE CHOICES, IMPORTANT CHANGE

Once you feel comfortable with The BASIC Plan (Steps 1, 2, and 3), you can choose to add Heart Health–Enhancing Options, one at a time. Each Enhancing Option is designed to further reduce your insulin levels and your body's insulin resistance. The more options you add, the greater the probability of reducing insulin-related high blood pressure, risk-related blood fats, adult-onset diabetes, obesity, and heart disease.

Enhancing Options target the powerful hidden triggers that you may not even know are in your body and threatening your heart health. These options are simple to follow and can easily be adapted to your lifestyle and preferences.

The order in which you choose your Enhancing Options and when you choose them are unimportant. What is important is that you choose as many as suit your particular circumstances. The choices are yours: you will decide which Enhancing Option you want to add, and you will decide when, and in what ways, you want to add it.

> You choose the options you want to add, one at a time, as well as *when* and *in what way* you want to add each one.

A CHOICE TO LISTEN—TO YOURSELF

When you choose an Enhancing Option, you are in essence making a choice to continue to increase your commitment to your own health and longevity. Take a moment to consider how important a change you are making and let yourself feel the pride and appreciation we feel for you.

As you select your Enhancing Options, continue to follow The BASIC Plan. We have found that some people prefer to start with simpler Enhancing Options, such as The Over-the-Counter Remedy Timing Option. Others choose Enhancing Options that implement a change that they "have been wanting to do anyway" such as The Stress-Reduction Option. Still others prefer to begin with an Enhancing Option that is likely to have the most powerful influence on heart health—for instance, The Food Frequency–Reducing Option.

> **Do not choose an Enhancing Option simply because it fits someone else's idea of what you should be doing.**

As you add option after option, you will be surprised at how easy and rewarding each turns out to be.

Do not choose an Enhancing Option simply because it fits someone else's idea of what you should be doing. Most of us are influenced by the opinions of others far more than we realize. You would not choose an eyeglass prescription for yourself simply because a friend thought it would be right for you or because it was right for your husband. In the same way, it is essential that you concentrate on you—your health, your preferences, your needs. Before choosing your first Enhancing Option, take a few moments to read through all of them, then pick the one that is most appealing to you.

After you have made your selection, read through its description carefully, reading it a second time if necessary, so that you fully understand what is expected. Think through your day and plan how you might best incorporate your first Enhancing Option into your routine. You might, for example, decide on a private place where you can do some of your stress-reduction exercises without fear of being interrupted.

Remember, it is important that you continue The BASIC Plan as you add the Enhancing Option of your choice.

> **Your Enhancing Option choice selection is not carved in stone. Options can change as your needs and preferences change.**

If, in the days to come, you find that your first Enhancing Option fits comfortably into your life, then most certainly continue. On the other hand, if your first choice does not feel quite right or if you find that it is more demanding than you had anticipated, if you find yourself resenting it or "cheating," then drop it. The success of a program must be based on the reality of your needs and your willingness and ability to continue to follow the guidelines. Our experience tells us that if you are free to drop an Enhancing Option should you find that it isn't right for you, you will be far more likely to select another Enhancing Option that is better suited to you. The better suited the option, the more likely you will be to incorporate it into your heart health program and your life.

If an Enhancing Option falls somewhere in between—that is, if you are not sure whether you want to continue it—give it a two-week trial period. At the end of two weeks, make a decision to continue or drop it.

As time goes on, Enhancing Option selections can be changed to meet your changing needs and preferences. Your choice of options is not carved in stone. You may choose an Enhancing Option that seems appealing at one time in your life, for instance, then find that at another time new demands prevent you from continuing that particular option. Should such changes occur, you are most certainly free to drop that option, without guilt or self-blame (none!). Remember, if it is to bring about any lifestyle change, your program must be livable. This is not a contest that requires perfection in order to win the prize. This is a program that is designed to last and to help you do the same.

Remember to add only one Enhancing Option at a time and, for best results, stay with an option for at least two weeks before adding another. With your physician's approval, you are free to add as many Enhancing Options as you like (always one at a time), but at all times be sure to pay attention to your own feelings and thoughts. Listen to yourself. You'll probably be surprised at how good your own advice can be!

> **Add each new option as you continue to follow The BASIC Plan.**

Once again, we must remind you that it is absolutely essential that you continue The BASIC Plan as you add Enhancing Options. The options are meant to supplement The BASIC Plan; they are never meant to replace it.

If you do not want to add any new Enhancing Options, don't. It's as simple as that. If there are Enhancing Options that you have tried in the past but dropped for various reasons, you can try them again at any time.

> This program does not push you to be perfect.
> Perfectionism will only cause you to rebel
> or to feel angry and resentful.

You may find that as time goes by, the physical improvements that come from following the Program make options that might have seemed challenging easier to follow or more appealing than they had been in the past. So if you have tried an option and decided not to continue it, you may want to try it again at some later date and see whether it might have become a bit more to your liking.

One last word: An Enhancing Option should be selected only when you feel comfortable and ready to incorporate it into your life. This program is designed to be livable and usable. Contrary to what you may have experienced in other endeavors, this program does not push you to be perfect. Perfectionism will only cause you to rebel in the future or to feel angry and resentful, neither of which is likely to contribute a great deal to a healthy heart.

So give yourself the right to make changes at an easy, comfortable pace. You will most likely find that as your body comes into balance naturally, change will come easily. We have found that when things are easy and pleasurable and when they give us what we want, there is little need to "motivate" ourselves to do them. In the same way, if you are caring and sensitive to yourself and your needs, you will find that you will be far more likely to stay on your program indefinitely—without struggle.

If an Enhancing Option says, "Skip a meal or snack only when you don't really want it," take heed of the entire message—not just the first few words. If you keep yourself from pushing past what feels right and natural, you may find that the option will move you in the right direction, at the right time, without struggle. So give the Program your best, follow The BASIC Plan guidelines, and choose appropriate Enhancing Options, but at the same time be realistic and treat yourself considerately, sensitively, and lovingly.

> Give yourself the right to make changes
> at an easy, comfortable pace.

FIVE HEART HEALTH–ENHANCING OPTIONS FOR LIFE

THE OVER-THE-COUNTER REMEDY TIMING OPTION

It is important to understand that although *what* you consume is certainly important in determining your cravings, weight, and risk for insulin-related heart disease, *when* and *how* you consume it may be equally important.

Imagine how you might feel after not eating all day and then consuming three shots of liquor within five minutes' time. Now picture how you would feel if you had consumed the same amount of liquor diluted in mixed drinks and sipped over several hours accompanied by food. Although the amount of alcohol is the same, differences in how and when the alcohol is consumed make for big changes in the way our bodies handle it.

> Carbohydrates are prime stimulators of insulin release.
> The more often you consume them,
> the more your insulin levels spike.

Although in a reverse fashion, a similar process takes place with the consumption of carbohydrates and carbohydrate act-alikes. Carbohydrates are prime stimulators of insulin release, and the more often you consume them, the more your insulin levels spike. So when it comes to any food or drink, or anything else that can lead to an insulin surge, it is important to take it in less frequently and, when feasible, to take in all insulin releasers at once.

In this Enhancing Option you will learn how to change the timing of many over-the-counter remedies so that you may cancel out both their insulin-evoking power and your body's tendency toward insulin resistance.

There are two basic ways in which over-the-counter remedies can raise insulin levels. First, some of these remedies can cause a general metabolic shift that slows the body's ability to use energy. Nonsteroidal anti-inflammatory medications—such as acetaminophen, ibuprofen, and aspirin, packaged under the brand names Bayer, Tylenol, and Advil, among others—fall into this category. These over-the-counter anti-inflammatories may affect your insulin levels by affecting your metabolic rate, though the exact mechanism is still unknown.

> Taking aspirin, Tylenol, or Advil several times a day could significantly raise your insulin levels.

Their impact makes sense when you consider the fact that the body's by-product of "burning" energy is the heat it produces. The more heat you release, the more energy (and the greater the number of calories) you are burning. Anti-inflammatories reduce the heat your body produces, which is why they are used to bring down fevers.

By reducing the heat output, anti-inflammatories appear to reduce the amount of energy (and the number of calories) your body burns, putting you into an "energy-saving" mode, for which it requires higher levels of insulin. Yet at times, despite their tendency to increase your insulin levels, these heat-reducing medications can prove an important ally for home health care, reducing uncomplicated fevers, headaches, body aches, and so forth. The good news is that there is a way to get the periodic benefits of these over-the-counter remedies while reducing their insulin-raising impact.

> Sweet-tasting cough remedies will raise your insulin levels. Some people become addicted to cough drops.

A second group of over-the-counter remedies is those that taste sweet. These remedies appear to raise your insulin levels much more directly than do anti-inflammatories. The good news is that the effects of these remedies can easily be reduced or eliminated entirely. Any sweet taste will cause the body to release high levels of insulin. Sweet-tasting over-the-counter remedies often contain sugar and/or sugar substitutes (including artificial sweeteners). No matter what they contain, however, if they taste sweet, they are almost sure to cause an insulin surge.

Examples of sweet-tasting over-the-counter medications include:

- Antacid tablets and liquids (Tums, Rolaids, Mylanta, and so on)
- Breath fresheners (liquid, mints, tablets, sprays, and so on)
- Cough drops, syrups, and lozenges (for cough or sore throat)
- Stool softeners (Metamucil, Konsyl, and so on)

You may not realize that many of these nonprescription remedies contain at least one kind of sugar or sugar substitute because the sweetener is included among their inactive ingredients. Manufacturers tend to place the list of active ingredients in a far more obvious place on the label than the "nonactive" ingredients, so it may take a bit of persistence on your part to locate the sugar or sugar substitute (if it is listed at all).

It is not always necessary to identify "sweet" ingredients in over-the-counter remedies. For the purposes of this Enhancing Option, just assume that in all likelihood most over-the-counter remedies must contain some sort of sweetening agent, for if they were made without a sweetening agent, their taste would be intolerable—and they would never be marketable.

In order to incorporate this Enhancing Option into your program, begin by eliminating as many *nonessential* over-the-counter remedies as possible. It is important that you never (never!) eliminate a remedy that your physician has recommended or that you think may be important to your health or well-being. On the other hand, nonessential over-the-counter remedies that you may be taking more by rote than out of need might be discontinued.

For example, although taking an antacid as per your physician's recommendation should not be stopped, you might consider having a glass of cool water or taking a minute to brush your teeth and tongue rather than using a commercial breath freshener.

Whenever possible, take as many over-the-counter remedies as you can with your Reward Meal. Some of these remedies (stool softeners, for instance) can easily be taken at the Reward Meal. Many of our patients and research participants tell us that the remedy's effectiveness is unchanged by the time of day it is taken. Helping to reduce your insulin levels by scheduling these remedies to coincide with your Reward Meal can provide a welcome benefit.

Some remedies, such as cough medication, may, by their very nature, need to be taken at times other than Reward Meals. If you cannot combine them with your Reward Meal, try to combine them with a low-carbo meal, so that the protein and fiber-rich foods in those meals may help reduce the remedies' insulin impact.

If it is not possible to combine a remedy with either a Reward Meal or a low-carbohydrate meal, then you will simply have to take it at a more appropriate time with the comforting knowledge that the Program's BASIC Plan and other Enhancing Options can help correct the insulin imbalance that these remedies can cause.

If you can, always try to correct the need for the remedy. If you cannot, just stay with your program and be patient until the remedy is no longer needed.

The Over-the-Counter Remedy Timing Option: Easy Alternatives

Antacids: Tums, Rolaids, Mylanta, and so forth.
Breath fresheners: Bianca, all brands of mouthwashes, rinses, and so forth
Cough and cold medications: cough drops and syrups of all kinds
Stool softeners: Metamucil, Konsyl, and so forth

> EFFECTS: When you take these remedies, your body may interpret them as "sweet foods," which can bring about an increased release of insulin and an increase in insulin resistance. When taken on a regular and ongoing basis, these remedies may increase your risk for insulin-related heart problems.

Nonsteroidal anti-inflammatories: aspirin, Tylenol, Advil, and so forth.

> EFFECTS: These remedies may decrease your body's ability to "burn" calories, putting your body into an "energy-saving" and insulin-producing mode.

What You Can Do:
- Continue all medically recommended over-the-counter remedies.
- Whenever possible, correct the underlying problem so that the remedy is no longer necessary.
- If the remedy is taken once a day, take all remaining remedies with Reward Meals.
- If the remedy is needed throughout the day, take it with or immediately after low-carbohydrate meals.
- If a remedy cannot be taken during or after a meal, take heart in knowing that The BASIC Plan and other Enhancing Options may help offset the remedy's insulin-increasing effects.

THE STRESS-REDUCTION OPTION

It is almost impossible to watch the evening news or pick up a magazine or newspaper without hearing about stress-related health problems, especially with regard to increasing your blood pressure or raising your risk for heart disease. (Some might say that the news itself could be considered a stress factor!) Everywhere the message is the same: Avoid stress in your life. One wonders about this advice.

By definition our lives are complicated and involved, and a multitude of everyday experiences is literally beyond our control. Eliminating stress is, for most of us, a seemingly unattainable goal, and attempts to do so can leave us more frustrated than when we started.

On the other hand, we can take positive action to try to reduce the unnecessary stress in our lives (such as perfectionistic expectations we may place on ourselves). In addition, there are many things we can do to reduce the effects that stress has on our bodies.

> **Stress hormones raise insulin levels**
> **(which explains why many people turn to food when under stress).**

For the carbohydrate addict, stress reduction is very important; stress hormones are known to raise insulin levels (which explains why many people turn to food while under stress or immediately after a stressful experience and why others may experience sudden elevations in blood pressure). Many carbohydrate addicts seem to be particularly sensitive to the stress response, and for them stress reduction is a valuable part of any heart health promotion program.

By choosing The Stress-Reduction Option, you are making a commitment to focus on the stressors in your life, learning to recognize them and to take appropriate steps to limit or reverse the effects that stress can have on your heart health.

In the best of all possible worlds, you would be able to avoid unnecessary stress. Whenever possible, without compromising integrity and priorities, walk away from the stressful situation. It is important to recognize, however, that there are times when stress is simply unavoidable. There are some situations from which you cannot readily walk away.

When you cannot avoid stress altogether, here are some suggestions for limiting and relieving stress' effects on your body.

Stress Talks

Most of us are so busy trying to avoid stress that we don't listen to the important messages it may be giving us. Your first task is to become sensitive to your body's response to stress, to listen to your feelings rather than running from them. Many of us fail to realize that we are feeling pressured or stressed until we simply cannot stand it anymore. Then we retreat emotionally or, more likely, explode. To make matters worse, we may feel guilty and/or angry and, in so doing, stress ourselves even more.

> **The key to becoming sensitive to your body's stress response is learning to trust yourself.
> Trust comes hard for carbohydrate addicts, whose bodies have led them astray.**

When you are able to listen to your feelings, however, your body's early responses to stress will tell you what you need to know, and you will find yourself much more in control.

The stress-reducing techniques that follow may help you find it easier to limit or avoid stress' hold and its insulin-releasing power as well.

Most people do not realize that stress comes not from without but from within. The key to becoming sensitive to your body's stress response is learning to trust yourself. Rather than trying to suppress the feelings and thoughts that fill you with anger, fear, frustration, resentment, self-recrimination, or blame, it is essential that you stop the process in midstream and focus on the very ideas and experiences that are making you unhappy and uncomfortable. Don't let the tension build to the point where you "blow up," internally or externally.

Stop for a moment and think about it. Is the tightness that you feel at the base of your skull coming from impossible demands that your boss is making on you? Is the churning in the pit of your stomach related to the prospect of going home and dealing with unfinished family business? Are you really hungry, or have you found that eating makes you feel calmer? Or perhaps the full feeling gives you an excuse to go to sleep and thereby avoid some unpleasant task.

> **You can't always avoid stress.
> We have three effective ways to help you reduce its impact.**

To incorporate The Stress-Reduction Option, begin by making a concerted effort to pay more attention to your body's stress signals. In this way you can better learn what your body is trying to tell you. You may find it more effective to work backward: if you lose your temper (even though you hold it all inside), try to recapture what you were feeling or thinking right before the emotional buildup. Make note of your thoughts or feelings, especially if a theme recurs. Don't judge it; just be on the lookout for the same feelings or thoughts the next time. Let that be your signal that you need to be attended to—that you are experiencing stress and that you need to take an appropriate action that will reduce stress's impact on your body.

Small Actions, Big Change

As you begin to recognize when you are under stress, you have three basic choices to help reduce the stress and/or its effect on your life: (1) avoid argument escalation, (2) limit the duration of stress, and (3) remove the impact of stress.

Avoiding argument escalation entails refraining from the back-and-forth emotional escalation that often accompanies disagreements. Outbursts can include crying, screaming, fighting, or the fury that almost all of us have experienced. Sometimes the escalation never shows, and in many cases internal escalation can be the most stressful. It is important to understand that the avoidance of escalation does not entail "holding in" your feelings but, rather, choosing to avoid a useless and stressful verbal war.

In most cases you will need some help and support to avoiding argument escalation. You may choose to get some guidance from a professional counselor or discuss with your friends alternative argument-avoiding strategies. There are several good books and audiotapes by reputable authors as well as many helpful websites and on-line support groups. Keep in mind that you are the focus. Do whatever you need to do to find the right "noncombative" way for you to deal with highly charged conversations that are filling your life with stress.

Limiting the duration of stress involves taking charge of the moment and minimizing how long you are involved in a stressful situation. Chances are you will have to give up on "winning." By realizing that the real victory in any stressful moment involves taking care of your body and your health, you are more likely to find yourself able to calmly and effectively extricate yourself from stressful situations.

There are several innovative ways that can help you directly or indirectly limit the duration of stress. Some people find it helpful to state their limits, in a clear and direct manner, *before* they are pushed to the end of their emotional rope.

Some of our patients have found it helpful to set the stage. "I know you don't want this to end in a screaming match, and neither do I," they begin. "But since this is a difficult area for me to discuss without getting emotional, I may need to stop for a bit if I feel things getting out of control for me." Then, with an explanation of why they need to leave until they sort out their feelings and get some clarity and control, they follow through, walking away calmly before they are overcome by the need to storm out. Changes in your fighting behavior may be met with some resistance, especially if the other person is caught up in his or her emotions, but setting the scene before you begin and repeating the reason for limiting the stress-filled interaction (without escalating) will leave others with little chance to continue the interaction at some future time.*

Some people find a more indirect approach preferable in limiting the duration of stress. It really does not matter which tactics you employ; what matters is finding the technique that is appropriate for you. Your goal is to eliminate or reduce the physical toll that stress can take on your heart health and to remain focused on continuing to take care of yourself and your health.

Removing the impact of stress is a third alternative to stress reduction. Certainly, whenever possible, it is best to avoid stress or limit your exposure to a stressful situation, but when these options are not feasible, you may find it helpful to learn to remove stress's impact. Focusing on your own body through exercises (such as jogging or dancing) or by stress-relieving techniques (like yoga or tai chi) can be helpful; a warm and relaxing bath, a good nap, or fine companionship can do the trick. Whatever works to relax you and remove the impact of stress (while staying on your Program) should be planned for and incorporated into your life.

Planning for stress reduction, giving it priority in your life, is very important for heart health. If you fail to make effective provisions for de-stressing yourself, it is likely that your body will experience many of the stress hormone consequences—in particular, excess release of insulin—that can easily compromise your heart health and increase your risk for insulin-related heart disease. We encourage you to take the time and energy to be good to yourself. Just as you would take care of anyone or even

---

*As appropriate, professional counseling and advice may be advisable in some situations. Always consult a professional as needed.

anything you love, your mind, your body, and your soul need to be spared the unnecessary bumps, bruises, and wear and tear of everyday life.

> Reducing the impact of stress often means
> actively focusing on yourself.

THE COMPLEX-CARBOHYDRATE OPTION

All carbohydrates are not created equal. In general, the carbohydrates that are found in high-carbohydrate foods fall into two categories: simple sugars and complex carbohydrates. Some typical examples of simple sugars include table sugar, honey, fruit sugar (fructose), lactose (milk sugar), corn syrup, and high-fructose corn syrup (which actually contains mostly glucose).

Foods that contain simple sugars are often themselves referred to as "simple sugars." You might hear someone say that fruit and fruit juice, candy (including chocolate), cookies, ice cream, sugar-sweetened soda, and the like are simple sugars. Actually, they aren't simple sugars themselves; they just contain great amounts of simple sugars.

Complex carbohydrates, on the other hand, are starches—long chains of the simple sugar glucose that are bonded together chemically. Foods rich in complex carbohydrates are generally referred to as complex carbohydrates or as starches. Some typical examples of complex carbohydrates include grain and grain products like breads and crackers, as well as rice, pasta, and starchy vegetables like peas, potatoes, and corn.

> For many carbohydrate addicts, complex carbohydrates
> cause less of an insulin release than do simple sugars.

Although your body releases insulin whenever you eat food that contains either simple sugars or complex carbohydrates, chances are you will release far less insulin and your insulin resistance will decrease when, in the carbohydrate portion of your Reward Meal, you eat primarily complex carbohydrates (as opposed to simple sugars). Findings from more than a decade of research indicate that both frequency—how often you eat carbohydrates—and type of carbohydrate consumed can strongly affect insulin responses.

The Complex-Carbohydrate Option entails replacing simple sugars with complex carbohydrates for the carbohydrate portion of your daily Reward Meal. To fulfill this Enhancing Option, simply read over the "Complex-Carbo Option" chart later in this subsection. Then, during your Reward Meal, as much as possible, choose foods from the left-hand column (the complex carbohydrates) rather than the right-hand column (the simple sugars) for the one-third carbohydrate portion of that meal.

> **There will be times when you want a special treat, and once in a while an "indulgence" is certainly to be expected. You don't have to go "off Program" to have it.**

Sometimes you will want a special treat, and even though it contains simple sugars, you should allow yourself to have it as part of your Reward Meal. Just remember that, as much as possible, to fulfill this option, choose complex carbohydrates rather than simple sugars at your Reward Meal. Many people use the following guideline: when they really want a sweet, they have it as part of their Reward Meal, but when a complex carbo will do, they make an effort to choose a starchy goody (such as a bagel, chips, popcorn, or pretzels) rather than a concentrated sweet.

It is important to remember to keep your Reward Meal balanced: all carbohydrates (complex and simple) in that meal should equal one-third of the total meal and should be balanced with one-third protein and one-third low-carbohydrate vegetables in addition to a premeal salad. (For more details on balancing your Reward Meal, see Chapter 5.) Remember, on this program, even if you choose complex carbohydrates over simple sugars, you should not have high-carbohydrate foods at more than one meal each day.

In the "Complex-Carbo Option" chart, you may notice that fruits are not listed. Fruit contains the simple sugar fructose, which has been shown by many researchers to raise insulin levels and put the body into a fat-making mode. Furthermore, according to Dr. J. Hallfrisch of the National Institute on Aging, fructose can lead to "greater elevations in triglycerides and sometimes cholesterol." Dr. Hallfrisch goes on to note that people who have high blood pressure, high levels of insulin, or high triglycerides or who have adult-onset diabetes or are postmenopausal appear to be more susceptible to fructose's adverse effects.

We would certainly agree that, in its extracted state—in particular in foods that use fructose in place of sucrose (table sugar)—fructose can raise heart disease–related risks, but packaged as it was meant to be eaten, in its natural state, fruit contains a great amount of fiber as well. For some people the fiber balance in whole fruit may help reduce the insulin release.

> Fructose can raise insulin-related risks,
> but when it is consumed as part of the whole fruit,
> nature's fiber balance may help reduce the insulin release.

The verdict, then, is still out when it comes to including fruit in your Reward Meal. Watch how your body responds to it. If you find that after you eat fruit you want more and more fruit or that although you feel good at first, an hour or two after eating fruit you show signs of blood sugar swings (including sweats, weakness, headache, fatigue, or cravings), discuss with your physician the possibility of replacing fruit with a high-fiber complex carbohydrate. Also discuss with your doctor the other foods you eat and/or vitamins you take to be certain that you are getting all the nutrients that fruit might otherwise provide. In any case, do not eat fruit other than at your Reward Meal.

> Fruit juice does not contain fiber to balance its high sugar content;
> it can pack a powerful insulin punch.

In contrast to fruit, fruit juice does not contain fiber to balance its high sugar content. All of the calories in fruit juice come from fructose. So unless otherwise instructed by your physician, when choosing this option, eliminate fruit juice from your program. If fruit is not a problem, you might replace all fruit juice with the whole fruit from which it was made or eliminate it altogether.

Remember that nature made the whole fruit, neatly packaged with fiber, and further, made it available only a few weeks each year. Your body was never made to drink the equivalent of six oranges in a tall glass of juice, with no blood sugar–balancing fiber, nor were you meant to sugar-shock your body with intensely sweet juices every day all year long. So pass on the juices and, whenever possible, choose complex carbos rather than reaching for the sweets. Chances are you will be helping to reap the sweet rewards of a healthier heart.

> ### The Complex-Carbo Option
>
> Choose any of the following foods containing complex carbohydrates:
>
> > Bagels and other breads (preferably whole-grain)
> > Beans (legumes)
> > Chips° (low-fat or regular)
> > Corn
> > Crackers
> > Nuts° and seeds (low-fat or regular)
> > Pasta
> > Popcorn (dry)
> > Potatoes
> > Pretzels
> > Rice
>
> Instead of any of these foods that contain simple sugars:
>
> > Cake
> > Candy
> > Chocolate
> > Cookies
> > Doughnuts
> > Fruited yogurt
> > Ice cream or ice milk
> > Pie
> > Pudding
> > Sherbet
> > Snack bars
>
> °Always follow your physician's guidance regarding low-fat or low–saturated fat alternatives.

THE CAFFEINE-REDUCING OPTION

Research exploring the effects of caffeine on heart health has produced a wide variety of findings. Some researchers, such as Dr. D. Robertson and his colleagues, reporting in the *New England Journal of Medicine*, have found that caffeine can lead to rises in blood pressure as well as changes in neurotransmitters (biochemicals in the body that communicate with the sympathetic and central nervous systems). Other researchers have reported that the body "adjusts" to caffeine intake and that long-term consumption of caffeine can decrease the likelihood of caffeine-induced high blood pressure.

Still other researchers have reported that caffeine consumption can lead to nervousness, tremors, heart palpitations, and insomnia. Excessive intake of caffeine has been found to result in gastrointestinal problems, including diarrhea, whereas withdrawal of caffeine has been found to cause headaches and other neurological symptoms.

> Scientists at the National Institute of Mental Health
> found that caffeine consumption can cause
> a fivefold increase in the release of stress hormones.

Of all the research related to caffeine, perhaps of most importance to the carbohydrate addict are the findings by researchers such as Dr. T. W. Uhde and his colleagues at the National Institute of Mental Health, who have observed that caffeine consumption can lead to an increase in the "stress hormone," cortisol, of up to 500 percent! That is five times the normal amount of this insulin-releasing hormone.

A postcaffeine insulin release may go unnoticed, however. It can be hidden by caffeine's temporary stimulant effect. Caffeine is sometimes referred to as a drug, and perhaps with good reason. Caffeine's stimulatory effect may make you feel more energetic for a while, and when you hit a slump two hours later, you may never attribute it to caffeine's ability to trigger insulin-related blood sugar swings. You may simply sense that you need another "cup of coffee" or diet soda and reach for one, only to begin the cycle again.

We have seen amazing changes in many of our patients who have chosen to reduce their caffeine intake or eliminate it from their diets. The initial headaches and feelings of tiredness that some attribute to "caffeine withdrawal" may be minimized or eliminated on this program while following the BASIC Plan. The Enhancing Options found in this chapter constitute important adjuncts to The BASIC Plan.

> The BASIC Plan and other Enhancing Options can help greatly
> reduce symptoms of "caffeine withdrawal."

Many people report that the elimination or reduction of caffeine has given them a new sense of peace and clarity. This benefit, combined with the knowledge that you may be giving your heart a healthy boost by eliminating its daily caffeine ration, will most likely give you a far greater reward than the caffeine ever could.

If you would like to select the Caffeine-Reducing Option, look over the list of foods, beverages, and remedies that follow. As much as possible, and where appropriate, choose caffeine-free alternatives or avoid caffeine-added foods and drinks altogether.° On food and beverage labels, look over lists of ingredients carefully; and before you take over-the-counter remedies, read both the active and nonactive ingredient lists.

Caffeine-Rich Foods, Beverages, and Over-the-Counter Remedies

Choose decaffeinated or caffeine-free alternatives or, if appropriate, eliminate:°
    Chocolate
    Coffee
    Colas and other soft drinks
    Cough, cold, and flu remedies
    Over-the-counter "diet" pills
    Pain relievers (some aspirins and other anti-inflammatories)
    Tea (regular and some herbal teas)

°Never eliminate a remedy that your physician has recommended or that you think may be important to your health.

THE FOOD FREQUENCY–REDUCING OPTION

Because this program has been specifically designed to help balance your insulin levels and reduce insulin resistance, it is likely that you have noticed a significant decrease in cravings and hunger. Even though you may not crave food as intensely, nor need it as often, you may not have thought to change your basic eating pattern (of three meals—perhaps in addition to snacks—each day).°° Or you may be eating more out of habit than because of hunger.

You may be eating often, throughout the day, because you are used to eating "by the clock"—routinely eating at regular times. It's easy to understand why so many carbohydrate addicts get used to eating at specified times rather than in response to their bodies' hunger signals. When you stop to

---

°Unless otherwise directed by your physician.
°°If your physician has recommended that you eat frequently or on a regular schedule, skip this option and, as always, follow your doctor's advice.

think about it, most carbohydrate addicts no longer trust their bodies' requests for food, for fear that if they did, they would be eating all the time.

On this program, however, the reduction or elimination of carbohydrate cravings and the increase in control you experience with your eating will probably make it easier for you to trust yourself and to respond to your body's true hunger.

> Some carbohydrate addicts find that the more they eat, the more they want. Some have trained themselves to "eat by the clock," allowing themselves food only when it's "time to eat."

The Food Frequency–Reducing Option asks you to respond to your body's need for food rather than listening to the old rules that dictate when you should eat. When your insulin and blood sugar levels are in balance, you can more easily trust your body's signals and stop eating by the clock.

In this Enhancing Option, if it is "time" for a low-carbohydrate meal and you are simply not hungry, put it off—or skip it altogether. You may choose to have it later in the day or in the evening. If you don't want to skip the meal entirely (even though you are not hungry), you may choose to take smaller portions (enjoying a low-carbo snack instead of a full meal). In any case, if you are not hungry, unless otherwise directed by your physician, don't eat (or at least eat less).

> On this program, as your cravings subside, it is likely you will lose the need to nibble and snack throughout the day.

If skipping or delaying a low-carbohydrate meal or having a small snack rather than a full meal makes you a bit nervous, remember this: if you don't eat your usual low-carbohydrate meal at your typical time and get hungry or for any reason want it later, you can have it! So don't be concerned that if you don't have the food now, you may be sorry later. If you get hungry later, make yourself the same meal, out of the same low-carbohydrate foods you would normally include. Likewise, if you have a low-carbo snack rather than a meal and later find that you are hungry or sorry that you did not have your usual meal, you can still have the rest of the meal at that time. So if you are not particularly hungry, nothing is lost by skipping, delaying, or "downsizing" a low-carbohydrate meal.

> You can always have a low-carbohydrate meal or snack
> as you need it.

The one exception to skipping meals relates to your Reward Meal. If you find that you are not hungry when it is time for your Reward Meal, do *not* skip it altogether. You may choose to postpone your Reward Meal for a while, but it is important to remember that carbohydrates are essential to both your health and satisfaction and that they should be enjoyed (in a balanced meal) every day. If you are not hungry for your Reward Meal and you cannot or do not want to postpone it, simply eat a smaller meal.

If you prefer to have a small Reward Meal, make certain that you maintain your usual one-third, one-third, one-third balance of carbohydrates, protein, and low-carbohydrate vegetables along with a small premeal salad. Do not have a carbo-loaded snack in place of your well-balanced meal. Whenever you have carbohydrates, you need protein and fiber as well, to help balance your insulin and blood sugar levels. Some patients and readers prefer to go lightly on their high-carbohydrate foods at some Reward Meals. As long as your physician agrees, you can do so, but be sure to include enough carbohydrates to maintain your good heath. Remember, if you want to skip, reduce, or delay any low-carbohydrate meal or snack, you can—just be certain not to skip your Reward Meals on a regular basis.

> You can postpone your Reward Meal or have smaller portions,
> but do not regularly skip Reward Meals.

Some carbohydrate addicts are afraid to skip their low-carbohydrate meals. They are concerned that they might experience the typical symptoms of hypoglycemia (low blood sugar) that they knew in the past (including sweats, headaches, shakes, inability to concentrate or think clearly, tiredness, irritability, mood swings, and the like). These concerns are usually based on experiences that occurred at a time when they were eating carbohydrates often throughout the day—most likely, when their insulin levels were high and their blood sugar levels low. Although we do not recommend that you do without food until you feel faint, and you should never skip meals or delay them if your doctor has recommended otherwise, we do offer you the choice of skipping a meal when you aren't really hungry. You will probably be very surprised at how little you miss it.

Many of the patients and research participants with whom we have worked ask whether they can skip breakfast. If you don't really want breakfast, you may find it preferable to skip it. Instead of a full low-carbohydrate breakfast, you may prefer just a cup of coffee or tea (decaffeinated if you like) with milk.° After you have been on The BASIC Plan for a few days, you may be surprised at your lack of cravings and hunger and may feel very comfortable and able to hold off until lunch. Or you may choose to postpone your breakfast until late morning (eleven o'clock, for instance) and combine your breakfast and lunch. You may choose to skip one meal or another during weekdays and not on weekends, or vice versa.

Stay focused on your body and your hunger; listen to your body's messages rather than the rules in your mind. Do not push yourself. Give yourself "permission" to skip or delay a low-carbohydrate meal, but do not pressure yourself to give up any meal or snack. Let the desire come naturally as your cravings are reduced.

Some people use a meal or snack as a "pleasure break," a chance to get away from work. If you normally use meal or snack time as a chance to give yourself some time off, continue to do so even though you may not be eating then. You do not have to eat in order to have a reason to leave your desk or take a break. Choose some other pleasurable activity, besides eating, during these mealtimes. Bring headphones to work and, during the time you would normally be eating, listen to some music you enjoy. You may want to bring a book on tape to listen to or a favorite book to read. You may choose to indulge in a phone call to a friend or start a diary (perhaps your own book). Bring some knitting or puzzles you enjoy. Take a walk and/or a nap. You can choose any alternative you like, but do take the time that you would have used to consume a meal and "give" it to yourself in the form of some other pleasurable activity. (Running errands or making task-related phone calls is not an acceptable substitute unless you *really* want to do it.)

Just because you aren't eating does not mean you don't have the right to make yourself unavailable to others. During your "lunch hour," you

---

°At times other than your Reward Meal, you should have milk with only one cup of coffee each day. Limit your intake of milk (regular or low-fat) or cream (if appropriate) to a total of two ounces in one cup of coffee, consumed within fifteen minutes. Do not use nondairy creamers or sugar substitutes; both can stimulate an insulin release.

might want to take the phone off the hook or put it on voice mail or activate the answering machine. If you have your own office, you might want to lock the door and take a short nap (bring a dependable and quiet alarm clock). If you work at home, get away from your duties and take time for yourself. Go watch your favorite television show or part of a movie on videotape or take a relaxing bath. You might even take a nap.

When it comes to using your well-earned work break, give yourself the option of a non–food-related pleasurable alternative to eating. If you give yourself only two choices, work or eating, you know which one will win. So when you feel like delaying or skipping a low-carbohydrate meal, do so, but be certain to provide yourself with some other fun or pleasurable pastime in its stead.

9

ON THE HORIZON

EMERGING WARRIORS IN THE BATTLE FOR HEART HEALTH

The future is not something we enter. The future is something we create.
—*Leonard I. Sweet*

Tomorrow. It holds so many exciting breakthroughs, new approaches, new solutions, important changes on the horizon, all showing signs of new and vital heart health protection. Although their effectiveness is still being investigated, we thought you would like to learn a bit about the warriors who may someday help you in your noble battle for heart health.

Some of these breakthroughs may be familiar to you, yet we have placed them in the "emerging" category because we feel that further research is needed before their heart-related benefits can be assured. Other breakthroughs may be new to you, awaiting only additional research to confirm their exciting potential.

In either case they cannot be given a wholehearted stamp of scientific approval, so at this time we will only touch on their importance. We certainly do not expect or recommend that you begin incorporating them into your diet until their efficacy has been proved. Still, we wanted you to know what promises lie just ahead so that you may be on the lookout for trustworthy research that supports their usefulness. Then, in consultation with your physician, choose those that are most appropriate for you.

Here, then, are some of the exciting discoveries that lie just over the horizon.

SENSATIONAL SOY

Soy protein, in the form of tofu, is emerging as one of the leading breakthroughs in health nutrition. The role of vegetable proteins in the reduction of coronary artery disease risk was postulated as long ago as 1909 in Russia by Vladislov Ignatowski. Since that time generations of scientists have studied the possible role of animal versus vegetable protein in the modification of blood fat levels and thus cardiovascular disease risk. Only recently, with media attention being drawn to the possible role of soy in reducing the risk for cancer, have the heart healthy benefits of soy protein come to the fore.

Although researchers disagree as to whether it is the presence of phytoestrogens (plant-based naturally occurring estrogens) in soy protein or the replacement of saturated fats in animal protein by soy that causes the improvement in blood fat levels, soy protein holds great promise in the war on heart disease.

> **Soy protein has been found to lead to lower levels of insulin release.**

Most exciting for the carbohydrate addict is the discovery of the soy protein–insulin link. Researchers in the Department of Nutrition, School of Public Health, Loma Linda, have reported that the type of protein you eat in a mixed meal and the building blocks that your protein choice contains influence the insulin release that follows. As we would expect, soy protein was found to lead to lower levels of insulin release in those with both normal and elevated levels of blood cholesterol. Furthermore, these scientists hypothesized that the resultant amino acids in the blood and insulin reduction that followed the intake of the soy protein could be expected to reduce cholesterol levels contributing to heart disease.

Though all the research is not yet in, it just may be that soy, like the biblical white manna that fell from heaven and was all foods to all people, provides a wonderful, healthful, potentially insulin-reducing, and heart healthy source of protein. For some exciting low-carbohydrate recipes that include soy protein (tofu) and can be enjoyed at any meal, see Chapter 12, "Eating Hearty, Part I: Low-Carbohydrate Recipes."

One word of caution, however. Soy, in any form, contains free glutamates and may present problems along with the benefits for those who are particularly sensitive (see page 140 for information on carbohydrate act-alikes). The jury is still out on soy, but it looks very promising, so keep up on all the pros and cons.

A NEW DIRECTION IN DIETARY FAT

Most scientific discoveries go through a predictable series of changes. First, there is a flurry of excitement. Advocates herald the breakthrough; opponents discount it. In time both points of view are seen to hold some kernel of truth, and a differentiation process occurs, replacing the all-or-nothing position that each side held at the outset. The new understanding that emerges generally supplants the one-size-fits-all viewpoint that often accompanied the first flush of discovery.

An example of this differentiation process can be seen in the area of blood fats. At first the discovery of cholesterol's connection to heart disease was heralded by some as a supremely important breakthrough. Others disagreed, claiming that total cholesterol did not offer the trustworthy predictive power that advocates claimed. In the end, both were right.

Cholesterol's connection to heart disease did prove to be important, but only after different types of cholesterol (HDL, LDL, VLDL, and other lipids) had been researched and their actions defined. In the near future new findings related to insulin's impact on each cholesterol subtype will once again change science's understanding of cholesterol's connection to heart disease.

> **Not all dietary fat is bad.**
> **Some dietary fats may be more protective against heart disease than is a very low-fat, high-carbohydrate diet.**

In this same way dietary fat's connection to heart disease is undergoing a differentiation process. Scientists are learning that not all dietary fat is bad and indeed that some dietary fats are more protective against heart disease than are previously recommended in low-fat, high-carbohydrate diets.

Remember, trans fatty acids are unsaturated fats that have been chemically transformed from their normal room-temperature liquid state into solids.° You may see them referred to as hydrogenated or partially hydrogenated fats. Food processors prefer to include trans fatty acids in your

°For more information on dietary fats, see page 79.

food because these solid fats can be used as margarine or in other food products without fear that they will become an oily mess. In addition, trans fatty acids have a longer shelf life than other fats. Unfortunately trans fatty acids have a very dark side healthwise.

In order to make an unsaturated fat into a trans fatty acid, extra hydrogen atoms are pumped into unsaturated fat. This process is called hydrogenation. With hydrogen atoms added, the formerly unsaturated fat has been turned into a saturated fat, obliterating any benefits it had as a polyunsaturated fat. Food manufacturers prefer to use the term *trans unsaturated fat* instead of the equally correct term *trans fatty acids* because the former contains the word *unsaturated*. Though "trans unsaturated fat" sounds as if it would be good for you, it is not. Hydrogenation of unsaturated fat can spell real problems for your heart. In fact, scientists are finding evidence that hydrogenated fats may be far more damaging than naturally saturated fats.

Dr. F. B. Hu and his team of researchers studied the diet and heart health of more than 80,000 women during a fifteen-year time period. Reporting in the *New England Journal of Medicine*, Dr. Hu and his team found that trans unsaturated fats caused the greatest increase in risk for heart disease. They found that replacing only 2 percent of daily caloric intake of carbohydrates with trans unsaturated fats increased the risk for heart disease by a whopping 93 percent. The good news is that replacing a tiny amount of trans fatty acids with monounsaturated or polyunsaturated fats reduced heart disease risk by more than half.

In addition, Dr. Hu's team found that replacing only 5 percent of daily caloric intake of carbohydrates with unsaturated fats reduced the risk for heart disease by 19 percent for the monounsaturated fats and 38 percent for the polyunsaturated fats. Replacing saturated fat with monounsaturated and polyunsaturated fats had an even greater calculated effect, reducing heart disease risk by 38 and 55 percent, respectively. Dr. Hu's conclusion: when it comes to reducing heart disease, replacing trans unsaturated fats with monounsaturated and polyunsaturated fats is more effective than reducing overall fat intake.

**Hydrogenated fats may be far more damaging
than naturally saturated fats.
Replacing a tiny amount of trans fatty acids
with unsaturated fats cuts heart disease risk by more than half.**

Other scientists, physicians, and laypersons have known these fat facts for years. Reports indicate that only one person in five gets the health benefits promised by low-fat diets. In our research and clinical practice, we, too, have been witness to the fact that, for some, low-fat diets do not reduce individual risks for heart disease. In particular, in the case of the carbohydrate addict, for whom lower overall fat intake can mean higher carbohydrate intake and higher insulin levels, an overall low-fat diet may not be as beneficial as one that simply stresses polyunsaturated and monounsaturated fats.

It is important to add two thoughts to this new wave of research: (1) At this time both monounsaturated and polyunsaturated fats are being hailed as "good" fats. It is possible, we believe, that as research continues, polyunsaturated fat may not prove as beneficial a choice as monounsaturated fat. By its very chemical structure, polyunsaturated fat is less stable and more likely to participate in oxidative injury along arteries than are monounsaturated fats. Some researchers recommend supplementing with extra vitamin E and C to help reduce oxidative injury. Our choice would be to use monounsaturated fats whenever possible. (2) Never apply research findings to your own lifestyle choices without discussing this matter with your physician prior to making any changes. Your needs may be special, and you deserve the time required to make an informed decision. (For more detailed information, see pages 223–225 as well as our easy-to-read charts, "Simple Fat Facts" and "Fast Fat Facts," which begin on this page.

Scientists have also found that eating enough fat for your body's needs is essential for heart health. When you do not eat enough dietary fat, your body compensates by making its own, and the fat your body produces (endogenous lipids) poses far more of a threat to your heart health than does the fat you eat (exogenous lipids).

Now, armed with your fair share of fat facts, you can be on the lookout for a change in attitude regarding dietary fats and heart health, and in keeping with your physician's recommendations, you may find new, fear-free fats coming your way.

Simple Fat Facts

Fat is one of the body's basic nutrients (the others being carbohydrates and protein). All forms of fat are made up of a combination of building blocks called fatty acids. These building blocks can remain unattached as single molecules (free fatty acids) or may be assembled into groupings that form larger molecules (fats). When each molecule in the group of molecules that makes up a fat is filled to capacity with hydrogen, it is said to be a saturated fat. When there is one opening for an atom in each molecule, the fat is said to be monounsaturated. When there are several openings for hydrogen in each molecule, the fat is said to be polyunsaturated.

To illustrate the differences between saturated, monounsaturated, and polyunsaturated fat, imagine a fat molecule as a train of passenger cars. Each car is a carbon atom. If every seat on the train is filled by a "passenger" (a hydrogen atom), then this is a saturated fat molecule. If there is one seat open in one car of the entire train in which a hydrogen-atom passenger can sit, this train is like a monounsaturated fat; if there are several seats open in the cars of the train, it is very much like a polyunsaturated fat.

Saturated fats usually come from animal sources and are solid enough to hold their shape at room temperature and remain solid. Tropical oils, such as coconut oil and palm oil, are exceptions to the rule about saturated fats being solid. These two saturated oils are semisolid at room temperature and come from plant sources.

Saturated fats are of special importance to the carbohydrate addict because they have been shown to increase insulin levels and total cholesterol and have been associated with some forms of cancer as well. Recent research indicates that replacing even small quantities of saturated fats with monounsaturated or polyunsaturated fats reduced heart disease risk by 38 and 55 percent, respectively. Replacing trans fatty acids with monounsaturated or polyunsaturated fats can cut heart disease risk even more.

Research is currently under way that may someday reveal that replacing saturated fat with polyunsaturated fat is not as beneficial a choice as changing to monounsaturated fat. Polyunsaturated fat is less stable and more likely to participate in oxidative injury along arteries than is monounsaturated fat. Our choice would be to use monounsaturated fat whenever possible.

It is important to remember that it is not advisable to apply research findings to your own lifestyle choices without discussing this matter with your physician prior to making any changes.

Fast Fat Facts

Fats and oils are composed of varying proportions of all types of lipids: trans fatty acids, saturated fats, polyunsaturated fats, and monounsaturated fats. In each category below, fats are listed in descending order according to their concentrations of the specified type of lipid.

High in Trans Fatty Acids°	High in Saturated Fats	High in Polyunsaturated Fats	High in Monounsaturated Fats°°
Vegetable shortening	Butterfat	Safflower oil	Olive oil
Hydrogenated fats	Beef fat	Soybean oil	Canola oil
Margarine	Lard	Corn oil	Peanut oil
	Milk fat	Sunflower oil	
	Coconut oil	Sesame oil	
	Chicken fat	Cottonseed oil	
	Palm oil	Omega-3 oils	
	Cocoa butter		

Although trans fatty acids are also known as trans unsaturated fats, processing removes any unsaturated fat benefits, converting an unsaturated fat into a saturated fat. Trans fatty acids appear to be the most health-damaging of all fats. Trans fatty acids may also be listed as partially hydrogenated or hydrogenated fats. By any name, trans fatty acids are clearly not good for your heart health.

To reduce the potential for and repercussions of oxidative injury, some researchers indicate that the preferential use of monounsaturated fats whenever possible would seem to be an ideal choice. Additional research may further change our understanding of the relationships between dietary lipids and heart health.

Always remember to check with your physician before making any dietary changes.

°Worst for heart health.
°°Best for heart health.

Good Cholesterol, Bad Cholesterol—Explained in Eight Sentences

When people refer to "good cholesterol" and "bad cholesterol," they are not really speaking about cholesterol at all. Rather than cholesterol, these are carrier proteins (called lipoproteins, or fat-carrying proteins) that act like "baskets," transporting cholesterol between the blood and the liver. The "bad" form is a low-density lipoprotein (LDL), which picks up cholesterol from the liver and carries it around in the blood. LDL is considered bad because a high level of this lipoprotein is a sign that the liver is in a fat-making mode and the high level of cholesterol it produces may cause plaque buildup in the arteries, eventually leading to heart disease.°

The "good" form of cholesterol refers to high-density lipoproteins (HDL), which transport cholesterol in the blood to the liver. High levels of HDL usually indicate that the liver is in a fat-burning mode. When your body is hyperinsulinemic, you are far more likely to have high levels of "bad" LDL lipoproteins and low levels of "good" HDL lipoproteins because your liver is being told to go into a fat-making mode. When your insulin levels are balanced, chances are your body is far more likely to burn excess blood fat, so that your "good" HDL levels rise while your "bad" LDL levels drop.

°At this time, for those with established heart disease, the American Heart Association has advised reducing LDL levels to below 100 milligrams per deciliter.

INFLAMMATION, GUM DISEASE, AND *HELICOBACTER PYLORI*: A NEW AGE

Helicobacter pylori (*H. pylori*) is quite a mouthful, and although it may be difficult to pronounce, you are going to be hearing a great deal more about it. *H. pylori* as well as other infectious organisms—such as *Chlamydia pneumoniae,* cytomegalovirus, and herpes—are being studied intensively to determine their roles in heart disease.

H. pylori was first described almost a hundred years ago, but it was not given serious attention at the time. In the late 1970s an Australian pathologist, Dr. John Robin Warren, noticed that *H. pylori* were often found in the inflamed areas of the stomach lining. In the years that followed, Dr. Warren, working with Dr. Barry Marshall, revolutionized the treatment of stomach ulcers and laid the foundation for the prevention of stomach cancer, too.

Marshall's tale of courage and commitment is a wonderful story in itself. When facing overwhelming criticism by the medical community that threatened the acceptance and use of his findings (such criticism is typical with all new discoveries), Marshall self-administered *H. pylori* and, after contracting an acute infection, which resulted in severe gastritis and ulceration, cured himself of it with a few weeks' course of antibiotics and bismuth salts.

Since that time *H. pylori* has been confirmed to be involved not only in the inflammation of the lining of the stomach but in the formation of dental plaque and full immunologic responses to these inflammations as well. The story is still unfolding, and for a while there may be quite a bit of confusion about all the medical problems associated with *H. pylori*. In time, however, when the supporting research is assembled in the right order, *H. pylori* and its link to dental plaque, gum disease, inflammation, and hyperinsulinemia may provide science with the biggest heart disease connection since the discovery of insulin.

H. pylori is a species of spiral-shaped bacteria. It appears to be present in the stomach linings of between 20 and 50 percent of Americans, and unless you are specifically tested for this infection, you will probably never suspect its presence—until it may be too late. Its link to stomach ulcers and cancer was established by the National Institutes of Health in 1994. Its connection to insulin and heart disease is just emerging.

For the carbohydrate addict *H. pylori*'s most important connection is about to emerge. For a while a scientific debate regarding *H. pylori* and its role in infection and disease raged. Although some scientists had found *H. pylori* to be a strong risk factor for high blood pressure and risk-related blood fat levels, as well as for heart disease itself, other researchers denied this connection. At the same time, other scientists claimed that gum disease increased the risk for heart disease. Yet none of the scientists seemed to understand the connections (if any) among these seemingly discrepant risk factors for heart disease.

**For the carbohydrate addict,
H. pylori's most important connection is about to emerge.**

Recent research conducted by Dr. O. A'cbay and his team, however, has provided that valuable link. Discovering that *H. pylori* increases insulin production by stimulating stomach release of the hormone gastrin, which in turn stimulates the pancreas to release insulin, has afforded scientists the one essential piece of information that is needed to connect *H. pylori,* gum disease, and inflammation to heart disease.

> *H. pylori* increases insulin production.

H. pylori, as a stomach-based infection, can be spread upward through the esophagus. As the bacteria find a new home in the mouth, they encourage gum disease through the bacterial buildup of plaque on the teeth. The linings in the stomach and mouth become inflamed. At the same time, the *H. pylori*–gastrin–insulin release can greatly increase the risk for heart disease. It appears obvious that neither the gum disease nor the plaque nor the stomach inflammation are themselves responsible for the ensuing heart problems but rather that the resulting hyperinsulinemia brings about the changes that may put your heart at risk.

Very shortly, as the pieces of the puzzle fall into place, it will become clear to physicians and scientists alike that gum disease, dental plaque buildup, and gastric inflammation are not the cause of heart disease but rather the signs that *H. pylori* is present. Furthermore, they will come to understand that *H. pylori* and the hyperinsulinemia it encourages are the real heart disease culprits.

If this sounds a bit scientific, just think of it this way: if, within your stomach, you are harboring *H. pylori* bacteria (and the chances may be as high as fifty-fifty that you are), your body may well be releasing high levels of insulin due to the presence of that bacteria. The bacteria and the hyperinsulinemia it encourages can set you up for heart-related problems as well as for heart disease.

> *H. pylori* and the hyperinsulinemia it encourages
> can set you up for heart disease.
> But help is on the way.

Help is coming. Being on The Carbohydrate Addict's Healthy Heart Program can help you in two ways. First, by being on a program that is designed to help lower and balance your insulin levels, you are likewise making choices to help reduce insulin-related heart disease. So most likely you are that much better off right now.

Second, even as you read these words, diagnostic tests are being perfected and a treatment that is relatively easy and risk-free (a combination of three weeks of antibiotics and bismuth salts) is under development. Although the testing and treatment are still in the research stages, when it comes to applying them to heart-related factors, the work is moving quickly.

So stay informed. This is an important discovery, and once the "wrinkles" are ironed out, this new treatment may offer a world of hope and help. In the meantime understand that you may hear a great deal of debate as well as criticism from those who have little or no knowledge of the insulin connection. Stick with your program and keep your eyes and ears open. In the not-too-distant future, we trust that this potential lifesaver will make its way into everyday good medical care.

NOTHING FISHY ABOUT OMEGA

Omega-3 oils are a particular classification of unsaturated fats. They are found in some plants (such as flaxseed) and in the tissues of all fish. There is a growing body of compelling research evidence that points to the particularly beneficial effects of omega-3 oils on heart health. They appear to lower the "bad" cholesterol (LDL) and raise the "good" cholesterol (HDL). Popular fish that are particularly good sources of omega-3 oils include:

Bluefish	Salmon
Herring	Sardines
Mackerel	Tuna

It is important to remember that cooking fish at high temperatures can destroy almost half the omega-3, although microwave cooking doesn't appear to have an adverse effect on it. Canned salmon, tuna, and sardines can be excellent sources of omega-3 oils. Unfortunately, the addition of mayonnaise (which contains saturated fat) to canned tuna can offset some of the benefits of the omega-3 oils.

There is one particularly important concern that should make you think twice about running out and stripping the supermarket shelves or fish stores of their omega-3–rich products. Some omega-3 fish oils may be contaminated with mercury. High levels of mercury have the capacity to increase oxidant injury, thereby negating or reversing the health benefits that the omega-3s confer.

At this time researchers are unclear as to whether supplemental omega-3 fish oil provides the same benefits observed in omega-3 oils consumed as part of a fish-rich diet. Be on the lookout for scientific reports from dependable sources that will let you know whether omega-3 lives up to its promise of providing heart health benefits.

> Although they appear to reduce risk-related blood fats, some omega-3 fish oils may be contaminated with mercury.

AN ANTIOXIDANT WAITING TO HAPPEN

Nature has provided us with more than six hundred plant pigments, called carotenoids, that give carrots, sweet potatoes, winter squash, apricots, papaya, and many other fruits, vegetables, and flowers their rich yellow and orange colors. (By the way, flamingos get their vibrant color from diets rich in carotenoids.) Carotenoids can also be found in broccoli and dark leafy vegetables.

One carotenoid that is currently being studied intensively is beta-carotene. Found in many vegetables (including carrots, kale, collard greens, broccoli, squash, spinach, and sweet potatoes), beta-carotene accounts for approximately one-quarter of all edible carotenoids, which the body needs to make vitamin A. Scientists are now researching the possibility that in order for beta-carotene to do its health-promoting work, the body needs other carotenoids working together with beta-carotene.

Many reports indicate that beta-carotene is a powerful antioxidant with properties that can contribute to greatly reducing the incidence of heart disease.

There has been some controversy regarding the possibility that beta-carotene supplementation may reduce levels of vitamin E, but as yet this has not been established. In addition, it is important to note that oral contraceptives have been shown to reduce levels of beta-carotene in the body. The final word is not yet in, and safety and recommended levels must always be established, but once these are in hand, beta-carotene may become part of the heart healthy supplementation program.

> Oral contraceptives have been shown to reduce levels of the antioxidant beta-carotene in the body.

TAURINE: A PROMISING BLOOD VESSEL ALLY

Like magnesium,* taurine shows promise in improving insulin sensitivity as well as lessening the risk for the blood vessel complications of diabetes. Taurine appears to lower blood pressure and protect against cholesterol-induced atherosclerosis. It may also cooperate to prevent the formation of blood clots within vessels. All these effects parallel those of magnesium. Magnesium itself appears to act as an antiarrhythmic, helping to keep the heartbeat regular and strong.

Whether this "dynamic duo" work their heart healthy magic through their reduction of insulin levels and insulin resistance or by other means is still unknown, but in any case taurine—perhaps in combination with magnesium—shows early signs of becoming a good choice for carbohydrate addicts who seek enhanced heart health.

THE POTENTIAL POWER OF VANADIUM

One of the most exciting of the emerging nutrients in the fight for your heart's health is unfortunately the one that needs the most continued investigation. This nutrient is vanadium, a naturally occurring element. The early findings on vanadium are so promising that we wanted you to know about it so that you might look forward to its potential lifesaving benefits.

Vanadium is actually part of the earth's crust. Two forms of vanadium, vanadyl and vanadate, have been found to have many properties similar to insulin, so much so that vanadium is said to "mimic" insulin's actions. This might sound like the opposite of what those with high levels of insulin should seek, but an interesting effect occurs. When given orally, vanadyl and vanadate dramatically lower insulin levels and blood pressure and improve or normalize blood glucose. Although much of the research to date has been done with animals, scientists are currently hoping to find the same results in humans.

*For more information on magnesium, see page 180.

In studies performed at the Joslin Diabetes Center, Dr. A. B. Goldfine and her colleagues have found that oral vanadyl sulfate treatment resulted in improved insulin sensitivity in humans with adult-onset diabetes. Dr. Goldfine concluded that "[v]anadium salts, or some related compound, may provide a new [and] effective oral treatment for patients with diabetes mellitus." Serum cholesterol levels as well were lowered in research participants.

> Vanadyl and vanadate dramatically lower insulin levels and blood pressure and improve or normalize blood glucose.

The Joslin Diabetes Center has also noted that "[o]ngoing studies are now in progress to evaluate the efficacy and safety of oral vanadium salts in glycemic control and, more importantly, on insulin sensitivity, as well as on blood pressure and cholesterol in people with diabetes and other insulin resistant medical conditions, such as hypertension."

In the future, perhaps the very near future, vanadium may be recognized as an essential element for insulin-related heart disease risk reduction and thereby become an important supplement for the carbohydrate addict, who can benefit from its potentially powerful protection.

L-CARNITINE: AN EMERGING RESISTANCE FIGHTER

In those with heart-related medical problems, deficiencies in L-carnitine are certainly not uncommon, and researchers have found that increasing carnitine in patients with carnitine deficiency can improve heart function. Recently the underlying process responsible for the improvement in heart health has been identified as L-carnitine's ability to furnish the heart with needed glucose without elevating insulin levels by decreasing insulin resistance. Research still under way may soon add L-carnitine to the growing list of heart health–enhancing supplements.

SELENIUM: A POTENTIALLY ILLUMINATING LINK

Among other common nutrient deficiencies found in the general population, a shortage of selenium has been connected to risk-related blood fat levels and ultimately to cardiovascular disease. Low selenium levels have been found to be linked to a number of ischemic heart disease risk factors, including cigarette smoking, alcohol consumption, total cholesterol, hypertension, age, and physical inactivity. It is interesting to note that all of these risk factors have been shown to exhibit a strong link to hyperinsulinemia, and it appears logical to hypothesize that as selenium deficiency has been linked to each of them, selenium deficiency may indeed be linked directly to increased levels of insulin. At this time the nature of the insulin-selenium connection is not understood.

Selenium is part of an antioxidant complex, and although it is unclear how many people may be selenium-deficient, this important nutrient may soon be proved to be critical in the achievement and maintenance of heart health—and therefore perhaps of particular importance for the carbohydrate addict.

LIPOIC ACID: A DOUBLE-DUTY HEART SAVER IN DISCOVERY

Lipoic acid is a nutrient that may be found to be doubly beneficial for your heart health. It appears to be a metabolic antioxidant, helping replenish other antioxidants needed to reduce oxidant injury.

> Research indicates that lipoic acid reduces insulin resistance and may prove helpful in lowering insulin levels.

In addition, research indicates that lipoic acid reduces insulin resistance in some cells and may prove helpful in lowering insulin levels. A full body of research confirming lipoic acid's importance in heart health is not yet in, and we await with interest the scientific findings on this potentially important supplement.

THE COENZYME Q-10 DEBATE

Sometimes referred to by its nickname, *CoQ10*, or by its scientific name, *Q-ubiquinone*, this antioxidant is at the center of a heated debate regarding its heart health–enhancing capabilities. Coenzyme Q-10 has been shown to facilitate energy movement within cells, and research has verified that many patients suffering from heart failure not only show coenzyme Q-10 deficiencies but benefit greatly from its supplementation.

The debate continues regarding its efficacy in the prevention of heart disease and the enhancement of heart health. One well-established scientific finding is that coenzyme Q-10 has been shown to be an important antioxidant companion to vitamin E. From the findings we have reviewed, at this time we think more research is needed to verify or discount its contribution to heart disease prevention.

ON THE OTHER HAND: CAUSE FOR CONCERN

One up-and-coming nutrient, L-arginine, is still in debate, and we did not feel we could include it in the "emerging warriors" category. It is likely that in the near future you will be hearing a great deal about this nutrient. Indeed, you may have heard about it already. We have reason to be concerned about its long-term effects and wanted you to know why we think that it may *not* be an appropriate adjunct to your heart health program, either now or in the future. As always, check with your physician.

> Although it may help open blood vessels, L-arginine has also been shown to raise insulin levels.

L-arginine—an amino acid that is used by the body to make nitric oxide, a potent vasodilator—appears to be the most mysterious and complex of the emerging nutrients. Although L-arginine has beneficial properties, in many ways extreme caution must be exercised with its use.

Scientists and physicians alike have been impressed by L-arginine's ability to open blood vessels and increase blood flow. Increasing blood flow to the heart itself is important in the treatment of heart disease. At the same time, however, other research has uncovered a great concern for the carbohydrate addict: in addition to its ability to help open blood vessels, L-arginine has been shown to lead to elevated insulin levels.

In the short term L-arginine may provide some important heart health benefits, but in the long run, for the carbohydrate addict in particular, the insulin-related effects may negate the heart health–related advantages.

10

HEART AND SOUL

THE MYSTERIOUS POWER OF PRAYER

Prayer is a healing power that cannot be prescribed.—*Ben Franklin*

A HEARTBEAT AWAY FROM GOD
DR. RACHAEL HELLER'S STORY

I was no more than five years old, barely able to describe the sound I heard crashing in my own ears as I lay silent in my room. It frightened me, that swooshing, pounding, rhythmic noise. The more I listened, the louder and faster it seemed to get.

I made my way out of my darkened bedroom and headed for the kitchen, where I knew I would find my babysitter, Angela, reading the "good book" and enjoying a cup of tea. I sought her comfort and wisdom as naturally as I sought food and water.

I climbed onto her lap and described the sound that had so distressed me. She kissed me gently on top of my head, swept the plastered tendrils of hair off my sweaty forehead, and explained that it was only the sound of my heartbeat that had disturbed my rest. She went on to explain that by lying with one ear pressed up against the pillow, I could always hear the sound of my heart.

"Your heart is far more than just a muscle that is made to pump blood," she explained. "Certainly, that is what keeps you alive, and that is a miracle in itself. But even more, your heart is the sanctuary of your soul, and each beat is a prayer to God."

I sat in silent wonder. "Each time your heart beats," she went on, "you are praying."

"Praying?" I asked.

"Yes," she explained. "You see, whatever you do and think and say, all that you are, can be heard in your heartbeat. When you are unhappy, your heartbeat tells God how you feel. And when you are ashamed of something you have done, your heart beats differently, and God can tell. So you have to be the best little girl you can be, so that when God hears your heartbeat, he will know that your prayers are coming from the heart of a very good child."

"God can really hear my heartbeat?" I asked, fascinated by this new revelation.

"He can hear everyone's heartbeat," Angela assured me. "And every heartbeat is different," she added, "just like your fingerprints. That's how he keeps track of you." I looked down at my fingers, and in her inimitable way she raised my tiny hand and kissed it. I smiled and snuggled in to hear more.

"When God listens to your heartbeat, he knows everything that you feel, and he answers you the same way, through your heart."

I must have cast her a somewhat cynical look. "You don't believe me?" she asked laughingly. "Well, I'm going to prove it to you. When you do something bad, you know that feeling you get all over your body, even though no one has said anything to you, even though maybe no one knows you did it?"

I gave in to a nod, even though I had intended to hold back, afraid of confirming the fact that I ever did anything bad; after all, this might have been a trick question. But Angela hugged me at my admission and smiled her reassurance.

"Well, that feeling you get when you've done something wrong, that's God's answer to you. He's saying, 'That wasn't a good thing to do, my child. I forgive you, but don't do it again.' Now it's time for bed," she concluded, setting me on my feet and gently pushing me toward the door.

"But Angela," I added as I headed for my room, "if every heartbeat is a prayer to God, why do I have to say my prayers before I go to sleep?"

"That's the last question," Angela declared, then in a few sentences gave me an answer I would never forget. "You see, child, your heartbeat may tell God everything that he needs to know, but your prayers, ahh, they tell you what you need to know. Right now you pray with the words that others have taught you, but as you grow up, you will learn to pray with your own words, and when you do, you will learn to be humble and open to God.

In each prayer you will see all that you are, all that you are not, and all that you hope someday to be. And," she added, "if you are living right, God will know it, and so will you."

I lay awake for a long time that night, thinking about what Angela had said, pressing my ear against the pillow, listening to my heartbeat, wondering if I had been a good girl and what I would say when I was old enough to make up my own prayers. When my parents came home, I pretended to be asleep. Even then, I knew they would be irritated at another of "Angela's stories," so I kept it as our little secret: mine, Angela's, and God's.

Yet even to this day, as I lie awake in the darkness, pressing an ear up against my pillow, listening to the sound of my heartbeat in the night, I think over the day that has just passed, and I consider whether I have been living right. Then I fall off to sleep with the knowledge that each beat of my heart is a silent prayer to God.

BEYOND THE LIMITS OF OUR UNDERSTANDING

Throughout this book you have read about the scientific discoveries and breakthroughs that can help you in your quest for optimal heart health. In this chapter, however, you will discover all that we do not know about the spiritual connection to heart health, and you will hear testimony about why, in any case, the power of prayer may help bring peace and health to your heart.

WHAT SCIENCE KNOWS

In a fascinating article published in the *Journal of Holistic Nursing*, C. E. Hughes concluded that "[t]he apparent healing that results from prayer mystifies researchers. Numerous theories may be offered as to the mechanism by which this healing occurs. The belief of the praying person in the power of the prayer itself may stimulate healing[;] . . . the act of praying may enhance the immune system." And Hughes adds that "there sometimes exists a facet of prayer and healing that defies rational explanation and seems to suggest the existence of a higher power." We could not agree more. Yet it has taken science a very long time to verify what so many people have known for so many centuries: that prayer offers hope, help, and healing.

WHAT SCIENCE DOES NOT YET KNOW

The health of your heart is equal to far more than the sum of the chemicals, impulses, and muscle that can be observed, identified, dissected, and labeled. Against all scientific logic, much about your heart—its beat, strength, vitality, and endurance—springs from something beyond our limited understanding.

We have seen it with our own eyes. Men and women who have had little upon which to draw except their own will to live, the devotion of their friends and family, or their belief in a higher power or purpose have outlived others who, though strong in heart, have had little else in their lives.

Heart to heart, heartfelt, speaking from the heart, heart and soul—in all ways the heart connects to that which lies at our core. How many of us, in great pain or torment or having lost a loved one, have felt as if our hearts had been ripped from our very chests? And at these times how many of us have turned to a power greater than ourselves for guidance and help? It is as natural as inhaling and exhaling. In times of need and times of joy, our hearts reach out to something greater than ourselves. Only in that connection do so many of us find comfort, peace, health, and happiness.

We can tell you that scientists have confirmed two things we've known all along: that those whose faith is strong are far less likely to suffer from heart disease, and that prayer has a healing effect. We can say that it doesn't seem to matter whether you pray as you were taught to pray or whether you communicate through more unconventional methods. An open, ongoing connection with God seems to reap a wide variety of heart health–related benefits.

Health-related spiritual benefits do not come solely to those whose idea of a higher power is in keeping with society's; your higher power may be something less easily defined and still bring you peace of mind and perhaps a healthier heart as well. Prayer need not be spoken with words (although this method seems very effective). It may instead, or in combination, include meditation, guided imagery, joyous and soul-enriching work, music, dance, or other artistic creations.

Of great importance, however, is that your prayer, communication, celebration be right and true for you and that it, one might say, come from the heart. It is within this special connection that a healing can come forth, one that goes beyond all that humanity or science can explain.

This chapter contains no guidelines or options. It simply confirms what so many of us already know, that prayer, silent or spoken, through word or action or celebration, is important. The stories that follow are testaments to the mysterious power of prayer and will hopefully confirm and inspire you to embrace your own spiritual connections that lie within.

TRUST AND CARE

After interviewing a wide variety of participants in their research study, Dr. L. B. Bearon and Dr. H. G. Koenig concluded that "prayer and medical help-seeking are not mutually exclusive."

We agree completely. Although prayer and connection to a higher power may offer you help and hope, it is essential that you never choose prayer as a substitute for good medical care. Certainly it may be a good idea to use prayer in all its many forms as a wonderful adjunct, a helpful addition to your usual heart healthy program, but it should never replace more traditional approaches to diagnosis and treatment.

An old Middle Eastern truism advises, "Trust in God and tie your camel, too." We might rephrase it to read, "Talk to God, reach for the faith and hope that will keep you strong and focused, then do all that you can to keep your heart healthy."

Remember that God does indeed help those who help themselves.

FROM THE HEART: DEEPLY PERSONAL STORIES OF DISCOVERY, HEALTH, AND HOPE

A GIFT FROM MY FATHER: NINA'S STORY

My parents were not particularly religious people. They believed in God but were of two different religious backgrounds, so they exposed me to both. They also made certain that I experienced a whole variety of other beliefs and views, from Orthodox Judaism to Zen Buddhism. They figured that if I was exposed to many different religions, I would settle on the one that called to me and that perhaps might provide me with more of a spiritual connection than either of them experienced. I know that my father felt more strongly about my having a faith I could believe in, but I never got around to discussing it with him. And now I never will.

As I teenager, I figured that my parents' "experiment in religion" was more about making up for their own alienation and guilt than about providing me with spiritual guidance, but I went along with it because I found it interesting. I wrote award-winning essays comparing the creation myths common to several religions; detailed the similarities in the laws of Judaism, Christianity, and Islam; and likened the paths of Zen enlightenment to popular psychology guidelines for self-empowerment. Yet I never knew God. Religion was an intellectual pursuit that I understood but never felt. It was something that other people needed, but it meant nothing to me. My parents were disappointed, but they never talked about it, and in my teenage rebellion I reveled in showing them that their "experiment" had failed.

My only regret is that my father will never know how successful he had been and that it was his death that brought me the faith he had longed to instill in me when he was alive.

I was almost forty years old when I was given Dr. Vagnini's name and number. "He's terrific," a friend had told me. "You know, you can talk to him. He's really nice, and he might be a good person to see about your father." I took the slip of paper and flashed a fake smile.

"Thanks. I'll go give him a call," I said, and never let on to what I was really thinking. "Great," I thought. "A nice doctor. That's the last thing we need. My father doesn't need a nice doctor, he needs a smart doctor. If he needed nice, I'd get him a puppy. What he needs is smart." Placing the paper in my coat pocket, I said good-bye and headed for the hospital where my father was recovering from heart surgery. Two days later that paper saved my life.

I hadn't slept for more than forty-eight hours. We had been told that my father's operation had been a success and that with some lifestyle changes he would be just fine. But he wasn't, and as I walked through his hospital room door, I knew he wasn't going to make it. I did everything I could; so did my mother—but a lifetime of smoking, overindulgence, and stress had taken their toll. And he died in his sleep with my mother on one side of his bed and me on the other.

I sprang into action and began making all the plans my mother was not prepared to handle. My mind was amazingly clear, and I felt very little emotion. I was in shock, but I was so busy congratulating myself on holding it all together, I never suspected a thing.

I probably slept no more than a total of twelve hours over the next four days, on top of not having had any sleep before my father's death. I got ready for his funeral in a complete fog. I felt sick from overeating. I was already fifty or sixty pounds overweight, and I must have gained another twenty. I couldn't think, I couldn't sleep, I couldn't work, and I couldn't feel anything. I was off from work for the week, and after all the relatives had been called and the plans had been made, I just watched television and continued to eat.

In the short time between my father's heart attack and the funeral, I had gained so much weight that my clothes no longer fit. I didn't realize how bad things were until I tried to put on my black dress for the funeral. I suddenly realized that the buttons up the front were pulling and the material was gaping. I had nothing to wear. In desperation I pulled on my coat and wrapped it around me.

The coat felt surprisingly comforting, warm and soft. I had been alternately cold and hot for two days, and though I didn't want to think about it, my blood pressure was probably high. I had been battling it for a couple of years, but I had not wanted to give in and take the drugs my doctor had recommended. Now a pounding headache, probably from the blood pressure, made me want to crawl into a dark corner and stay there.

My mother's sobs sounded as if they were coming from far away. They had barely started the funeral service when the first pain shot across my chest. I felt as if I had been struck by lightning. Without a second thought, I knew I was having a heart attack.

My first thought was "No, dear God. Don't do this. Please don't do this. It will kill my mother. Please, dear God, don't do this." The stream of words coming from me surprised me, me who was so nonreligious. I had no time to give it any thought. I was sweating profusely, but I would not let them take my coat off, and, as if I had rehearsed it a hundred times before, when they did convince me to take it off, I carefully removed the paper with Dr. Vagnini's number.

Now it was my mother's turn to be calm. I had half expected her to go to pieces, but she never did. She had called an ambulance, and when they said it would be at least fifteen minutes before it would arrive, she had called Dr. Vagnini. "He said he would meet us at the hospital," she told me. "He was very nice and told me that he would be waiting there for us. He said not to worry." I almost made a wisecrack when another pain shot through me. "He said to keep you comfortable and . . ."

"What?" I demanded. "What else did he say?"

"He said to pray," she responded calmly.

"Who?" I asked. "You or me?"

"Both of us."

I laughed out loud. "Oh, Mom. He's incredible!"

But my mother didn't answer. There next to me, in front of everyone, with her head bent and eyes closed, my mother sat and prayed.

The hushed conversations came to a halt. And one by one, family and friends joined her in prayer. I wanted to tell them to stop, to say that this was crazy, but my eyes filled with tears and the lump in my throat stopped me from speaking.

Then I felt it; a cool hand on my forehead, a certainty in my being, and suddenly the invisible hand that was squeezing the life out of my heart loosened its grip. As my vision cleared, I saw a scene I will never forget. There in front of me were about a hundred people, all silent and praying and beseeching God on my behalf. Behind them was my father's closed casket and in the distance the sound of the approaching ambulance. My mother's face, so old and sad this morning, looked young and beautiful, and when I told her that I was going to be all right, she smiled and told me that she already knew.

Dr. Vagnini was waiting for us at the hospital. I thought that we must have seemed strangely serene, but he later told us that we were not the first to take his advice and to literally find the answer to our prayers.

It's been three years since that day. I celebrate it as my rebirth-day. With Dr. Vagnini's help I have turned my life around. I eat carbohydrates only once a day. I mall-walk three times a week, and I take the chromium he recommends. I have lost more than forty pounds, and my blood pressure is normal. I sustained no permanent damage from the heart attack, and Dr. Vagnini, God bless him, has taught me a lot about the unity of medicine and faith.

I no longer take my health or my life for granted. I eat right, I live right, and I have found a faith in God that would have made my father very happy.

MY FAITHFUL HUSBAND: ELLEN'S STORY

Somebody once said, "If you want to make sure your youngster doesn't become Catholic, send her to Catholic boarding school." Well, apparently my father never heard that piece of wisdom. While I was in grade school, my parents divorced. My father, who had custody of me, sent me off to Catholic boarding school within days of the divorce becoming final. By the time I was twelve, I hated everybody—my father, my mother, my sister (who was imprisoned in this snake pit with me), the nuns, and most of all a God who would have allowed nuns to beat me and shame me so much that I wished I were dead.

I lived the rest of my life in secrecy. My husband, Chris, and my kids rarely saw me unprotected. I decided what I would reveal and what was all for myself, and I guarded my real thoughts like a mother lion protecting her cubs. My husband was not Catholic, and it didn't take much for me to pull him away from his own church, which I attended for a limited time, more out of duty and guilt than out of love of God.

Chris never said much about religion. He didn't join in when I put it down, but he didn't defend it either. That's just the way he is: unless you push him, he doesn't say anything. That's why when he came home one night and said he wasn't feeling well, I got very scared.

We had not been to a doctor for longer than I liked to admit. We took the girls to their doctor whenever they were sick or needed a physical exam for school or camp, but for ourselves, well, that was something else.

Chris had been adopted, and we knew nothing about his natural parents. He had been overweight all his life, and now, as he approached fifty, his belly had become really big. I didn't care so much for myself, but I didn't like his labored breathing. At night he would keep me awake with his snoring—something he had never done when we were first married. He also had become a heavy snacker. On weekends it seemed as if he was eating from morning 'til night. We all teased him and he laughed about it, but I knew that he wasn't happy with his weight. But he was a salesman, and he didn't get any chance to exercise and was always eating on the road, so I let it go.

When Chris's old company started downsizing (a fancy word for firing people), he jumped ship and quickly got another job with its biggest competitor. It was a smart move, because within a few months all the available jobs had been taken. The one problem that he faced was the physical exam the new company required for insurance purposes. I remember Chris's joking that when his old company downsized, he should have, too.

The company doctor gave Chris the bad news on a Monday, and Chris didn't tell me until the following Friday morning. "I knew you'd put me on another diet," he told me later, and he was right.

Chris had been on more diets than anyone I had ever met. He would always go into it with all this enthusiasm, then start to give in and then give up. They coined the term *yo-yo dieting* just for him. But I knew it wasn't his fault. Some of his diets required counting calories; others would withhold foods; others made him measure or weigh his food. That just isn't Chris. He was hungry all the time, and sometimes I would give in and let him eat whatever he wanted. What I didn't even imagine was how close he was to a heart attack.

The company doctor had been shocked by Chris's blood pressure. He said that not only couldn't he okay him for the job, he thought that Chris should really be put into the hospital. The doctor had also taken blood tests. In the middle of Chris's telling me about the high blood pressure problem, the phone rang. It was the company doctor, and he informed us that the test results were not good. Chris's cholesterol was over 300, and the good and bad cholesterols were the opposite of what they should be. The doctor told us that Chris was heading straight for a heart attack. We thought he was going to give us the same old diet sheet, with portions and exchanges. But instead, he recommended a book on carbohydrate addiction.

Chris was out of the house in a flash. He said he wanted to get started right away, but I think he just wanted to avoid talking about it. When an hour had passed without his coming home, I began to get frightened. It was only a five-minute drive to the bookstore. I couldn't imagine what was keeping him. I figured that he had stopped to get a last meal before starting the diet, and I felt a lot better.

When he got home, Chris seemed different. He had the book under his arm and a smile on his face. He laid down the book and took me into his arms. He stroked my hair like he used to do when we were just married. His clothes smelled strange, and I could not figure out what was going on.

"I stopped into St. Barnabas's," he explained. I could hardly believe it, but I shrugged it off, attributing it to the bad medical news we had just received. If Chris needed a crutch right then, I could be big enough not to make fun of it. What I saw in the weeks that followed, however, was far more than a crutch.

As the weeks went by, Chris remained faithful to his diet and his faith. I did everything in my power to make it work. I didn't want to lose him. He read the book religiously, worked his program, and went to church. He began helping around the house and woke up early to spend some time with the children before they left. He religiously took his new morning walk, too. He was a changed man, and although I waited patiently for the old Chris I knew to reemerge, it never happened.

Instead, slowly but surely, he lost more than fifty pounds. He never complained about the diet, explaining that he wasn't hungry anymore. As his blood pressure went down, another position opened in the company, and this time he passed his physical exam with flying colors. It turned out to be a sweetheart of a job, and his territory was within driving distance of home. Church remained an important focus in his life, and it still is. I cannot join him in that part of his life; the scars I have are still too raw. But I can see in Chris the joy and peace his faith brings him. He prays every night.

I once asked Chris what he asked for when he prayed. He looked at me with a puzzled expression and shook his head.

"I don't ask for anything," he explained. "I just say 'thank you.'"

A PRAYER OF OUR OWN: THE AUTHORS' WISH

You hold in your hands the manifestation of our knowledge, our experience, and our prayers as well. These pages have turned our pain into purpose, and our struggles into resolve. The one wish that remains is our wish for you—for your health, well-being, and happiness.

From the depths of our souls, we send to you love and courage; in the years ahead may you discover all that you are and all that the gift of life holds for you. May you use your health in the pursuit of good and truth; may you never forget the power and importance of simple kindness; and may you live well and serve God and humanity, in a life of righteous and honorable pursuit.

11

HELPING HANDS
YOU ARE NOT ALONE

> Help, like food and wine, is sweetest when it is most needed.
> —*Benjamin Disraeli*

The Carbohydrate Addict's Healthy Heart Program is a tool to be used as part of an ongoing, heart health–enhancing relationship between you and your physician. Each of us has different needs, health concerns, and challenges, so before starting this program (as with any new program), you must consult with your physician.

Sometimes, however, your physician may not have the time, knowledge, or expertise to answer your questions, offer you ongoing encouragement, or provide the resources you need.

This chapter, the first part of which is in simple question-and-answer format, provides the names, contact addresses, phone numbers, and website addresses of resources that can offer you guidance, information, products, support, and encouragement. Where possible, in an effort to meet individual needs, more than one resource is specified. At the time this book was written, we found the resources that follow to be the very best. Because quality of service, availability, and consistency may change over time, however, we cannot take responsibility for any changes that may occur.

Many of the resources shown here are free; others are offered on a fee basis. In each case we have provided contact information and indicated whether a fee is required or a cost is involved. Please be aware that, over time, details change and may no longer reflect those resources available at the time this book was prepared.

Also, in addition to the resources that follow, at times you may be directed to other pages in this book. Referring you to these pages will ensure that, as a first step, you have read the information we have included. If you have already read the page(s) indicated, choose from among the other resources offered.

As always, begin with a visit to your physician, then move to other helping hands that may offer additional assistance as needed. Many of our research participants and patients have found that the circle is completed when they can return to their own physicians and share their newly discovered information as well as their personal experiences of improved heart health.

Some final words of encouragement: Your health is your most precious possession. With it, everything else is possible; without it, nothing is. Do not be afraid to speak out in defense of your health. Do not let others devalue your health or what you know in your heart to be valid and true. Guard your health and cherish it. And never, under any circumstances, be shamed or pressured into compromising it on someone else's behalf.

How can I incorporate low-fat and low-salt health agency dietary recommendations into my program?

Step-by-step suggestions for incorporating the health agency dietary guidelines of the U.S. Department of Health and Human Services (Department of Agriculture) and the American Heart Association's guidelines can be found on pages 307–312. As always, decisions should be made in consultation with your physician.

Where can I get more information on the program? Where can I get my questions answered?

The BASIC guidelines and Heart Health–Enhancing Options of The Carbohydrate Addict's Healthy Heart Program are contained within the pages of this book, but on occasion you might want additional information or clarification, or have questions you would like answered. Once you have read *the entire book*, if you feel you would like more information or still have questions, you may:

- Visit The Carbohydrate Addict's Official Website at www.carbohydrateaddicts.com, where you will find more than forty pages of

clear, up-to-date, and interesting information. (No cost involved; you must have internet access; to reach The Carbohydrate Addict's Official Website, see page 249.)
- Speak with a licensed nutritionist, by phone or in person, at The Cardiovascular Wellness Centers. (Fee involved; to contact The Cardiovascular Wellness Centers, see page 251.)
- Additional information can be found in other books on hyperinsulinemia by Drs. Richard and Rachael Heller. (Cost of book involved; for a full list of books by the Hellers and easy, discount ordering information, see page 250.)
- A listing of scientific articles and books that form the basis for The Carbohydrate Addict's Healthy Heart Program can be found beginning on page 313.
- For further information on the scientific basis for the Program, use free Medline, which enables you to do an internet data search of the best-known and most respected scientific publications. Search on the keywords *hyperinsulinemia* and *heart disease*. (No cost involved; must have internet access; for information on how to reach free Medline, see page 253.)

Where can I purchase supplements?
Supplements described in Chapter 6 can be purchased by phone or in person through The Cardiovascular Wellness Centers or at your local pharmacy, supermarket, or health food store. (Cost of supplement involved; to contact The Cardiovascular Wellness Centers, see page 251.)

Do you have any other books that might be helpful? Where can I get them?
Drs. Richard and Rachael Heller have written six other books on hyperinsulinemia and its impact on weight as well as a wide variety of health concerns, including adult-onset diabetes and cancer. They have focused on the psychological aspects of carbohydrate addiction in their workbook. They have also written books that focus on the needs of carbohydrate-addicted children as well as the needs of adults in their forties, fifties, sixties, and beyond. For a full list of books by the Hellers and easy, discount ordering information, see page 250.

Where can I go for testing and treatment to reduce my risk for insulin-related heart disease or to bring about insulin-related restoration of heart health?

Dr. Vagnini's Cardiovascular Wellness Centers, located in New York City and Long Island, New York, offer state-of-the-art testing and the latest in complementary, evidence-based medical treatment. (Fee involved; must be able to travel to New York; for contact information or to arrange for an appointment, see page 251.)

Where can I learn more about preventive medicine, particularly in relation to my heart health? How can I learn about important new heart-related breakthroughs?

- Subscribe to *Cardiovascular Wellness*, the monthly newsletter of Dr. Frederic J. Vagnini. (Subscription cost involved; to subscribe, see page 252.)
- Dr. Frederic J. Vagnini's *The Heart Show*, on WOR radio, 710 AM (New York), provides the latest in information on preventive medicine and heart health. If you live in the greater New York City tri-state area, you can hear Dr. Vagnini live on the radio on Sundays, 4–5 P.M. (Eastern). (No cost involved; must live in the New York City area or tri-state for radio access.)
- For additional information on research on preventive medicine and summaries on medical breakthroughs, use free Medline, which enables you to do an internet data search. (No cost involved; must have internet access; for information on how to reach free Medline, see page 253.)
- The American Heart Association offers information and guidelines related to a wide variety of heart diseases and heart disease risk factors. You can reach the AHA by phone or through the internet. (No cost involved; for contact information, see page 253.)

RESOURCES

THE CARBOHYDRATE ADDICT'S OFFICIAL WEBSITE

The Carbohydrate Addict's Official website offers more than forty pages of information, quizzes, personal stories, recipes, frequently asked questions, on-line support and chat groups, and books at discount. Links guide you through the website, and many visitors return again and again to learn more and share their discoveries with friends and family. (No cost involved;

internet access required.) You can find The Carbohydrate Addict's Official Website at:

http://www.carbohydrateaddicts.com

OTHER BOOKS BY DRS. RICHARD AND RACHAEL HELLER

All of the Hellers' books are available at your local bookstore. All titles are usually in stock, but if they are temporarily out of stock, you can simply ask someone at the store to order you a copy. Titles are available within only a few days. If you have internet access, you can order their books at a substantial discount through The Carbohydrate Addict's Official Website at http://www.carbohydrateaddicts.com (scroll down the page until you come to the link to books at discount).

- *The Carbohydrate Addict's Diet* (Signet, 1993, paperback): the original jump-start program for weight loss only.
- *The Carbohydrate Addict's Program for Success* (Plume, 1993, paperback): an interactive workbook for breaking free of the power of painful experiences, feelings, and thoughts so often connected to an addiction to carbohydrates.
- *The Carbohydrate Addict's Gram Counter* (Signet, 1993, paperback): pocket-sized powerhouse of food counts especially designed for the carbohydrate addict.
- *Healthy for Life* (Plume, 1996, paperback): a step-by-step program for weight loss and health enhancement.
- *The Carbohydrate Addict's Lifespan Program* (Signet, 1998, paperback): a jump-start program for weight loss and health enhancement with updated information on the impact of sugar substitutes, MSG, medications, and stress.
- *Carbohydrate-Addicted Kids* (HarperCollins, 1998, paperback): struggle-free, step-by-step, and jump-start programs for children and teens addicted to starches, junk foods, snack foods, and sweets.
- *The Carbohydrate Addict's Cookbook* (Wiley, 2000): 250 all-new low-carb recipes that will cut your cravings and keep you slim for life.

THE CARDIOVASCULAR WELLNESS CENTERS

The Cardiovascular Wellness Centers are located in New York City and Long Island, New York. Here, in state-of-the-art testing facilities, Dr. Frederic J. Vagnini offers the latest in complementary, evidence-based medical treatment. Patients are evaluated and given the newest in individualized approaches in the prevention and aggressive treatment of high blood pressure, adult-onset diabetes, obesity, risk-related blood fats, atherosclerosis, heart disease, and stroke.

Advanced testing procedures offered at The Cardiovascular Wellness Centers include blood vessel imaging for detection of arteriosclerosis and evaluation of change, high-resolution imaging of twenty-four blood vessel sites in order to detect and evaluate potential plaque problems, and advanced blood studies to detect a wide variety of heart disease risk factors.

Many insurance plans are accepted, and patients are offered pharmaceutical (drug), nutritional, and lifestyle treatments as appropriate.

Locations:

Cardiovascular Wellness Center
944 Park Avenue, New York, NY 10028
(212) 517-2500 or (888) HEART90 ([888] 432-7890)

Cardiovascular Wellness Center
1600 Stewart Avenue, Westbury, NY 11590
(516) 222-2288 or (888) HEART90 ([888] 432-7890)

(Fee involved; potential patients must be able to travel to the New York City area.)

Nutritional Counseling
For those who have questions or seek more information, individualized counseling, or motivational enhancement, a licensed nutritionist on staff at The Cardiovascular Wellness Centers is available for support and guidance. Consultations may be conducted in person or by phone. Appointments must be made in advance by calling The Cardiovascular Wellness Center at (516) 222-2288 or toll-free at (888) HEART90 ([888] 432-7890). (Fee involved; all major credit cards accepted.)

Supplements

Although the supplements discussed in Chapter 6 are available at your local pharmacy, supermarket, or health food store, you can also obtain these supplements directly from The Cardiovascular Wellness Centers. To order by phone, call (516) 222-2288 or (888) HEART90 ([888] 432-7890) toll-free. Or if you are near either of the centers (whose addresses were shown above), you can purchase your supplements in person. (Cost of supplement involved.)

The Cardiovascular Wellness Website

If you need more information about The Cardiovascular Wellness Centers, supplements, or Dr. Vagnini's newsletter, you will find all of this and more via the internet at www.vagnini.com.

Cardiovascular Wellness: Your Monthly Newsletter Link to Heart Health

Subscriptions to *Cardiovascular Wellness*, an informative monthly newsletter with features by Dr. Frederic J. Vagnini and his nutritionist, will keep you up to date on the newest in traditional and complementary breakthroughs in the prevention and treatment of heart disease. To subscribe for a fee, call (516) 222-2288 or call (888) HEART90 ([888] 432-7890) toll-free. You can also write to:

>Healthstar Publishing
>146 Sterling Avenue
>Greenport, NY 11944

The Heart Show

The Heart Show, on WOR radio, 710 AM, features Dr. Frederic Vagnini and provides the latest in information on preventive medicine and heart health. If you live in the New York City tri-state area, you can hear him live from four to five P.M. eastern standard time on Sundays. Dr. Vagnini's wide breadth of knowledge, fascinating in-studio experts, and call-in guests make this a not-to-be-missed experience. (No cost involved, but you must live in the New York City tri-state area.)

THE AMERICAN HEART ASSOCIATION

The American Heart Association can be reached by phone at (800) AHA-USA1 ([800] 242-8721) or through the internet at: http://www.amhrt.org. The AHA's mailing address is:

>The American Heart Association
>National Center
>7272 Greenville Avenue
>Dallas, TX 75231

FREE MEDLINE

Free Medline is a window on the world of science and medicine that will afford you access to the same studies that researchers and physicians use to keep up on the latest breakthroughs, techniques, and treatments. To reach free Medline, go to http://www.infotrieve.com and click the "free Medline" link. The site will guide you in searching summaries of relevant articles (choose all fields on the right for an optimal search). If you need assistance, a link is provided to help you perfect your search technique.

Although only summaries (called abstracts) are included in the free search, you can order the entire article for a fee, or if the medical journal is fairly recent, you can track down the journal on-line and see whether it offers the entire article (called full text) free on-line. Other options include checking with your local library, which can get you the article free or for a fee. In any case, even without the entire article, the abstracts will give you a starting point that familiarizes you with the most up-to-date research in the area of your choice and can help you begin a good dialogue with your physician. By the way, while you are on free Medline, try searching on the keywords *hyperinsulinemia* and *heart* and see what research scientists are learning each day about this vital link.

If the website address above is not working, you can find some suggestions by searching on the keywords *"free Medline"* with an internet search engine. Be careful never to choose fee-based links or alternatives unless that is your intent. (As described, no fee but must have internet access.)

THE TWO BEST RESOURCES OF ALL

This book would not be complete without our reminding you that you have within you the two best resources of all: your commitment to your own health and your connection to your higher power. Your willingness to learn new strategies, keep up on the latest in research findings, and seek your physician's advice, wisdom, and guidance, together with your strength and commitment, will serve you well. In addition, your connection to a higher power—be it spiritual, human, or nature—can likewise provide you with a vital source of strength and guidance that can bring you help, hope, and healing.

Our wish for you is simple: May you find all that you need in the pages you hold, in the world around you, and of course, within that most precious of places we call the soul. May you seek what you need and share in the process. May you find that health, happiness, hope, and freedom can be synonymous. Most of all, may you never forget that it is the joy of the journey that makes the adventure worthwhile.

PART FOUR

RECIPES FOR SUCCESS

12

EATING HEARTY, PART I:
LOW-CARBOHYDRATE RECIPES

By now, you are quite aware that The Carbohydrate Addict's Healthy Heart Program has been designed to reduce your release of insulin and, in so doing, to cut your risk for high blood pressure, obesity, risk-related blood fat levels, adult-onset diabetes, and heart disease.

At this point it should be clear that it is important for you to keep insulin levels balanced throughout the day. It is also important for you to have, and to enjoy, carbohydrates daily. Your daily Reward Meal provides you with high-carbohydrate foods in a balance with nutritious low-carbohydrate foods,* while your other daily meals and snacks contain only low-carbohydrate foods. In this way you can enjoy all the food you need and love while still reducing your insulin release and your risk for insulin-related heart disease as well as related illnesses and risk factors.

Chapter 12 includes many wonderful examples of low-carbohydrate recipes. Remember that only low-carbohydrate foods should be included in your low-carbohydrate meals or snacks. At your Reward Meals, however, low-carbohydrate foods should be combined with high-carbohydrate foods in an exciting and nourishing balance.

The low-carbohydrate recipes in this chapter are only examples of some of the many low-carbohydrate combinations that are possible. Here is an opportunity for you to play and use your creativity. You can devise an unlimited number of other low-carbohydrate recipes by combining foods

---

*For more information on Reward Meal balancing, see page 124.

> ## Low-Fat, Low–Saturated Fat, and Low-Salt Recommendations
>
> The Carbohydrate Addict's Healthy Heart Program is compatible with the low-fat, low–saturated fat, and low-salt health agency dietary recommendations of the U.S. Department of Health and Human Services (Department of Agriculture), the American Heart Association, and the American Cancer Society. As appropriate, and as recommended by your physician, choose low-fat, low–saturated fat, and/or low-salt alternatives as part of your daily meal plan.
>
> In the recipes that follow, you will find some suggestions for the inclusion of low-fat, low–saturated fat, and low-salt alternatives. Detailed recommendations related to low-fat, low–saturated fat, and low-salt substitutions can be found in "Incorporating Low-Fat, Low–Saturated Fat, Low-Salt, and Other Health Agency Dietary Recommendations into Your Program" (pages 307–312). Individualized dietary fat and salt recommendations should always be discussed with your physician.

found in the "Low-Carbohydrate Foods List," on page 132. When you plan your low-carbohydrate meals, remember to choose only those items found in the "Low-Carbohydrate Foods List."

As the name implies, low-carbohydrate foods are low in simple sugars and starches, so they do not stimulate your insulin release (and insulin resistance), thereby reducing your risks for insulin-related heart disease.

In this chapter, you will find some of our favorite low-carbohydrate recipes for:

- Breakfasts (page 261)
- Dressings and dips (page 264)
- Appetizers (page 267)
- Salads (page 269)
- Proteins: meats, poultry, and seafood (page 271)
- Vegetarian (nonmeat) alternatives (page 275)

All low-carbohydrate foods may be baked, boiled, broiled, poached, roasted, fried, or sautéed as per your physician's recommendations. Remember, for low-carbohydrate meals, it is important that you not use breading or batter of any kind.

We have included low-fat alternatives for those who are concerned about fat in their diets, and whenever possible, we have chosen recipes that feature olive oil (a source of monounsaturated fats) rather than butter or other foods that contain significant amounts of saturated fats. For suggestions on incorporating low-fat, low–saturated fat, low-salt, and other health agency dietary recommendations into The Carbohydrate Addict's Healthy Heart Program, see page 307.

Recipes can always be adjusted to desired change of the number of servings. If you were eating alone, for example, you might wish to reduce a recipe by half or by three-quarters, or you might choose to make the full recipe and refrigerate the remainder for the next day or freeze the leftovers for future meals. (It's always fun to have a delicious meal waiting in the freezer or refrigerator; just be certain to date all packages and eat these meals in a timely fashion.)

We actually keep an inventory of frozen foods, cooked and uncooked, on small Post-it notes pinned to a corkboard in the kitchen. Each shelf is color-coded, and colored pushpins holding the content cards help us easily locate frozen items and watch their dates to avoid leaving foods in the freezer for too long.

Important note: Remember that the low-carbohydrate recipes that follow provide dishes that can be enjoyed not only at your low-carbohydrate meals and snacks but, when balanced with high-carbohydrate foods, at Reward Meals, too.

HOW SWEET IT IS, UNFORTUNATELY

If you decide to include mayonnaise at any of your low-carbohydrate meals, make certain that you choose "regular" varieties only. Do not have any "low-fat" variety of mayonnaise at low-carbohydrate meals.

Low-fat varieties of mayonnaise often contain several forms of sugar in place of the fat that has been removed. These added sugars can increase your insulin release and in turn your insulin resistance.

Here's a trick we use to turn "regular" mayonnaise into a lower-fat alternative: simply "thin" regular mayonnaise with a small amount of water.

By adding cool water, a little at a time, and mixing well, you can reduce the fat content of regular mayonnaise by one-quarter to one-third—without adding any sugar. And you will be surprised at how little effect it has on the consistency of the mayonnaise.

THE CARBOHYDRATE ADDICT'S MAGIC BOX

Microwave ovens can be a real blessing to those who love good cooking but find themselves very short on time (sounds like most of us!).

You can use your microwave to warm up refrigerated or frozen leftovers, at home or at work. In a matter of minutes, you can serve up a wonderful, homemade treat. Once you try it and find out how easy it is to plan a bit ahead, you will find yourself making double and triple portions of your favorite recipes, just so you can enjoy the leftovers in the days to come. We even know one woman who purchased her own microwave oven to use at work. She swears that her investment paid for itself within a few weeks by saving her the cost of ordering in from a local restaurant and that she "eats like a queen" while getting healthier at the same time. Her feasts are said to be the envy of the office, and she loves every minute of them.

So plan ahead and use your energy, creativity, and the conveniences available to take good (and delicious) care of yourself.

LOW-CARBOHYDRATE BREAKFASTS

FREEDOM FRITTATA
SERVES 3

Add your favorite leftover low-carbohydrate vegetables and protein and cook up a great start for your day. Wonderful for brunch, lunch, or as the mainstay of a light Reward Meal dinner as well.

6	eggs (or low-fat substitute)	Salt to taste
1½	tablespoons olive oil	Pepper to taste
2	cups diced, cooked low-carbohydrate vegetables (mushrooms, spinach, celery, cauliflower, green peppers, etc.) and protein (chicken, seafood, meat, or tofu)	

Beat the eggs well and pour into a heated, greased 10-inch frying pan. After the eggs set fully, forming a solid pancake, gently flip it over. Spoon the diced vegetable-protein combination on one half of the egg pancake and fold the other half over to cover.
Flip the egg pancake and cook fully on the other side.
Serve with cool slices of cucumber as a special wake-up treat.

HIGH-FIBER STUFFED MUSHROOMS
SERVES 3-4

A great low-carbo breakfast or brunch.

8	large mushroom caps, fresh	1	large green pepper, drained and finely chopped
4	teaspoons olive oil		
1	tablespoon minced garlic	4	large eggs (or low-fat substitute)
10	ounces clean, fresh spinach leaves, drained and coarsely chopped		Salt to taste
			Pepper to taste
¼	teaspoon sweet dried basil		

Preheat the oven to 400°F.

Arrange the mushrooms, rounded side down, in a medium glass baking dish and sprinkle with salt and pepper.

Bake until tender (12–15 minutes), then remove from the oven and place on a plate. Reduce oven temperature to 250°F.

Put 3 teaspoons of oil in a large skillet and place over medium heat. Add the garlic and sauté until brown (2–3 minutes).

Add the spinach and toss until wilted (2–3 minutes). Stir in the basil.

Arrange the spinach in the same baking dish. Carefully arrange the mushrooms, rounded side down, and fill each cap halfway with peppers. Place in the oven to keep warm.

Blend the eggs in a medium bowl. Sprinkle with additional salt and pepper.

Heat 1 teaspoon of oil in a medium skillet over medium heat. Pour the eggs into the skillet and stir until softly set (2–3 minutes).

Fill the mushroom caps with the scrambled eggs. Top each mushroom cap with 1 tablespoon of peppers. Divide the spinach and mushrooms among 3–4 plates.

BREAKFAST QUICHE SANS CRUST   SERVES 5–6

Breakfast was never so good as this wonderful treat, served hot or cold. Choose low-fat alternatives as appropriate.

1	teaspoon olive oil	2	teaspoons sweet dried basil
1	cup light cream (or low-fat milk)*	1/4	tablespoon dried paprika
1	cup grated cheese (American, cheddar, Parmesan, or Swiss, regular or low-fat varieties)	4	eggs (no low-fat substitutes)
			Salt to taste
			Ground black pepper to taste

Preheat the oven to 325°F.

Oil the bottom and sides of a 9-inch pie pan.

Put the cream (or milk) in a medium saucepan and heat until scalded. Reduce the heat and stir in the grated cheese.

---

*If this dish is included in a low-carbohydrate meal, refrain from adding non–Reward Meal milk to coffee or tea that day.

When the cheese is melted, add the basil and paprika.
Remove the saucepan from the heat and cool for 5 minutes. Then add one egg at a time and mix in thoroughly until all the eggs are used. Salt and pepper to taste and mix well.
Pour the mixture into the pie pan, place it in the oven, and bake until the quiche is set (45–50 minutes).
Serve hot or cold.

BREAKFAST TURKEY SAUSAGE TREAT   SERVES 5–6

Nothing like some tasty protein to start a busy day.

2	pounds ground turkey	1/2	teaspoon ground cloves
1	tablespoon dried sage	1/2	teaspoon nutmeg
1	tablespoon soy sauce	1	teaspoon olive oil for frying
1/2	teaspoon ground pepper		
1/2	teaspoon dried sweet basil		

Combine all the ingredients except the oil in a large bowl and mix well.
Divide the mixture into 20 equal portions and shape each into a patty about 1 1/2 inches in diameter.
Put the oil in a large frying pan and place the pan over moderate heat.
When the pan is hot, brown the patties on both sides (making sure that they are cooked thoroughly).
Serve with sliced cucumbers, celery stalks, or string beans.
Freeze any remaining patties for future use.

LOW-CARBOHYDRATE DRESSINGS AND DIPS

SUMPTUOUS CREAMY DRESSING **MAKES ABOUT 1 CUP**

Elegant enjoyment at any meal.

3	ounces cream cheese	1/2	teaspoon prepared mustard
1/4	cup olive oil		Salt to taste
1	tablespoon white vinegar		Coarse ground black pepper to taste
2	teaspoons garlic, finely minced		

Cut the cream cheese into small chunks, then beat until smooth.
Add the oil and vinegar gradually. Beat until blended.
Add the garlic, mustard, salt, and pepper. Beat until blended completely.
Chill and enjoy as a dip or dressing.

BASIC GARLIC DRESSING **MAKES ABOUT 1 CUP**

A dressing that will perk up any salad.

1/2	teaspoon mustard powder (mild or spicy, as desired)	1/3	cup white vinegar
		2/3	cup olive oil
			Salt to taste
2	garlic cloves, finely minced		Coarse ground black pepper to taste

Combine and mix the mustard, salt, and black pepper in a bowl or large jar.
Add the remaining ingredients to the mixture and shake or stir until thoroughly mixed.
Let sit for an hour before use.

GREEN GARDEN MAYONNAISE DRESSING MAKES ABOUT 1 CUP

An unusual dressing. Family and friends won't believe how easy it is.

1	stalk celery and leaves	1	tablespoon dried sweet basil
5	spinach leaves		
5	scallions, finely chopped	1/2	cup mayonnaise*

Chop the celery and leaves, spinach, and scallions in a blender or food processor.
Add the sweet basil and mayonnaise. Blend well.
Use as a topping on vegetables, fish, chicken, or fresh green salads.

TANGY CREAM CHEESE DIP MAKES 2 CUPS

Adds a spicy lift to raw vegetables.

8	ounces of cream cheese	1	teaspoon minced garlic
2	tablespoons sweet basil flakes	2	tablespoons olive oil
2	tablespoons prepared horseradish	1/2	cup water

Cut the cream cheese into medium chunks and place them in a mixing bowl.
Add the basil, horseradish, garlic, and olive oil and mix thoroughly.
Add the water and mix thoroughly. (If you prefer a thinner dip, add more water.)

---

*Do not use low-fat mayonnaise at low-carbohydrate meals or snacks; lower-fat varieties of mayonnaise often contain added sugars. For an easy low-fat, low-carbohydrate mayonnaise alternative, thin "regular" mayonnaise with a little water at a time and mix well. Using this method, you can reduce the fat up to one-half.

TANGY CLAM DIP

MAKES 1²/₃ CUPS

A dip that complements raw vegetables.

- 2 cans minced clams (6–8 ounces each), drained
- 1 cup sour cream (or low-fat substitute)
- 1/4 teaspoon garlic powder
- 1/2 teaspoon salt
- Cayenne pepper to taste

Combine the drained clams, sour cream, garlic powder, salt, and cayenne pepper in a large bowl and mix well.

Place the mixture in a serving bowl and chill for 1 hour.

If desired, garnish with a light sprinkle of paprika and parsley.

Surround with crisp, fresh vegetables, such as cauliflower, celery, green peppers, green beans, and raw mushrooms.

SPICY SPINACH DIP

SERVES 5–6

A piping hot dip that is a sparkling preview of things to come.

- 1 package (10 ounces) frozen, chopped spinach, defrosted and drained (retain water)
- 1 tablespoon chopped chives
- 2 tablespoons butter
- 3 ounces jalapeño pepper cheese, grated
- 1/4 cup sour cream (or low-fat substitute)
- 1/4 teaspoon ground black pepper
- 1/2 teaspoon garlic powder
- 1/4 cup spinach water
- 1/4 teaspoon celery seed
- Salt to taste

Cook the spinach following the instructions on the package.

Drain the cooked spinach and retain the water.

Cook the chives in butter in a medium saucepan until they are flaccid.

Add the spinach and the remaining ingredients and cook over low heat, stirring occasionally, until the cheese is melted and the mixture is creamy.

LOW-CARBOHYDRATE APPETIZERS

TANGY FILLED MUSHROOMS   SERVES 3–4

A special appetizer or snack requiring little work and easily prepared a day ahead of time.

8	medium-sized fresh mushrooms	1/2	teaspoon minced fresh chives
1	tablespoon butter	1/4	teaspoon salt
2	ounces cream cheese	1	tablespoon paprika
1	tablespoon horseradish	1	tablespoon olive oil
1/2	teaspoon dried sweet basil		Ground black pepper to taste
1/2	tablespoon heavy cream (or milk)		

Preheat the oven to 350°F.

Remove and discard the mushroom stems; wash and dry the caps.

Put the butter in a shallow baking pan (microwavable or conventional) and place it in the oven to melt.

Combine the cream cheese, horseradish, basil, cream, chives, salt, and black pepper to taste and blend thoroughly.

Spoon a generous amount of the blended ingredients into each inverted mushroom cap and sprinkle with paprika.

Coat a shallow baking dish with the olive oil, then place the mushroom caps into the dish and bake in the oven for 10–15 minutes.

Remove the mushrooms from the oven and place them on a serving tray, garnishing with parsley and toothpicks.

DEVILED EGGS

SERVES 6

A favorite standard.

12	eggs*†	1	tablespoon mild prepared mustard
1/4	cup mayonnaise*		
1	teaspoon horseradish	1	tablespoon paprika
2	tablespoons green pepper, diced		

Place a large saucepan 3/4 filled with water over high heat, bringing the water to a boil.
Using a spoon, lower the eggs one at a time into the boiling water.
Boil the eggs until they are hard (10 minutes).
Cool the eggs in cold water, then remove their shells and slice them in half lengthwise.
Scoop out the yolks, place them in a mixing bowl, and mash them.
Add the mayonnaise, horseradish, green pepper, and mustard and mix thoroughly.
Spoon the blended mixture into the egg white halves. Sprinkle with paprika and serve on a bed of lettuce.

*Eat only on occasion and at that time avoid other foods high in saturated fat.
†Do not use low-fat mayonnaise at low-carbohydrate meals or snacks; lower-fat varieties of mayonnaise often contain added sugars. For an easy low-fat, low-carbohydrate mayonnaise alternative, thin "regular" mayonnaise with a little water at a time and mix well. Using this method, you can reduce the fat up to one-half.

STUFFED CELERY

SERVES 2–4

An unusual twist on a savory appetizer or snack that is best prepared the day before.

2	tablespoons olive oil	6	celery stalks, trimmed and washed
1/4	pound chopped chicken or meat, raw	1	teaspoon dried basil
1	tablespoon horseradish		Salt to taste
2	ounces cream cheese, at room temperature		Ground black pepper to taste

Put the olive oil in a medium skillet and place it over medium heat.
Add the meat or chicken and sauté until browned.
Finely chop the meat or chicken and set it aside to cool.

Combine the horseradish and cream cheese with the meat or chicken and then add the remaining ingredients.
Spoon the mixture into the celery stalks.
Chill well before serving.

LOW-CARBOHYDRATE SALADS

FLAKE TUNA SALAD WITH DRESSING

SERVES 3–4

A good blend of fiber and protein that is fun to make and eat.

1	cup celery, diced	1	tablespoon mayonnaise
1	cup green peppers, diced	1/4	teaspoon thyme, dried
1	cup mushrooms, sliced	1/4	teaspoon dried sweet basil
1	can tuna in water, drained	1/4	teaspoon ground oregano
3	tablespoons white vinegar		Ground black pepper to taste
2	tablespoons olive oil		

Combine the celery, peppers, mushrooms, and drained tuna in a large salad bowl. Set the mixture aside.
Combine the vinegar, olive oil, mayonnaise, thyme, basil, and oregano in a separate bowl and blend thoroughly.
Pour the dressing mixture over the salad and toss until the mixture is uniformly distributed. Pepper to taste.
Serve immediately or chill first.

SEAFOOD SALAD

SERVES 3–4

Bounty of sea and land, this lunch or snack will delight anyone.

2	tablespoons olive oil	1/2	cup cucumber, coarsely chopped
1/2	teaspoon powdered garlic		
2/3	pound medium shrimp, cooked, cleaned, and deveined	1/2	cup celery, chopped
			Coarse black pepper to taste
1/4	pound sea scallops		
1/4	pound fresh fish of choice, cut into small pieces		

Place the olive oil, powdered garlic, shrimp, scallops, and fish in a large bowl and toss until garlic and oil coat all pieces.

Boil, broil, or sauté the mixture until all the seafood is cooked, then cool.

Combine the cooled mixture in a large bowl and then add the cucumber, celery, and pepper to taste.

Add your favorite dressing and toss lightly, cover, and chill for 2 hours.

Serve on a cool bed of large lettuce leaves.

CABBAGE DELIGHT

SERVES 3–4

Cabbage never tasted so good.

2 1/2	cups water	1/8	teaspoon dried sweet basil
1/4	teaspoon salt	1	bay leaf
4	cups red or green cabbage	1	large garlic clove, quartered lengthwise
1/8	teaspoon cumin	1	cup white vinegar
1/8	teaspoon dried oregano		

Combine 2 cups of water and the salt in a large bowl. Mix well.

Add the cabbage and soak 8–12 minutes. Drain and discard the liquid.

Combine the cabbage, cumin, oregano, basil, bay leaf, garlic, vinegar, and remaining water in a medium saucepan.

Cover and bring to a rapid boil.

Remove from the heat immediately, uncover, and allow to cool.

Serve with your favorite protein.

SPROUT 'N' CHEF SALAD

SERVES 3–4

A surprisingly satisfying salad topped off with any low-carbohydrate dressing.

2	cups fresh spinach, washed and drained	4	ounces real chicken breast, cut in julienne strips (not deli)
1	cup fresh bean sprouts or alfalfa sprouts	2	ounces hard cheese, such as Swiss or cheddar (regular or low-fat), cut in julienne strips
¼	cup chopped green pepper		
¼	cup chopped celery		
½	cup thinly sliced cucumber	1	sliced hard-boiled egg (optional)

Gently combine the spinach, sprouts, green pepper, celery, and cucumber in a large bowl.

Top with chicken, cheese strips, and egg slices, as desired.

Toss with low-carbohydrate dip or dressing.

LOW-CARBOHYDRATE PROTEINS: MEATS, POULTRY, AND SEAFOOD

PEPPERED FILLET OF CHICKEN

SERVES 3–4

A wonderful dish, warm or cold.

2	large boneless chicken breasts	1	tablespoon coarse ground black pepper
4	large garlic cloves, slivered	1	teaspoon dried sweet basil
1	tablespoon olive oil		
1	tablespoon paprika		

Preheat the oven to 350°F.

Cut down the center of each chicken breast with a sharp knife, forming four half breasts.

With the pointed tip of the knife tip, poke 1-inch slits into the surface of each half breast and insert a garlic sliver into each slit until all slivers are used. Try to distribute the slivers evenly over the surface.

Pour the oil over the surface and sprinkle with the paprika, black pepper, and basil.

Put the chicken breasts on a roasting rack in a shallow roasting pan, then place the pan in the oven.

Bake for 40–45 minutes or until the chicken turns golden brown.

CAULIFLOWER AND HAM SUPREME   SERVES 3–4

A once-in-a-while special treat.

½	cauliflower, cut into one-inch cubes	1	cup grated cheddar cheese° (or low-fat substitute)
4	very lean precooked ham steaks (approximately 4 ounces each)°	½	teaspoon salt
		1	tablespoon Dijon mustard
2	tablespoons olive oil		
4	tablespoons sour cream° (regular or low-fat)		

Preheat the oven to 350°F.

Put 1 inch of water in a deep skillet, add the cauliflower, and place it over high heat.

Cover and heat for 2–3 minutes.

Turn off the heat, pour off the water, and keep the skillet covered.

Arrange the ham steaks in a medium casserole dish and spread an equal amount of cubed cauliflower over each chop.

Heat the olive oil in a small saucepan, then reduce the heat and add the remaining ingredients, stirring until completely mixed.

Pour the sauce over the cauliflower and ham steaks.

Place the casserole dish in the oven and cook until hot (8–10 minutes).

°Eat only on occasion, and at that time avoid other foods high in saturated fat.

EGG FOO YUNG

SERVES 3–4

Delicious and satisfying at any meal.

- 2 tablespoons olive oil
- 1 slice gingerroot, minced
- 6 scallions, thinly sliced
- 1 stalk celery, thinly sliced
- 3 cups cooked meat, chicken, or seafood, finely chopped
- 6 eggs, beaten well (or egg substitute)
- 2 cups bean sprouts
- Salt to taste
- Fresh ground pepper to taste

Stir-fry the gingerroot, scallions, celery, and cooked meat, seafood, or chicken in 1 tablespoon of oil in a medium skillet or wok.

Cook until translucent and crisp. Remove from heat.

Fold in all the other ingredients except the remaining oil.

Oil a large skillet with the remaining oil and drop the mixture as small omelettes onto the hot surface.

Cook until golden brown on both sides.

If served as a Reward Meal, top with soy sauce.°

CLASSIC PORK ROAST

SERVES 5–6

Delightful to the eye and the nose, it is the palate that is the final test.

- 2 pounds boneless pork roast°
- 2 tablespoons olive oil
- 2 tablespoons sesame oil
- 1 tablespoon paprika
- 2 tablespoons garlic powder
- Ground black pepper to taste

Preheat the oven to 350°F.

Place a meat thermometer in the thickest part of the pork roast, then put the roast on a rack in a roasting pan with 1 inch of water on the bottom.

°For more information on soy sauce, see pages 139–143.

Combine the oils, mix, and pour over the top of the roast. Sprinkle on garlic powder and paprika to form a powder on the oil, which will turn to crust. Pepper as desired.

Roast about 2½ hours (until the appropriate temperature is reached on the meat thermometer).

Trim any visible fat and serve warm or cold with high-fiber vegetables.

BROILED FISH OF YOUR CHOICE   SERVES 3–4

Got a favorite fresh fish? Here's a simple recipe that will delight both you and others.

1½	pounds of your favorite fish	2	garlic cloves or powder equivalent (optional)
⅛	teaspoon paprika		Salt to taste
2	tablespoons mayonnaise*		Ground black pepper to taste
1	tablespoon dried basil		
1	tablespoon prepared mustard		

Place a greased broiler rack or broiling pan at a level about 2 inches below the broiler flame.

Preheat the broiler.

Wash the fish and sprinkle it with salt, pepper, and paprika.

Combine the mayonnaise, basil, garlic, and mustard in a mixing bowl.

Place the fish on the preheated broiler rack.

Coat the top of the fish with half the mixture of mayonnaise, basil, garlic, and mustard. Broil for 3 minutes.

Turn the fish and coat with the remaining mixture. Broil for 4–5 more minutes until thoroughly cooked but not overdone.

If desired, garnish with watercress. Delicious hot or cold.

*Do not use low-fat mayonnaise at low-carbohydrate meals or snacks; lower-fat varieties of mayonnaise often contain added sugars. For an easy low-fat, low-carbohydrate mayonnaise alternative, thin "regular" mayonnaise with a little water at a time and mix well. Using this method, you can reduce the fat up to one-half.

BROILED LAMB CHOPS

SERVES 4–6

A tasty dish with a delicate flavor.

2	large garlic cloves, crushed	6	thick loin lamb chops
2	tablespoons sage		Coarse ground black pepper to taste
2	tablespoons rosemary		Parsley sprigs
2	tablespoons thyme		

Combine the garlic, sage, rosemary, thyme, and pepper in a small bowl. Mix well.

Coat both sides of the chops with the mixture and press the mixture into the chops. Cover and refrigerate overnight.

Broil the chops about 6–7 minutes per side, until thoroughly done, and serve hot with a garnish of parsley sprigs.

LOW-CARBOHYDRATE VEGETARIAN (NONMEAT) ALTERNATIVES

THE ULTIMATE TOFU BURGERS

SERVES 3–4

Delight your family, friends, and relatives with this healthful dish.

2	medium garlic cloves, minced	1	pound of extra-firm tofu,* mashed
1/2	large green pepper, minced	2	large eggs
		1	teaspoon dried sweet basil
2	celery stalks, trimmed and minced	1/2	cup grated mild cheddar cheese (regular or low-fat)
2	tablespoons olive oil		

Preheat the oven to 350°F.

Combine the garlic, green pepper, celery, and olive oil in a medium skillet and mix well.

Place the skillet over medium heat and sauté the mixture for 1–2 minutes.

---

*For more information on tofu, see page 220.

Combine the vegetable mixture, tofu, eggs, basil, and cheese in a medium bowl.
Shape into 3-inch patties and place them on a greased cookie tray.
Place in the oven and heat for 25–30 minutes.
Serve warm on a bed of cucumber slices or lettuce.

TOFU WITH CABBAGE AND MUSHROOMS   SERVES 3–4

A marvelous meatless combination of low-carbohydrate foods.

2½	cups water	1	teaspoon white vinegar
1	small cabbage head, thinly sliced	1	teaspoon dried sweet basil
8	medium mushrooms, sliced	2	tablespoons prepared horseradish
1	pound firm tofu,° cut into ¼-inch cubes	4	large lettuce leaves
			Cucumber slices

Put 2 cups of water, cabbage, and mushrooms in a medium saucepan and place the pan over low heat.
Simmer until the vegetables are soft (8–10 minutes).
As the vegetables simmer, put the tofu cubes and the remaining water in a second saucepan and boil for 1–2 minutes.
Drain the boiled tofu and mash with a fork or potato masher.
Add the vinegar, dried basil, and horseradish and mix well.
Combine the drained vegetables and the mashed tofu combination in a large mixing bowl. Mix thoroughly.
Let sit for 5 minutes, then serve on a bed of lettuce leaves and garnish with cucumber slices.

°For more information on tofu, see page 220.

VEGETARIAN SAUTÉED "CHICKEN"   SERVES 5–6

Interesting contrasts in flavor highlight this unassuming but wonderful dish.

2	tablespoons olive oil	1	garlic clove, crushed
6	vegetable "chicken" slices, 3 inches in diameter*		Ground black pepper to taste
			Salt to taste
1	teaspoon dried sweet basil		Parsley sprigs

Put the oil and "chicken" in a large skillet and place over medium heat.
Brown the "chicken" on both sides (3 minutes each), remove from the skillet, and set aside.
Add the basil and garlic to the skillet and cook for 2 additional minutes.
Return the "chicken" to the skillet and simmer for 3 minutes.
Pepper and salt to taste. Garnish with parsley.
Serve with your favorite low-carbo.

VEGETARIAN "STEAK" CASSEROLE   SERVES 5–6

Your guests will never ask, "Where's the beef?"

2	tablespoons olive oil	1½	cups sour cream (or low-fat substitute)
6–8	vegetarian "steaklets"*	3	garlic cloves, crushed
1	large green pepper, chopped	2	teaspoons gingerroot, freshly grated
½	cup water		
6	sticks celery, chopped		

Preheat the oven to 350°F.
Coat the bottom of a deep casserole dish using 1 tablespoon of oil.
Add the remaining oil to a saucepan and place over medium heat.
Add the pepper, celery, garlic, and gingerroot and sauté over medium heat until light brown.

*Containing no more than 4 grams of carbohydrate per average serving.

Cut the "steaklets" into 1-inch squares and add them to the saucepan over medium heat, mix the contents thoroughly, and sauté for 4 minutes.

Pour the mixture into the casserole dish.

Combine the water and sour cream in a small bowl and pour the mixture over the casserole.

Cover and bake for 30–35 minutes.

13

EATING HEARTY, PART II
HIGH-CARBOHYDRATE, REWARD MEAL RECIPES

"What can I include in my daily Reward Meals?" The combinations are limitless! Since your Reward Meals are made up of a balance of low-carbohydrate vegetables and proteins along with high-carbohydrate foods, once each day you are free to enjoy your favorite foods, including fruit, fruit juice, bread, pasta, potatoes and other starchy vegetables, rice, and desserts (though not all on the same day!).

A balanced Reward Meal is essential to insulin balance and a lowered risk for insulin-related heart disease. Although many of the recipes that follow may be high-carbohydrate, the rest of your Reward Meal must include appropriate amounts of salad, low-carbohydrate vegetables, and protein (see page 125 for important details on balancing your Reward Meal). The Reward Meal is not a binge. The key word here is *balanced*. It is a balanced feast of celebration of the joys of eating for health. Never select high-carbohydrate foods exclusively as your entire Reward Meal; always include an appropriate balance of low-carbohydrate foods as well.

The high-carbohydrate recipes that follow are examples of foods that should be enjoyed only during your Reward Meals. Any of the foods that you enjoy during your Reward Meals may be baked, boiled, broiled, fried (with breading or batter if you like), poached, roasted, or sautéed. As always, keep your physician's advice regarding the amount of fat, types of fat, salt, and other dietary recommendations in mind. For suggestions on easy ways to incorporate dietary recommendations into this program, see

Making Low-Fat, Low–Saturated Fat, and Low-Salt Choices

In the recipes that follow, we have provided suggestions for low-fat, low–saturated fat, and low-salt alternatives. Detailed recommendations related to low-fat, low–saturated fat, and low-salt substitutions as per the U.S. Department of Health and Human Services (Department of Agriculture) and American Heart Association Guidelines can be found in "Incorporating Low-Fat, Low–Saturated Fat, Low-Salt, and Other Health Agency Dietary Recommendations into Your Program" (pages 307–312). Dietary fat and salt recommendations should always be discussed with your physician.

pages 307–312. You are free to include any recipe you like in your balanced daily Reward Meal. Here's where you get a chance to enjoy your "old favorites" or explore new recipes, and we have included some of our favorite Reward Meal recipes here as well.

Remember, an entire world of recipes is now open for inclusion in your (balanced!) Reward Meals, including recipes for:

- Breakfasts (page 281)
- Appetizers (page 283)
- Dressings and dips (page 286)
- Salads (page 288)
- Soups (page 290)
- Proteins: meats, poultry, and seafood (page 292)
- Desserts (page 297)
- Vegetarian (nonmeat) alternatives (page 301)

As with the low-carbohydrate meal recipes in Chapter 12, we have included low-fat alternatives for those who are concerned about fat in their diets.

Remember that you are free to adjust these recipes to change the number of servings. For example, if you are having guests, you may want to double a recipe, or if you are eating alone, you may wish to reduce a recipe by half or three-quarters. In most cases you can make the full recipe and refrigerate the remainder for the next day or freeze the "leftovers" for future meals. Unless otherwise indicated, leftover high-carbohydrate foods should be saved for your next Reward Meal only.

As always, you are free to go back for "seconds" or even "thirds" at times,* but each time you go back, be certain to balance your high-carbohydrate foods with the right proportion of low-carbohydrate foods as well.

> The Reward Meal is not a binge.
> It is a balanced feast of celebration of
> the joys of eating for health.

REWARD MEAL BREAKFASTS

Remember that Reward Meal breakfasts, like all Reward Meals, should be balanced. See page 124.

WHOLE-WHEAT TOAST BROIL　　　　　　　　　　　　　　　　SERVES 3–4

Light and surprisingly hearty.

- 8 slices whole-wheat bread
- 8 large slices tomato
- 8 slices cheddar cheese (or low-fat substitute)
- 2 tablespoons fresh scallions, diced

Preheat the oven to broil.
Lightly toast the whole-wheat bread slices.
Place the toasted bread slices on a cookie sheet, cover each with a tomato slice, and top with a slice of cheddar cheese.
Place the cookie sheet in the oven and broil until the cheese topping is light brown (2–3 minutes).
Remove from the oven, sprinkle the bread slices with scallions, and serve immediately.

---

*Always keep your own physician's recommendations in mind.

PANCAKES SUPREME

SERVES 3–4

A warm and wonderful breakfast treat, rich in protein.

4	large eggs°	1 1/2	tablespoons baking powder
1/2	cup sugar		
1/4	cup mild olive oil	1/4	teaspoon salt
2	cups all-purpose flour	1	apple, skinned and diced
1	cup milk (regular or low-fat)	2	cups ham steak,° diced
			Mild olive oil, as needed

Preheat the oven to 250°F.

Beat the eggs, sugar, and oil in a mixer or by hand until blended.

Add the flour alternately with the milk in 3 additions, blending after each addition. Blend in the baking powder and salt.

Add the diced apple and ham and mix gently.

Grease a skillet (or griddle). Place the skillet over medium heat until hot.

Ladle a scant 3/4 cup of batter into the skillet, rotating the skillet to spread the batter into a pancake about 6 inches in diameter.

Heat the pancake until bubbles form on the top and the bottom is brown (about 1 minute). Turn the pancake and brown the other side (about 1 minute).

Transfer the pancake to a large baking sheet and place it in the oven to keep warm. Repeat with the remaining batter to form 7 more pancakes, adding more oil to the skillet as necessary.

Serve with low-fat turkey bacon or low-fat sausage. Preserves or syrup is optional, depending on the rest of your balanced Reward Meal breakfast.

°Eat this combination only on occasion, and at that time avoid other foods high in saturated fat.

FRENCH WHOLE-WHEAT TOAST

SERVES 3–4

A high-fiber twist on an old favorite.

6	eggs, slightly beaten	8	slices whole-wheat bread
1	tablespoon salt	2	teaspoons ground cinnamon
7	tablespoons sugar		
1½	cups milk (regular or low-fat)		

Mix the eggs, salt, 3 tablespoons of sugar, and milk in a shallow dish or pie pan.

Soak the bread in the mixture until soft, turning once.

Cook on a hot, well-greased skillet or frying pan, turning to brown on each side.

Combine the remaining sugar and ground cinnamon and sprinkle the mixture on top of the French toast slices.

Serve the crusty slices with low-fat turkey bacon or low-fat sausage. Butter, preserves, or syrup is optional, depending on the rest of your balanced Reward Meal breakfast.

REWARD MEAL APPETIZERS

Appetizers should be enjoyed after you complete your Reward Meal salad.

MARINATED BEEF STRIPS

SERVES 3–4

More than just an appetizer served on toothpicks, these tasty little strips will disappear from the serving plate faster than you can bring them out.

1½	pounds lean beef steak	1	tablespoon minced chives
1	cup red wine or tarragon vinegar	2	garlic cloves, minced
2	tablespoons teriyaki sauce*	¼	cup sesame seeds
1	tablespoon sugar	1	tablespoon olive oil

Trim all fat from the steak and, if it is thick, split it once lengthwise. Then cut the steak diagonally into thin slices.

*For more information on teriyaki sauce, see page 143.

Combine all the remaining ingredients in a medium bowl and add the steak strips.
Cover and marinate in the refrigerator for 3–4 hours, basting and turning frequently.
Remove the steak from the refrigerator, drain, and set the marinade aside.
Oil a large skillet and preheat it over medium heat.
Place the steak strips into the skillet and brown on each side, until tender (5–8 minutes per side).
Add the marinade to the skillet and simmer for an additional 20 minutes, until cooked thoroughly.
Remove the steak strips and serve on cocktail toothpicks, with the marinade for dipping.

SALMON AND CHEESE CANAPÉS

SERVES 3–4

Simple but sumptuous.

1/2	cup grated Swiss cheese, imported (or low-fat substitute)	6–8	slices of bread (white or whole-wheat)
1/4	cup canned salmon, drained		Ground black pepper to taste
1	tablespoon cooking sherry (or other dry wine)		

Preheat the oven to 350°F.
Combine the cheese, salmon, and wine in a medium bowl. Pepper to taste and blend the mixture well.
Toast the bread lightly, spread the mixture on the toasted slices, and bake on cookie sheet for 5 minutes.

STUFFED AVOCADO HALVES

SERVES 6

A wonderful blend of flavors that will delight every guest (or you alone).

- 2 tablespoons chili or salsa sauce
- 2 tablespoons ketchup
- 1 tablespoon red wine vinegar
- 2 tablespoons brown sugar
- 1 teaspoon teriyaki sauce*
- 8 dashes Tabasco sauce
- 4 tablespoons lemon or lime juice
- 3 large, ripe avocados, chilled
- 3 cups cooked or canned crabmeat, drained

Combine the chili or salsa sauce, ketchup, vinegar, brown sugar, teriyaki sauce, Tabasco, and 2 tablespoons of lemon or lime juice in a medium bowl.

Refrigerate 3–4 hours.

When ready to serve, peel the avocados, cut them in half, and remove the pits. Brush the cut sides with the remaining lemon or lime juice, fill the cavities with the crabmeat, and shape it into a mound. Drizzle the sauce on top.

Serve cold with garnish.

EXQUISITE DEVILED EGGS

SERVES 3–4

An old standard with new appeal.

- 4 hard-boiled eggs
- 4 tablespoons chopped chicken or tuna
- 2 tablespoons olive oil
- 1 teaspoon teriyaki sauce*
- 1 tablespoon mayonnaise
- Salt to taste
- Ground black pepper to taste

Cut the eggs lengthwise and remove the yolks.

Arrange the egg white halves on a cake rack and put 1/8 of the chopped chicken or tuna in the cavity of each half.

Using a mixer, combine the egg yolks with the remaining ingredients. Beat until smooth. Salt and pepper to taste. (Optional additions: dried mustard, paprika, dried basil, or lemon juice.)

*For more information on teriyaki sauce, see page 143.

Spoon the mixture into a pastry bag with a large star tube. Holding the pastry bag close to each egg white cavity, force the mixture through the tube while moving the tube to form a zigzag pattern.

Place on a tray lined with large lettuce leaves and serve chilled.

REWARD MEAL DRESSINGS AND DIPS

SPICY VINAIGRETTE   **MAKES ABOUT 1 CUP**

A tangy vinaigrette that will add interest to any salad.

1/4	cup red wine or tarragon vinegar	1/2	tablespoon dried parsley
1	teaspoon sweet Marsala wine	1	garlic clove, minced
2	tablespoons water	1 1/2	tablespoons olive oil
1	tablespoon Dijon mustard		Salt to taste
			Ground black pepper to taste

Combine the vinegar, wine, water, mustard, parsley, salt and pepper (to taste), and garlic in a medium bowl.

Add the oil slowly and whisk continually.

Just before serving, whisk thoroughly.

SIMPLE HOMEMADE RUSSIAN DRESSING   **MAKES 1 CUP**

So easy, so fast, so good.

- 3/4 cup mayonnaise*
- 1/4 cup ketchup

Blend the mayonnaise with a fork until smooth.

Add the ketchup and stir well. (If desired, 2 tablespoons of sweet relish may be added along with the ketchup.)

*To lower the fat content, thin with water by up to 50 percent.

OIL AND VINEGAR DRESSING — MAKES 2/3 CUP

A quick and simple dressing that you will want to keep on hand.

1/2	cup olive oil	1	tablespoon water
4	teaspoons wine vinegar	1/2	tablespoon parsley, finely chopped
1/4	teaspoon dried thyme		
1/4	teaspoon dried marjoram		Salt to taste
1/2	teaspoon dried basil		Ground black pepper to taste
1	tablespoon onion, finely chopped		

Combine all the ingredients in a medium jar and cover with a tight-fitting lid. Shake well for 1 minute and then let stand.

Use as a great topping for any mixed green salad.

SPINACH YOGURT DIP — SERVES 3–4

Works as a nice accompaniment to spiced foods or a delicious dip.

4	ounces fresh spinach, washed and trimmed (or defrosted, drained equivalent)	1	teaspoon ground cumin
		1/4	teaspoon ground cardamom
1	medium cucumber, peeled, seeded, and chopped		Salt to taste
			Ground black pepper to taste
2	cups plain yogurt (regular or low-fat)		Paprika (mild or hot) to taste

If using fresh spinach, dry the leaves and place them in a large covered pot containing 1/8 cup of water.

Steam over medium heat until the leaves are wilted (3–4 minutes).

Remove the spinach from the heat, drain it in a colander, and cool it to room temperature. (If you're using frozen spinach, simply defrost and drain it and continue from this point as if you had cooked it fresh.)

Gently squeeze out the liquid and finely chop the spinach.

Place the cucumber on paper towels to drain the excess liquid.

Combine the yogurt, cumin, cardamom, and salt and pepper to taste in a medium mixing bowl.
Add the spinach and cucumber and mix until all the ingredients are blended.
Cover and refrigerate for at least 2 hours.
Sprinkle with paprika to taste and serve with vegetables or salad.

REWARD MEAL SALADS

VITAMIN-RICH SPINACH SALAD WITH DRESSING — SERVES 3–4

An unappreciated green vegetable that can't be beaten for good eating.

- 1/2 pound raw spinach leaves, washed well
- 1/2 garlic clove, peeled and cut in half lengthwise
- 1/2 garlic clove, peeled and diced
- 1 tablespoon lemon juice
- 3 tablespoons olive oil
- 2 tablespoons diced scallions
- 1/2 cup diced cheddar cheese (or low-fat substitute)
- 1 medium ripe tomato, cut into wedges
- 1/2 medium red onion, thinly sliced
- Ground black pepper to taste

Pat the wet spinach leaves between two pieces of paper towel, then tear the spinach into bite-sized pieces, removing any tough main veins and stems.
Rub the sides of a mixing bowl with the half cloves of garlic.
Add the diced garlic, lemon juice, olive oil, and scallions to the bowl and refrigerate for 1 hour.
Remove the bowl from the refrigerator, add the spinach, and mix until the spinach is coated thoroughly.
Sprinkle with pepper and cheddar cheese.
Garnish with tomato wedges and onion rings.
Toss lightly and serve.

GREEN PEPPER AND TOMATO SALAD WITH DRESSING   SERVES 3–4

This simple dish, with its uncompromising nutrition, is a wonderful addition to any Reward Meal.

4	tomatoes	1/4	cup wine vinegar
2	tablespoons fresh basil, finely chopped	1/2	cup olive oil
		1/2	teaspoon sugar
2	tablespoons fresh parsley, finely chopped	2	tablespoons capers
			Salt to taste
4	tablespoons onion, finely chopped		Fresh dill
1	cup green peppers, diced		
1/2	cup carrots, diced		

Peel the tomatoes and cut them into halves.
Combine the basil, parsley, and onion and sprinkle the mixture over the tomato halves.
Refrigerate the tomato halves and the diced green peppers for 1 hour.
When ready to serve, arrange the diced green peppers and carrots in the center of a large serving platter, and sprinkle with the capers and fresh dill. Arrange the tomato halves around the edge.
Combine the vinegar, olive oil, salt, and sugar and mix thoroughly to form a dressing.
Sprinkle the dressing over the salad and serve immediately.

GREAT CAESAR'S SALAD   SERVES 3–4

A wonderful standard for friends, family, and countrymen.

1	large head romaine lettuce, torn into bite-sized pieces and chilled	1 3/4	cups freshly grated Parmesan cheese
		1/2	cup croutons
3	tablespoons olive oil		Salt to taste
3	garlic cloves, chopped		Freshly ground pepper to taste
3	tablespoons fresh lemon juice		
8	anchovy fillets, chopped		

Place the lettuce in a large bowl.
Whisk the olive oil, garlic, and lemon juice in a small bowl to blend them.
Pour the oil mixture over the lettuce and toss until each leaf is thoroughly coated.
Add the anchovies and toss again.
Add the Parmesan cheese gradually, in several additions, and toss well between additions to coat the entire salad evenly.
Season the salad with salt and freshly ground pepper.
Sprinkle the croutons over the salad and serve it cold.

REWARD MEAL SOUPS

CREAM OF BROCCOLI–CARROT SOUP
SERVES 3–4

This unusual and refreshing soup can be served hot or cold. Either way, you will serve up enjoyment.

2	celery stalks with leaves	1/3	cup heavy cream (or milk)
1	medium carrot		Coarse ground black pepper to taste
1	cup broccoli florets		Salt to taste
1	garlic clove		Dash cayenne pepper
1/2	cup water		
2/3	cup chicken broth° (homemade only or use milk)		

Cut the celery stalks crosswise into 3 parts.
Combine the celery, carrot, broccoli, garlic, and water in a medium pot and simmer for 15 minutes.
Transfer the contents of the pot to a blender and add the salt and cayenne pepper. Cover and blend at high speed. Stop blender. Change to low speed.
Uncover while running and add the broth and heavy cream.
Add black pepper to taste and serve warm or chilled.

°Commercial chicken broths almost always contain glutamates. We think it best for carbohydrate addicts to avoid glutamates whenever possible.

OLD-FASHIONED SPLIT-PEA SOUP   SERVES 3–4

High in carbohydrates, so make sure you balance this wonderful treat with salad, low-carbohydrate vegetables, and additional protein.

1½	cups split green peas, quick-cooking	½	cup carrots, peeled, cut into coins
2½	pounds cooked ham shank*	½	teaspoon sugar
		⅛	teaspoon thyme, dry
4	cups chicken broth** (homemade or use skim milk)	2	garlic cloves, split
		1	bay leaf
			Salt to taste
1	cup onion, chopped		Coarse black pepper to taste
½	cup celery, chopped		

Put 1 quart of water in a large pot or kettle, add peas, and bring to a boil. Reduce heat, cover, and simmer for 45 minutes.

Add all the remaining ingredients, cover, and simmer for 1½ hours.

Remove the pot from the heat, take out the ham shank, and cool it. Then cut the meat from the bone, dice the meat, and set it aside.

Remove the vegetables from the pot (leaving the liquid in the pot), then press the vegetables though a coarse sieve and return them to the pot.

Add the diced ham to the pot and slowly reheat the uncovered pot until the soup has warmed (15–20 minutes).

Serve plain or with a garnish of croutons.

*To reduce saturated fat, choose turkey or other low-saturated fat fowl or meat.
**Commercial chicken broths almost always contain glutamates. We think it best for carbohydrate addicts to avoid glutamates whenever possible.

REWARD MEAL PROTEINS: MEATS, POULTRY, AND SEAFOOD

BEEF AND TOMATO STEW　　　　　　　　　　　　　　　　SERVES 5–6

A gourmet taste in a hearty recipe.

3	tablespoons olive oil	2	tablespoons parsley, fresh
2	tablespoons butter	1	cup green peppers, diced
2	pounds lean beef chunks	1/2	teaspoon garlic, minced
1	large can whole tomatoes (2 pounds), diced and drained	4	tablespoons flour
		3	tablespoons water
3/4	cup dry red wine	12	medium mushrooms, washed and cleaned
1	teaspoon dried oregano		Salt to taste
1	teaspoon dried sweet basil		Pepper to taste

Combine the oil and butter in a 6-quart pan and heat over medium heat.

Place the beef chunks on the bottom of the pan, brown them well on both sides, and remove them from the pan.

Add the canned tomato pieces, salt, pepper, wine, oregano, basil, parsley, green peppers, and garlic. Stir and bring to simmer.

Return the browned beef to the pan. Cover and simmer until the beef is tender (45–50 minutes).

Combine the flour and water in a small bowl. Pour them into the pan and stir.

Add the mushrooms and cook over low heat until the sauce is thickened (10–15 minutes).

Serve warm.

CHICKEN AND RICE CASSEROLE

SERVES 3–4

An old-fashioned treat.

1	pound ground chicken breast (or ground turkey)	2	teaspoons chili powder
1	tablespoon olive oil	1	teaspoon teriyaki sauce*
1/2	cup chopped onion	1/2	cup pitted ripe olives (either green or black), sliced in large pieces
1	cup sliced celery		Salt to taste
1/4	cup chopped green pepper		Ground black pepper to taste
1/2	cup raw rice		
1/2	cup water		

Preheat the oven to 325°F.

Heat the oil and brown the ground chicken in a large skillet over low-medium heat.

Remove the meat from the skillet and add the onion, celery, green pepper, and rice. Cook, stirring, until the contents are browned.

Add the water, seasonings, poultry, and olives and bring to a boil. Pour into a two-quart casserole dish and cover.

Bake until done (45–60 minutes).

Serve hot.

BREADED FISH FILLETS

SERVES 5–6

A healthful and satisfying main course.

2	pounds fish fillets, raw	1/2	cup seasoned bread crumbs, packaged
6	tablespoons olive oil	6	lemon wedges
1	egg (or low-fat substitute)		Parsley sprigs

Rinse the fillets, pat them dry on a paper towel, and cut them into serving-sized pieces.

---

*For more information on teriyaki sauce, see page 143.

Pour the bread crumbs into a large, high-sided bowl.
In a small dish beat the egg with a fork.
Dip the fish into the egg, moistening both sides, and then dip it into the crumbs, coating both sides well.
Heat the oil in a large skillet until hot. Add enough fish pieces to cover the bottom of the skillet. Reduce the heat to medium and fry until golden brown (4–5 minutes). Gently turn the pieces and fry on the other side (4–5 minutes).
Place on a serving platter, garnish with parsley and lemon wedges, and serve. Add some salsa or your favorite dipping sauce as a topping.

POTTED PORK ROAST

SERVES 5–6

A special roast that provides a welcome change and a taste delight.

3	pounds pork roast°
3	tablespoons olive oil
1/2	cup chopped onion
1	garlic clove, finely chopped
1/2	teaspoon basil
2	cups canned tomatoes and 2 cups liquid (add water if needed)
1/2	teaspoon powdered ginger
	Flour, for dredging
	Salt to taste
	Ground black pepper to taste

Combine the flour, salt, and pepper. Dredge the pork roast with the dry mixture.
Heat the oil in a Dutch oven, add the pork, and turn it until it is browned well on all sides.
Add the onion, garlic, and basil. Stir until the onions start to brown. Add the tomatoes and ginger. Cover tightly and simmer until tender (2 to 2½ hours). (Alternately, you may brown the pork, then cook it with the remaining ingredients in a slow cooker or Crock-Pot until fully cooked.)
Remove and place on a heated platter.

°To reduce saturated fat, choose lower–saturated fat meat or fowl.

CLASSIC FRIED CLAMS

SERVES 5–6

An ocean bounty of new tastes.

- 2 cups sour cream (or low-fat substitute)
- 1 quart medium clams, shucked
- 4 tablespoons sweet-pickle relish
- 1 egg (or low-fat substitute)
- 1 teaspoon salt
- 1/4 teaspoon paprika
- 1/2 teaspoon Tabasco sauce
- 1 cup flavored bread crumbs, packaged
- 2 teaspoons garlic, minced
- Olive oil

Combine the sour cream, sweet-pickle relish, salt, Tabasco sauce, and minced garlic in a small bowl and mix thoroughly.

Refrigerate the sauce for at least 2 hours.

Drain the clams and set them aside. Reserve 2 tablespoons of the clam liquid.

Combine the clam liquid, egg, and paprika in a small bowl and mix thoroughly.

Put the bread crumbs in another small bowl.

Cover the bottom of a large skillet with oil (1/4 inch deep) and heat over medium heat.

While the oil is heating, dip the clams in the egg mixture, then in the bread crumbs.

When the oil is hot, fry the clams until done (3–4 minutes per side).

Drain on paper towels and serve with the sour cream sauce.

VEAL MEDALLIONS WITH MUSHROOMS AND HERBS   SERVES 4–5

Elegant from start to finish.

1/2	cup shallots (or scallions), finely chopped	2/3	cup chicken broth* (homemade or milk)
2	garlic cloves, minced	1/2	cup heavy cream (or milk)
1	teaspoon dried sage		
5	tablespoons olive oil	4	tablespoons fresh parsley, minced
1/2	pound fresh mushrooms, cleaned and sliced		Flour, salt, and pepper to taste, for dredging
1	cup dry wine		
1	pound veal medallions (each about 1/8 inch thick)		

Cook the shallots, garlic, and sage in 2 tablespoons of the oil in a heavy skillet over moderately low heat, stirring, until the shallots and garlic have softened.

Add the mushrooms and salt and pepper to taste, and cook over moderate heat, stirring, until the mushrooms are tender and all the liquid they give off has evaporated.

Add 1/2 cup of the wine and simmer the mixture until the wine has evaporated. Transfer the mixture to a bowl.

Dredge the veal in flour, salt, and pepper.

Heat the remaining oil in a skillet over moderately high heat until it is hot but not smoking. Sauté the veal in the oil for 1 minute on each side, until golden brown.

Transfer the veal to a platter and keep it warm.

Add the remaining wine to the skillet and warm it over moderate heat, stirring and scraping up the brown bits, until the wine is reduced by half.

Add the broth mixture. Boil the combined liquid until it is reduced by half again.

Stir in the cream and the mushroom mixture, then salt and pepper to taste.

Simmer the creamy mixture until slightly thickened, stir in the parsley, and pour it over the waiting veal.

---

*Commercial chicken broths almost always contain glutamates. We think it best for carbohydrate addicts to avoid glutamates whenever possible.

BATTER-FRIED SCALLOPS

SERVES 3–4

A delightful home preparation with little muss or fuss.

1	teaspoon salt	1	tablespoon butter (or low-fat substitute)
1/3	teaspoon ground coarse black pepper	1	cup flat beer
1	garlic clove, minced	1	pound medium scallops
2	eggs, separated		Olive oil, for frying

Combine the salt, pepper, garlic, egg yolks, beer, and melted butter in a medium bowl. Mix thoroughly, cover, and refrigerate for at least 4 hours.

Just prior to use, beat the egg whites and fold them into the batter.

Add oil to a deep fryer or large skillet and preheat it to 370°F.

Coat each scallop with batter and deep-fry them until golden brown. Drain them on paper towels and arrange them on a platter.

If desired, serve them with lemon wedges, marinara sauce, tartar sauce, or your favorite relish.

REWARD MEAL DESSERTS

KEY LIME PIE

SERVES 6–8

This old favorite is sure to make family and guests sit up and take notice.

1	cup sugar		Standard Meringue Pie Topping:
1/4	cup flour	3	egg whites
3	teaspoons cornstarch	1/4	teaspoon cream of tartar
1/4	teaspoon salt	6	tablespoons sugar
2	cups water		
3	eggs yolks (whites used for meringue)		
1	tablespoon butter		
1/4	cup lime juice		
	Grated rind of one lime (or lemon)		
	Baked 9-inch pastry shell		

Combine the sugar, flour, cornstarch, and salt in a medium saucepan. Add water gradually, stirring continually.
Cook over low-medium heat, stirring constantly, until thickened.
Beat the egg yolks and gradually add them to the saucepan, stirring continually for 2 minutes.
Remove from the heat and stir in the butter, lime juice, and rind. Allow to cool for 5 minutes, then pour into the pastry shell and cool for 30 minutes.
Preheat the oven to 425°F.
Beat the egg whites in a mixing bowl until frothy and light. Add the cream of tartar and beat until the whites hold a peak. Gradually add the sugar and beat until the meringue is glossy and stiff.
Pile the meringue on top of the pie and spread the meringue to the edge to prevent shrinkage when browning. Place in the oven and bake until the meringue is brown on top (about 5–7 minutes).
Cool and serve.

MIXED FRUIT COMPOTE   SERVES 3–4

A mix of your favorite fruits any time of the year.

12	ounces assorted dried fruits	4	slices peeled and seeded fresh lemon, lime, or orange or mixed citrus
1/2	cup of sugar		
2	cups of water		
	Dash of cinnamon		

Thoroughly wash the fruit and place it in a large cooking pot. Add all remaining ingredients.
Cover the pot and cook on low heat for 1/2 hour.
Serve chilled.

EASY CREPES

SERVES 4–5

Simple, fun, delicious.

Crepes:
- 2/3 cup whole milk, room-temperature
- 1/2 cup all-purpose flour
- 2 medium eggs
- 1 1/2 tablespoons unsalted butter, melted
- 1/2 tablespoon sugar
- 1/8 teaspoon salt
- 3 tablespoons of unsaturated vegetable oil

Filling:
- 1 quart fresh blueberries (or frozen equivalent)
- 1/4 cup sugar
- 1/2 teaspoon ground cinnamon
- 1 teaspoon lemon juice
- 1/2 teaspoon cream of tartar

CREPES:

Mix the first 6 ingredients in a blender until just smooth. Cover the batter and chill it for 30 minutes.

Spread a thin film of unsaturated vegetable oil on a 7-inch-diameter nonstick skillet and heat it over medium heat. Swirl 2 tablespoons of the batter so it coats the bottom of the skillet.

Cook until the edge of the crepe turns light brown (about 1 minute).

Loosen the edges of the crepe gently with a spatula and carefully turn it.

Cook until the bottom of the crepe begins to brown in spots (about 30 seconds).

Transfer the crepe to a plate and cover it with a single paper towel to separate it from the crepe that will be placed on top of it. Repeat with the remaining batter, carefully respreading vegetable oil on a cooled skillet. Transfer each finished crepe to a cool plate, covering each crepe with a paper towel.

FILLING:

Rinse the berries in a colander, but don't dry them.

Put the dripping berries in a medium saucepan and place it over low-medium heat for five minutes, stirring gently so that the berries do not stick.

Add the sugar, cinnamon, and lemon juice and continue stirring gently until the berries burst open and liquid fills the bottom of the pan.

Cook on low heat until most of the berries have burst.

(continued on next page)

Add the cream of tartar, stir well, and remove from the heat immediately.
   The filling will thicken as it cools.
Spoon the filling into the crepes and roll them.
Top the crepes with the extra filling.

NATURE'S FRESHEST AND BEST   SERVES 3–4

Takes advantage of the "fruits" of nature, chock-full of vitamins and minerals.

2	oranges, peeled, sectioned, and cut into chunks	1	cup fresh strawberries
2	cups fresh pineapple chunks	2	pieces candied ginger, thinly sliced
2	bananas, peeled and sliced	1/2	cup coarsely grated coconut
2	peaches, peeled, pitted, and sliced	1/4	cup honey
		1/4	cup fresh lemon juice

Combine all the fruit in a large bowl and toss lightly.
Cover and chill.
Combine the honey and lemon juice in a medium bowl to form a dressing.
Just before serving, toss the fruit with the honey-lemon dressing.

FRUITY DUMPLINGS   SERVES 3–4

A wonderful dessert that is well worth the effort.

2	tablespoons salt	1/2	pound freestone peaches, peeled, pitted, and coarsely chopped
1	cup cooked and mashed potatoes		
1	egg, beaten	1/2	pound blueberries, washed
1	cup flour		
1/2	teaspoon baking powder	1/2	cup sugar
1	cup apple, peeled and sliced		

Fill a large pot 3/4 full with water, add 1 teaspoon of salt, set over low-medium heat, and bring to a very low boil.

While the water heats, combine the potatoes, remaining salt, egg, flour, and baking powder in a large bowl and mix until a firm dough is formed.

Flour a pastry board, roll out the dough until it is 1/8 inch thick, and cut it into 4-inch squares.

Combine the sliced apple, peaches, blueberries, and sugar in a medium bowl.

Place one tablespoon of the fruit mixture in the center of each dough square. Carefully fold the dough over the fruit and tightly pinch all the seams closed. Lightly flour the seams to tighten and dry the dough so boiling water will not seep in and the juices will not seep out.

Drop the dumplings into the boiling salted water, cover, and cook for 8–10 minutes. The dumplings will float to the surface. Remove them one by one with a slotted spoon.

Optional: Fruit-filled dumplings are especially good coated with a mixture of ground walnuts and a dollop of yogurt or sour cream (regular or low-fat).

REWARD MEAL VEGETARIAN (NONMEAT) ALTERNATIVES

VEGETARIAN "BEEF" WITH AVOCADOS AND FETTUCCINE   SERVES 3–4

A recipe that will become a favorite for you and your guests.

- 1/4 cup olive oil
- 6 vegetarian "beef" patties, chopped
- 1/4 teaspoon salt
- 4–6 ounces (by weight) fettuccine, packaged or fresh
- 1 teaspoon flour
- 1/2 cup heavy cream (or low-fat plain yogurt with 1/2 tablespoon of sugar)
- 2 avocados, chopped
- 1 avocado, sliced
- 4 cups water
- Parmesan cheese (or low-fat substitute), grated
- Ground black pepper to taste

Heat one teaspoon of olive oil in a medium skillet over medium heat. Add the chopped "beef" and cook until golden (4–5 minutes). Set aside.

Put the salt and 4 cups of water in a medium pot. Heat to a boil, add the pasta, and cook until the pasta is al dente. Drain the water and cover the pot to keep the pasta hot.

Pour the remaining olive oil in a small saucepan over medium heat. Add the flour and stir. Add the heavy cream or yogurt and stir constantly while cooking for 2 minutes.

Briefly reheat the chopped "beef" in the skillet.

Place the pasta on a serving platter. Pour the cream sauce over the pasta, add the chopped avocado, 3/4 of the "beef," and 3/4 of the Parmesan cheese, then pepper to taste.

Garnish with the sliced avocado and the remaining "beef" and serve with the remaining grated cheese.

VEGETARIAN "CHICKEN" LOAF

SERVES 3–4

An unusual "meat loaf" for the vegetarian. Rich in fiber and low in calories and fat.

1 1/2	teaspoons olive oil	1/2	teaspoon hot sauce
2	garlic cloves, chopped	1/2	pound vegetarian "chicken,"* broken into chunks
2	large scallions, chopped		
1	medium tomato, chopped, with juice		
		1/4	cup rolled oats
1/3	cup basil, fresh	3	tablespoons oat bran
1/2	teaspoon oregano, dry	2	large egg whites, beaten
4	tablespoons red wine, dry		Salt to taste
1	small zucchini, chopped		Coarse black pepper to taste
1	medium green pepper, chopped		

Preheat the oven to 350°F.

Coat a loaf pan with 1/2 teaspoon of olive oil and set it aside.

Combine the remaining olive oil, garlic, and scallions in a saucepan and cook over medium-low heat for 3 minutes, stirring several times during cooking.

---

*Containing no more than 4 grams of carbohydrates per average serving.

Add the tomato with juice, 2 tablespoons of basil, oregano, and wine. Simmer for 10 minutes, stirring occasionally.

Combine the contents of the saucepan in a large bowl with the zucchini, green pepper, hot sauce, "chicken," rolled oats, oat bran, and egg whites, and salt and pepper to taste. Mix thoroughly.

Transfer the mixture to the loaf pan and spread it uniformly.

Place the pan in the oven and cook until golden brown on top (about 1 hour).

Serve hot or cold.

VEGETARIAN "SAUSAGE" AND BEANS   SERVES 3–4

A dish that will delight both vegetarians and nonvegetarians alike.

1½	quarts water	Salt to taste
1	cup small white beans, dried	Ground black pepper to taste
1	medium onion, sliced	Paprika to taste
2	garlic cloves, minced	Grated hard cheese (or nondairy substitute) to taste
6	vegetarian "sausage"* slices	

Combine the water and beans in a large saucepan and soak overnight.

Drain the water and add fresh water to just cover the beans. Add the onion and garlic and cook over medium heat (1½ hours or until the beans are tender).

Sauté or bake the "sausage" slices per the package directions. Add salt, pepper, and paprika.

Place the "sausage" on a serving plate and top with the beans and grated cheese.

*Containing no more than 4 grams of carbohydrates per average serving.

MACARONI WITH TOMATOES

SERVES 3–4

A pleasure to prepare and a delight to eat.

1	medium can whole tomatoes	1	large green pepper, thinly sliced
1	small can tomato paste	1	pound elbow macaroni
1/2	tablespoon sugar	6–8	thin slices imported Swiss cheese (or meltable low-fat or nondairy substitute) to taste
1	garlic clove, minced		
1/8	teaspoon dried basil		
1/8	teaspoon chervil, dried		
1/8	teaspoon marjoram, dried		Salt to taste
			Ground black pepper to taste
1/8	teaspoon oregano, dried		
2	tablespoons olive oil		
1	large onion, thinly sliced		

Combine the tomatoes, tomato paste, sugar, salt and pepper (to taste), garlic, basil, chervil, marjoram, and oregano in a large frying pan. Cook uncovered over low heat for 1 hour.

Preheat the oven to 350°F.

Combine 1 tablespoon olive oil, onion, and green pepper in a small frying pan. Sauté over medium heat for 3 minutes.

Boil the elbow macaroni according to the package directions, then rinse in cold water.

Use the remaining olive oil to coat the inside of a large casserole dish. Add the macaroni, sauce, and cheese slices, in layers. Top with sauce and cheese.

Place in the oven and bake uncovered until the cheese melts (20–30 minutes).

Serve warm (but great cold, too).

APPENDIX

INCORPORATING LOW-FAT, LOW–SATURATED FAT, LOW-SALT, AND OTHER HEALTH AGENCY DIETARY RECOMMENDATIONS INTO YOUR PROGRAM

Based on the U.S. Department of Health and Human Services' *Dietary Guidelines for Americans*, 4th ed. (U.S. Department of Agriculture); the American Heart Association's guidelines, *Eating Plan for Healthy Americans* (1996); and the American Cancer Society's *1996 Guidelines on Diet, Nutrition, and Cancer Prevention.*

GENERAL HEALTH AGENCY RECOMMENDATIONS

HEALTH AGENCY RECOMMENDATION 1: EAT A VARIETY OF FOODS.

To incorporate recommendation 1 into your program:

Incorporate new foods into your low-carbohydrate meals and choose from a variety of salad ingredients, low-carbohydrate vegetables, proteins, and low-carbohydrate dairy items. In planning your Reward Meals, choose from a variety of both low- and high-carbohydrate foods, including a wide assortment of grains, starches, additional dairy choices, fruits, and "healthy" desserts. Try one new vegetable or fruit each week and experiment with new recipes. Keep things exciting while continuing to enjoy your longtime favorites.

> Before incorporating any dietary guideline into your program, you should consult your physician. Only your doctor can determine which recommendations are appropriate for you and your individual health needs and how best to incorporate health agency recommendations.

HEALTH AGENCY RECOMMENDATION 2:
BALANCE THE FOOD YOU EAT WITH PHYSICAL ACTIVITY. MAINTAIN OR IMPROVE YOUR WEIGHT.

To incorporate recommendation 2 into your program:

The Carbohydrate Addict's Healthy Heart Program incorporates physical activity recommendations as Step 3 of its BASIC Plan. Gradual changes go a long way toward healthy, lifelong habits, and beginning on page 191, you will find a wide variety of physical activity options that you can add to your routine. As appropriate, start with small steps.

When it comes to maintaining ideal weight levels, weight loss and the maintenance of ideal weight are natural outcomes of this program, typical responses to its insulin-balancing focus.

HEALTH AGENCY RECOMMENDATION 3:
CHOOSE A DIET WITH PLENTY OF GRAIN PRODUCTS, VEGETABLES, AND FRUITS.

To incorporate recommendation 3 into your program:

Include a wide variety of fiber-rich, low-carbohydrate vegetables at all meals and snacks. As your balance of high-carbohydrate foods at your Reward Meals, select whole-grain breads, cereal products, rice, pasta, potatoes, and other starchy vegetables and fruit.

HEALTH AGENCY RECOMMENDATION 4:
CHOOSE A DIET LOW IN FAT, SATURATED FAT, AND CHOLESTEROL.

To incorporate recommendation 4 into your program:

As per the American Dietetic Association (ADA) recommendations, make small changes you can live with. The ADA suggests choosing foods in the same food category with less fat. For example, you would not have to give up milk because of the fat content. Instead, you might choose 2 percent, low-fat, or skim milk. The ADA adds that the guideline is related to the fat in your total diet, not individual foods, and that foods with higher and lower amounts of fat should balance each other as part of a healthful eating plan.

Selecting low-fat foods is easy. Some examples of low-fat or low–saturated fat alternatives include selecting egg substitutes rather than whole eggs when possible, cooking sprays or nonstick cooking surfaces rather than butter, and low-fat cheese and sour cream rather than their high-fat counterparts. Instead of higher-fat meats, select fish or chicken or turkey without skin or choose very lean cuts of meat, trimmed of all fat. Substitute turkey for beef and pork in burgers and sausage.

To reduce saturated fats, choose olive oil instead of heavy tropical or other saturated oils and avoid saturated fats (found in butter, other dairy foods, and meats), hydrogenated fats (saturated or unsaturated), and trans fatty acids (often found in margarine). For information on identifying foods high in saturated fat and the best sources of unsaturated fats, see "Fast Fat Facts" (page 225).

HEALTH AGENCY RECOMMENDATION 5: CHOOSE A DIET MODERATE IN SUGARS.

To incorporate recommendation 5 into your program:

The basic guidelines of The Carbohydrate Addict's Healthy Heart Program will help you to reduce your intake of sugar naturally. Your low-carbohydrate meals will essentially be sugar-free, and if you wish to continue to keep your intake of sugar low, at your Reward Meals choose desserts made of complex carbohydrates like whole-grain breads, popcorn, pretzels, or low-fat whole-grain snacks rather than candy.

HEALTH AGENCY RECOMMENDATION 6: CHOOSE A DIET MODERATE IN SALT (SODIUM).

To incorporate recommendation 6 into your program:

Limit the amount of salt you add while cooking or at the table. At all meals choose low-salt varieties of canned and packaged foods as well as low-salt cheese and other dairy products. At restaurants ask for low-salt alternatives. When possible, avoid smoked and salted products.

HEALTH AGENCY RECOMMENDATION 7:
IF YOU DRINK ALCOHOLIC BEVERAGES, DO SO IN MODERATION.

To incorporate recommendation 7 into your program:

On The Carbohydrate Addict's Healthy Heart Program, alcoholic beverages are designated as "carbohydrate act-alikes," and when they are consumed, they are to be consumed only in moderation and only during Reward Meals. Balancing alcoholic beverages (as part of your high-carbohydrate choices) with the low-carbohydrate portions of your Reward Meal will naturally help keep your intake to a moderate level. Always consult your physician; diabetics and others may be advised by their physicians to abstain from all alcohol.

AMERICAN HEART ASSOCIATION RECOMMENDATIONS

In addition to the general health agency recommendations in the preceding section, the American Heart Association makes the following recommendations:

- Total fat intake should be no more than 30 percent of total calories.
- Saturated fatty acid intake should be 8–10 percent of total calories.
- Polyunsaturated fatty acid intake should be up to 10 percent of total calories.
- Cholesterol intake should be less than 300 milligrams per day.
- Sodium intake should be less than 2,400 milligrams per day, which is about 1¼ teaspoons of sodium chloride (salt).
- Carbohydrate intake should make up 55–60 percent or more of calories, with emphasis on increasing sources of complex carbohydrates.
- Total calories should be adjusted to achieve and maintain a healthy body weight.*

To incorporate the American Heart Association's recommendations into your program:

Again, we have designed The Carbohydrate Addict's Healthy Heart Program to be compatible with the American Heart Association's recommendations. To comply with the AHA's guidelines:

---

*Per the American Heart Association's guidelines, *Eating Plan for Healthy Americans* (1996).

- Select proteins that are lower in saturated fat—for example, choose tofu (soybean curd), soybean-based protein, and fish rather than fatty cuts of animal protein.
- When eating prepared foods, choose low-salt varieties and, at home, cook with very little salt.
- In order to be sure of including the recommended proportion of carbohydrates, choose fowl, fish, and tofu as your proteins. These lower-calorie proteins in combination with low-carbohydrate vegetables will enable you to maintain your percentage of carbohydrate calories at 55–60 percent without overloading the carbohydrate balance of your Reward Meal. If, in addition, you consume mostly high-quality complex carbohydrates, you will be complying with the American Heart Association's recommendations to keep calories low and to maintain an emphasis on complex carbohydrates while keeping sugar intake low.
- For easy guidance in recognizing polyunsaturated versus saturated fats and saturated fatty acids as recommended in the American Heart Association's guidelines, see "Fast Fat Facts" (page 225).

Important note: Not every single food you eat must be low-fat. According to the American Heart Association:*

Some people misinterpret the first guideline to mean that each food or each recipe should have less than 30 percent of its calories come from fat. The guideline applies to total calories eaten over several days, such as a week. If it is applied to single foods, the "30 percent of calories from fat" guideline will cause many foods that fit into a well-balanced eating plan to be excluded.

Examples of these foods include: oil and margarine (100 percent of calories from fat), regular and low-calorie salad dressings (75–100 percent of calories from fat), dark chicken meat without skin (43 percent of calories from fat), salmon (36 percent of calories from fat), lower-fat meats like turkey or ham (34 percent of calories from fat), as well as many nuts and seeds (75–90 percent of calories from fat).

Applying the 30 percent standard to single foods greatly limits the variety of foods in the diet and can be misleading. The only way to maintain balance, variety, and enjoyment of the AHA eating plan is to interpret the guideline with emphasis on the words "total calories."

*www.americanheart.org/Heart_and_Stroke_A_Z_Guide/dietg.html

So in keeping with the American Heart Association guidelines, select a wide and wonderful combination of foods, choosing carefully and finding an enjoyable and healthful balance.

AMERICAN CANCER SOCIETY RECOMMENDATIONS

The American Cancer Society makes the following recommendations:

- Choose most of the foods you eat from plant sources (fruits, vegetables, grains) and food made from them.
- Limit your intake of high-fat foods, particularly from animal sources.
- Be physically active; achieve and maintain a healthy weight.
- Limit consumption of alcoholic beverages, if you drink at all.°

To incorporate guidelines from the American Cancer Society into your program:

The Carbohydrate Addict's Healthy Heart Program is compatible with the guidelines of the American Cancer Society. To comply with these guidelines:

- Select tofu (soybean curd) and soybean-based protein in place of animal protein whenever possible and as appropriate.
- Incorporate as many of the activity choices in Chapter 7 (Step 3 of The Carbohydrate Addict's Healthy Heart Program) as are appropriate to your physical abilities.
- Follow the guidelines to reduce insulin-related cravings so that you will lose excess weight and maintain a healthy, constant weight level.
- At your Reward Meal limit your consumption of alcoholic beverages or, as appropriate, pass on alcoholic drinks altogether.

°Per the American Cancer Society's 1996 *Guidelines on Diet, Nutrition, and Cancer Prevention.*

REFERENCES

Abraham, A. S., M. Sonnenblick, M. Eini, O. Shemesh, and A. P. Batt. "The Effect of Chromium on Established Atherosclerotic Plaques in Rabbits." *American Journal of Clinical Nutrition* 33 (1980): 2294–98.

A'cbay, O., A. F. Celik, and S. Gündögdu. "Does *Helicobacter Pylori*–Induced Gastritis Enhance Food-Stimulated Insulin Release?" *Dig Dis Sci* 41, no. 7 (1996): 1327–31.

Alemany, M. "The Etiological Basis for the Classification of Obesity." *Prog Food Nutr Sci.* 13, no. 1 (1989): 46–66.

Altomare, E., G. Vendemiale, D. Chicco, V. Procacci, and F. Cirelli. "Increased Lipid Peroxidation in Type 2 Poorly Controlled Diabetic Patients." *Diabete Metab* 18, no. 4 (1992): 264–71.

American Cancer Society. *Prevention and Detection Guidelines: 1996 Guidelines on Diet, Nutrition, and Cancer Prevention.*

American Dietetic Association. "ADA Offers Americans Tips on Putting Revised Dietary Guidelines into Practice." Press release, January 2, 1996.

American Heart Association. *Eating Plan for Healthy Americans, 1996.* Based on AHA medical/scientific statement: *Dietary Guidelines for Healthy American Adults: A Statement for Health Professionals from the Nutrition Committee, American Heart Association.* R. M. Krauss, R. J. Deckelbaum, N. Ernst, E. Fisher, B. V. Howard, R. H. Knopp, T. Kotchen, A. H. Lichtenstein, H. C. Mcgill, T. A. Pearson, T. E. Prewitt, N. J. Stone, L. Van Horn, and R. Weinberg (1996).

American Heart Association Journal report. "High Blood Levels of Insulin Possible Independent Predictor of Heart Attack Risk." (Circ/Pyorala) NR 98-4937 (1998).

American Psychiatric Association. *Diagnostic and Statistical Manual of Mental Disorders*, 3d ed. Washington, D.C.: American Psychiatric Press, 1987.

Anderson, J. W. "Nutrition Management of Diabetes Mellitus." In *Modern Nutrition in Health and Disease*, 7th ed., edited by M. E. Shils and V. R. Young, 1204–29. Philadelphia: Lea & Febiger, 1988.

Anderson, R. A. "Chromium Metabolism and Its Role in Disease Processes in Man." *Clin Physiol Biochem* 4 (1986): 31–41.

———. "Essentiality of Chromium in Humans." *Sci of the Tot Environ* 86, nos. 1–2 (1989): 75–81.

———. "Nutritional Role of Chromium." *Sci of the Tot Environ* 17 (1981): 13–29.

———. "Selenium, Chromium, and Manganese: (B) Chromium." In *Modern Nutrition in Health and Disease*, 7th ed., edited by M. E. Shils and V. R. Young, 268–73. Philadelphia: Lea & Febiger, 1988.

———. "Trace Elements and Cardiovascular Diseases." *Acta Pharmacol Toxicol* (Copenh) 59, suppl. 7 (1986): 317–24.

Anderson, R. A., N. A. Bryden, M. M. Polansky, and S. Reisner. "Urinary Chromium Excretion and Insulinogenic Properties of Carbohydrates." *American Journal of Clinical Nutrition* 51, no. 5 (1990): 864–68.

Anderson, R. A., N. Cheng, N. A. Bryden, M. M. Polansky, N. Cheng, J. Chi, and J. Feng. "Elevated Intakes of Supplemental Chromium Improve Glucose and Insulin Variables in Individuals with Type 2 Diabetes." *Diabetes* 46, no. 11 (1997): 1786–91.

Anderson, R. A., M. M. Polansky, N. A. Bryden, S. J. Bhathena, and J. J. Canary. "Effects of Supplemental Chromium on Patients with Symptoms of Reactive Hypoglycemia." *Metabolism* 36, no. 4 (1987): 351–55.

Anderson, R. A., M. M. Polansky, N. A. Bryden, and J. J. Canary. "Supplemental-Chromium Effects on Glucose, Insulin, Glucagon, and Urinary Chromium Losses in Subjects Consuming Controlled Low-Chromium Diets." *American Journal of Clinical Nutrition* 54, no. 5 (1991): 909–16.

Anderson, R. A., M. M. Polansky, N. A. Bryden, and H. N. Guttman. "Strenuous Exercise May Increase Dietary Needs for Chromium and Zinc." In *Sports, Health and Nutrition*, vol. 2, edited by F. I. Katch, 83–88. 1986.

Anderson, R. A., M. M. Polansky, N. A. Bryden, E. E. I. Roginsk, K. Y. Patterson, and D. C. Reamer. "Effect of Exercise (Running) on Serum Glucose, Insulin, Glucagon, and Chromium Excretion." *Diabetes* 31 (1982): 212–16.

Anke, M. "Role of Trace Elements in the Dynamics of Atherosclerosis." *Z Gesamte Inn Med* 41, no. 4 (1986): 105–11.

Anselmo, J., F. Vaz, L. G. Correia, E. Pereira, F. Lima De Silva, M. T. Pires, and J. C. Nunes-Correa. "Influence of Body Fat Topography on Glucose Homeostasis and Serum Lipid Levels." *Acta Med Port* 3, no. 6 (1990): 341–46.

Aparicio, M., H. Gin, L. Potaux, J. L. Bouchet, D. Morel, and J. Aubertin. "Effect

REFERENCES

of a Ketoacid Diet on Glucose Tolerance and Tissue Insulin Sensitivity." *Kidney Int* 27, suppl. (1989): S231–35.

Aronow, W. S., C. Ahn, I. Kronzon, and M. Koenigsberg. "Congestive Heart Failure, Coronary Events and Atherothromic Brain Infarction in Elderly Blacks and Whites with Systemic Hypertension and with and without Echocardiographic and Electrocardiographic Evidence of Left Ventricular Hypertrophy." *Federation of American Societies for Experimental Biology Journal* (1991): 295–99.

Assimacopoulos, F., and J. B. Jeanrenaud. "The Hormonal and Metabolic Basis of Experimental Obesity." *Clin Endocrinol Metab* 5, no. 2 (1976): 337–65.

Astrup, A., S. Toubro, S. Cannon, P. Hein, and J. Madsen. "Thermogenic Synergism between Ephedrine and Caffeine in Healthy Volunteers: A Double-Blind, Placebo-Controlled Study." *Metabolism* 40, no. 3 (1991): 323–29.

Atrens, D. M. "The Questionable Wisdom of a Low-Fat Diet and Cholesterol Reduction." *Social Science Medicine* 39, no. 3 (1994): 433–47.

Bagdade, J. D., and F. L. Dunn. "Effects of Insulin Treatment on Lipoprotein Composition and Function in Patients with IDDM." *Diabetes* 41, suppl. 2 (1992): 107–10.

The Bantam Medical Dictionary. New York, London: Bantam Books, 1982.

Barrett-Connor, L. "Obesity, Atherosclerosis, and Coronary Heart Disease." Part 2. *Annals of Internal Medicine* 103, no. 6 (1985): 1010–19.

Bearon, L. B., and H. G. Koenig. "Religious Cognitions and Use of Prayer in Health and Illness." *Gerontologist* 30, no. 2 (1990): 249–53.

Beck-Nielsen, H., O. H. Nielsen, P. Damsbo, A. Vaag, A. Handberg, and J. E. Henriksen. "Impairment of Glucose Tolerance: Mechanism of Action and Impact on the Cardiovascular System." Part 2. *American Journal of Obstetrics and Gynecology* 163, no. 1 (1990): 292–95.

Berne, C. "Insulin in Hypertension—A Relationship with Consequences?" *Journal of Internal Medicine* 735, suppl. (1991): 65–73.

Beverly, C. "Sugary Foods May Be Hazardous for Those Who Have Breast Cancer." *Natural Healing Newsletter* 3, no. 1G (1991): 5.

Bhathena, S. J., P. Aparicio, K. Revett, N. Voyles, and L. Recant. "Effect of Dietary Carbohydrates on Glucagon and Insulin Receptors in Genetically Obese Female Zucker Rats." *Journal of Nutrition* 117, no. 7 (1987): 1291–97.

Bhathena, S. J., E. Berlin, J. T. Judd, J. Jones, B. W. Kennedy, P. M. Smith, D. Y. Jones, P. R. Taylor, and W. S. Campbell. "Dietary Fat and Menstrual-Cycle Effects on the Erythrocyte Ghost Insulin Receptor in Premenopausal Women." *American Journal of Clinical Nutrition* 50 (1989): 460–64.

Bierman, E. L., and A. Chait. "Nutrition and Diet in Relation to Hyperlipidemia and Atherosclerosis." In *Modern Nutrition in Health and Disease*, 7th ed., edited by M. E. Shils and V. R. Young, 1283–97. Philadelphia: Lea & Febiger, 1988.

Bjorntorp, P. "Obesity and Adipose Tissue Distribution as a Risk Factor for the Development of Disease: A Review." *Infusionstherapie* 17, no. 1 (1990): 24–27.

Black, H. R. "The Coronary Artery Disease Paradox: The Role of Hyperinsulinemia and Insulin Resistance and Its Implications for Therapy." *Journal of Cardiovascular Pharmacology* 15, suppl. 5 (1990): S26–38.

Blackburn, G. L. "Medical Treatment of Obesity." In *Treatment of Obesity: A Multidisciplinary Approach*, edited by G. L. Blackburn, P. N. Benotti, and E. A. Mascioli. Presented through the Department of Education at Harvard Medical School, November 7–9, 1991.

Bland, J. *Nutraerobics*. San Francisco: Harper and Row, 1983.

Blendis, L. M., and D. J. A. Jenkins. "Nutrition and Diet in Management of Diseases of the Gastrointestinal Tract." In *Modern Nutrition in Health and Disease*, 7th ed., edited by M. E. Shils and V. R. Young, 1182–1200. Philadelphia: Lea & Febiger, 1988.

Block, G., C. Dresser, H. Hartman, and M. D. Carol. "Nutrient Sources in the American Diet: Quantitative Data from the HANES II Survey. I Vitamins and Minerals." *Am J Epidemiol* 122 (1985): 13–40.

Boden, G., F. Jadali, J. White, Y. Liang, M. Mozzoli, X. Chen, E. Coleman, and C. Smith. "Effects of Fat on Insulin-Stimulated Carbohydrate Metabolism in Normal Men." *Journal of Clinical Investigation* 88, no. 3 (1991): 960–66.

Bogardus, C., S. Lillioja, J. Foley, L. Christin, D. Freymond, B. Nyomba, P. H. Bennett, Reaven, and L. Salans. "Insulin Resistance Predicts the Development of Non–Insulin Dependent Diabetes Mellitus in Pima Indians." *Diabetes* 36, suppl. 1 (1987): 47A (abstract).

Bottermann, P., and M. Classen. "Diabetes Mellitus and Arterial Hypertension: In Search of the Connecting Link." *Z Gesamte Inn Med* 46, no. 15 (1991): 558–62.

Brands, M. W., and J. E. Hall. "Insulin Resistance, Hyperinsulinemia, and Obesity-Associated Hypertension." *J Am Soc Nephrol* 3, no. 5 (1992): 1064–77.

Bray, G. A. "Obesity—A Disorder of Nutrient Partitioning: The MONA LISA Hypothesis." *Journal of Nutrition* 121 (1991): 1146–62.

———. "Obesity: Historical Development of Scientific and Cultural Ideas." *International Journal of Obesity* 14, no. 11 (1990): 909–26.

Brindley, D. N. "Mode of Action of Benfluorex: Recent Data." *Presse Med* 21, no. 28 (1992): 1330–35.

Brindley, D. N., and Y. Rolland. "Possible Connections between Stress, Diabetes, Obesity, Hypertension and Altered Lipoprotein Metabolism That May Result in Atherosclerosis." *Clin Sci* 77, no. 5 (1989): 453–61.

Broderick, T. L., G. Panagakis, D. Didomenico, J. Gamble, G. D. Lopaschuk, A. L. Shug, and D. J. Paulson. "L-Carnitine Improvement of Cardiac Function Is Associated with a Stimulation in Glucose but Not Fatty Acid Metabolism in Carnitine-Deficient Hearts." *Cardiovasc Res* 30, no. 5 (1995): 815–20.

REFERENCES

Brought, D. L., and R. Taylor. "Review: Deterioration of Glucose Tolerance with Age: The Role of Insulin Resistance." *Age Aging* 20, no. 3 (1991): 221–25.

Bruning, P. F., J. M. Bonfrer, P. A. Van Noord, A. A. Hart, M. De Jong-Bakker, and W. J. Nooijen. "Insulin Resistance and Breast Cancer Risk." *Int J Cancer* 52, no. 4 (1992): 511–16.

Buchanan, T. A. "Glucose Metabolism during Pregnancy: Normal Physiology and Implications for Diabetes Mellitus." *Isr J Med Sci* 27, nos. 8–9 (1991): 432–41.

Buhler, F. R. "Cardiovascular Risk Factors—An Integrated Sympathetic Viewpoint." *Schweiz Med Wochenschr* 121, no. 49 (1991): 1793–1802.

Bunker, V. W., M. S. Lawson, H. T. Delves, and B. E. Clayton. "The Uptake and Excretion of Chromium by the Elderly." *American Journal of Clinical Nutrition* 39 (1984): 797–802.

Butler, P., E. Kryshak, and R. Rizza. "Mechanism of Growth Hormone–Induced Postprandial Carbohydrate Intolerance in Humans." Part 1. *American Journal of Physiology* 260, no. 4 (1991): E513–20. (Pub erratum appears in *American Journal of Physiology* 261, no. 6, part 1 [1991]: E677.)

Cabrijan, T., S. Levanat, P. Pekic, J. Pavelic, R. Spaventi, H. Frahm, V. Zjacic-Rotkvic, V. Goldoni, D. Vrbanec, M. Misjak, et al. "The Role of Insulin-Related Substance in Hodgkin's Disease." *J Cancer Res Clin Oncol* 117, no. 6 (1991): 615–19.

Campbell, W. W., and R. A. Anderson. "Effects of Aerobic Exercise and Training on the Trace Minerals Chromium, Zinc and Copper." *Sports Med* 4, no. 1 (1987): 9–18.

Capaldo, B., R. Napoli, P. Di Bonito, G. Albano, and L. Saccà. "Carnitine Improves Peripheral Glucose Disposal in Non–Insulin-Dependent Diabetic Patients." *Diabetes Res Clin Pract* 14, no. 3 (1991): 191–95.

Ceriello, A., A. Quatraro, F. Caretta, R. Varano, and D. Giugliano. "Evidence for the Possible Role of Oxygen Free Radicals in the Abnormal Function of Arterial Vasomotor in Insulin Dependent Diabetes." *Diabete Meta* 16, no. 4 (1990): 318–22.

Chandrasekhar, Y., J. Heiner, C. Osuamkpe, and M. Nagamani. "Insulin-Like Growth Factor I and II Binding in Human Myometrium and Leiomyomas." Part 1. *American Journal of Obstetrics and Gynecology* 166, no. 1 (1992): 64–69.

Chaouloff, F., D. Laude, D. Merino, B. Serrurier, and J. L. Elghozi. "Peripheral and Central Consequences of Immobilization Stress in Genetically Obese Zucker Rats." Part 2. *American Journal of Physiology* 256, no. 2 (1989): R435–42.

Clark, M. G., S. Rattigan, and D. G. Clark. "Obesity with Insulin Resistance: Experiential Insights." *Lancet*, November 26, 1983, 1236–40.

Comings, D. E., S. D. Flanagan, G. Dietz, D. Muhleman, E. Knell, and R. Gysin. "The Dopamine D2 Receptor (DRD2) as a Major Gene in Obesity and Height." *Biochem Med Metab Biol* 50, no. 2 (1993): 176–85.

Contreras, R. J., and V. L. Williams. "Dietary Obesity and Weight Cycling: Effects on Blood Pressure and Heart Rate in Rats." Part 2. *American Journal of Physiology* 256, no. 6 (1989): R1209–19.

Conway, G. S., R. Agrawal, D. J. Betteridge, and H. S. Jacobs. "Risk Factors for Coronary Artery Disease in Lean and Obese Women with the Polycystic Ovary Syndrome." *Clin Endocrinol* (Oxf) 37, no. 2 (1992): 119–25.

Conway, G. S., P. M. Clark, and D. Wong. "Hyperinsulinemia in the Polycystic Ovary Syndrome Confirmed with a Specific Immunoradiometric Assay for Insulin." *Clin Endocrinol* (Oxf) 38, no. 2 (1993): 219–22.

Coulston, A. M., C. B. Hollenbeck, A. L. M. Swislocki, Y-D. I. Chen, and G. Reaven. "Deleterious Metabolic Effects of High-Carbohydrate, Sucrose-Containing Diets in Patients with Non–Insulin-Dependent Diabetes Mellitus." *American Journal of Medicine* 82 (1987): 213–20.

Coulston, A. M., G. C. Liu, and G. M. Reaven. "Plasma Glucose, Insulin and Lipid Responses to High-Carbohydrate Low-Fat Diets in Normal Humans." *Metabolism* 32, no. 1 (1983): 52–56.

Creutzfeldt, W., R. Ebert, B. Willms, H. Frefichs, and J. C. Brown. "Gastric Inhibitory Polypeptide (GIP) and Insulin in Obesity: Increased Response to Stimulation and Defective Feedback Control of Serum Levels." *Diabetologia* 14 (1978): 15–24.

Daly, P. A., and L. Landsberg. "Hypertension in Obesity and NIDDM: Role of Insulin and Sympathetic Nervous System." *Diabetes Care* 14, no. 3 (1991): 240–48.

Defronzo, R. A., and E. Ferrannini. "Insulin Resistance: A Multifaceted Syndrome Responsible for NIDDM, Obesity, Hypertension, Dyslipidemia, and Atherosclerotic Cardiovascular Disease." *Diabetes Care* 14, no. 3 (1991): 173–94.

Del Prato, S. "Hyperinsulinemia: Causes and Mechanisms." *Presse Med* 21, no. 28 (1992): 1312–17.

Devlin, J. T., and E. S. Horton. "Hormone and Nutrient Interactions." In *Modern Nutrition in Health and Disease*, 7th ed., edited by M. E. Shils and V. R. Young, 570–84. Philadelphia: Lea & Febiger, 1988.

Dietz, W. H. "Obesity." *J Am Coll Nutr* 8, suppl. (1989): 13S–21S.

Di Pietro, S., and C. Suraci. "Metabolic Abnormalities in First-Degree Relatives of Type 2 Diabetics." *Boll Soc Ital Biol Sper* 66, no. 7 (1990): 631–38.

Djurhuus, M. S., P. Skøtt, O. Hother-Nielson, N. A. Klitgaard, and H. Beck-Nielsen. "Insulin Increases Renal Magnesium Excretion: A Possible Cause of Magnesium Depletion in Hyperinsulinaemic States." *Diabetes Medicine* 12, no. 8 (1995): 664–69.

Doeden, B., and R. Rizza. "Use of a Variable Insulin Infusion to Assess Insulin Action in Obesity: Defects in Both Kinetics and Amplitude of Response." *Journal of Clinical Endocrinological Metabolism* 64, no. 5 (1987): 902–8.

REFERENCES

Dorner, G., A. Plagemann, J. Ruckert, F. Gotz, W. Rohde, F. Stahl, U. Kurschner, J. Gottschalk, A. Mohnike, and E. Steindel. "Teratogenic Maternofoetal Transmission and Prevention of Diabetes Susceptibility." *Exp Clin Endocrinol* 91, no. 3 (1988): 247–58.

Drash, A. "Relationship between Diabetes Mellitus and Obesity in the Child." *Metabolism* 22, no. 2 (1973): 337–34.

Du Cailar, G., J. Ribstein, J. L. Pasquie, V. Simandoux, and A. Mimran. "Left Systolic Ventricular Function and Metabolic Disorders in Untreated Hypertensive Patients." *Arch Mal Coeur Vaiss* 85, no. 8 (1992): 1071–73.

Dustan, H. "Obesity and Hypertension." Part 2. *Ann Int Med* 103, no. 6 (1985): 1047–49.

Dyer, K. R., and A. Messing. "Peripheral Neuropathy Associated with Functional Islet Cell Adenoma in SV40 Transgenic Mice." *J Neuropathol Exp Neurol* 48, no. 4 (1989): 399–412.

Dzurik, R., J. Malkova, and V. Spustova. "Essential Hypertension and Insulin Resistance." *Cor Vasa* 33, no. 4 (1991): 294–300.

Eaton, S. B., M. Konner, and M. Shostak. "Stone Agers in the Fast Lane: Chronic Degenerative Diseases in Evolutionary Perspective." *American Journal of Medicine* 84, no. 4 (1988): 739–49.

Eaton, S. B., and M. J. Konner. "Stone Age Nutrition: Implications for Today." *ASDC J Dent Child* 53, no. 4 (1986): 300–3.

Einhorn, D., and L. Landsberg. "Nutrition and Diet in Hypertension." In *Modern Nutrition in Health and Disease*, 7th ed., edited by M. E. Shils and V. R. Young, 1277. Philadelphia: Lea & Febiger, 1988.

Ellis, E. N., S. K. Kemp, J. P. Frindik, and M. J. Elders. "Glomerulopathy in Patients with Donohue Syndrome (Leprechaunism)." *Diabetes Care* 14, no. 5 (1991): 413–14.

Ellison, R. C., J. W. Newburger, and D. M. Gross. "Pediatric Aspects of Essential Hypertension." *J Am Diet Assoc* 80 (1982): 21–25.

Epstein, M., and J. R. Sowers. "Diabetes Mellitus and Hypertension." *Hypertension* 19, no. 5 (1992): 403–18.

Eriksson, L. S., A. Thorne, and J. Wahren. "Diet-Induced Thermogenesis in Patients with Liver Cirrhosis." *Clin Physiol* 9, no. 2 (1989): 131–41.

Facchini, F., Y. D. Chen, C. B. Hollenbeck, and G. M. Reaven. "Relationship between Resistance to Insulin-Mediated Glucose Uptake, Urinary Uric Acid Clearance, and Plasma Uric Acid Concentration." *Journal of the American Medical Association* 266, no. 21 (1991): 3008–11.

Farquhar, J. W., A. Frank, R. C. Gross, and G. M. Reaven. "Glucose, Insulin, and Triglyceride Responses to High and Low Carbohydrate Diets in Man." *Journal of Clinical Investigation* 45, no. 10 (1966): 1648–56.

Feraille, E., M. Krempf, B. Chabonnel, J. B. Bouhour, and G. Nicolas. "Arterial

Hypertension in Patients with Obesity: Role of Hyperinsulinism and Insulin Resistance." *Rev Med Interne* 11, no. 4 (1990): 293–96.

Ferrannini, E., G. Buzzigoli, S. Bevilacqua, C. Boni, D. Del Chiaro, M. Oleggini, L. Brandi, and F. Maccari. "Interaction of Carnitine with Insulin-Stimulated Glucose Metabolism in Humans." Part 1. *American Journal of Physiology* 255, no. 6 (1988): E946–52.

Ferrari, P., P. Weidmann, S. Shaw, D. Giachino, W. Riesen, Y. Allemann, and G. Heynen. "Altered Insulin Sensitivity, Hyperinsulinemia, and Dyslipidemia in Individuals with a Hypertensive Parent." *American Journal of Medicine* 91, no. 6 (1991): 589–96.

Fisher, J. A. *The Chromium Program.* New York: Harper and Row, 1990.

Flack, J. M., and J. R. Sowers. "Epidemiologic and Clinical Aspects of Insulin Resistance and Hyperinsulinemia." *American Journal of Medicine* 91, no. 1A (1991): 11S–21S.

Flodin, N. W. "Atherosclerosis: An Insulin-Dependent Disease?" *J Amer Coll Nutr* 5 (1986): 417–27.

Fontbonne, A., M. A. Charles, N. Thibult, J. L. Richard, J. R. Claude, J. M. Warnet, G. E. Rosselin, and E. Eschwege. "Hyperinsulinemia as a Predictor of Coronary Heart Disease Mortality in a Healthy Population: The Paris Prospective Study, 15-Year Follow-Up." *Diabetologia* 34, no. 5 (1991): 356–61.

Fontbonne, A., and E. Eschwege. "Diabetes, Hyperglycemia, Hyperinsulinemia and Atherosclerosis: Epidemiological Data." Part 2. *Diabete Metab* 13, no. 3 (1987): 350–53.

———. "Insulin and Cardiovascular Disease: Paris Prospective Study." *Diabetes Care* 14, no. 6 (1991): 461–69.

Foreyt, J. P., and G. K. Goodrick. "Factors Common to Successful Therapy for the Obese Patient." In *Treatment of Obesity: A Multidisciplinary Approach*, edited by G. L. Blackburn, P. N. Benotti, and E. A. Mascioli. Presented through the Department of Education at Harvard Medical School, November 7–9, 1991.

Foster, D. W. "Insulin Resistance—A Secret Killer?" *New England Journal of Medicine* 320, no. 11 (1989): 733–34.

Friedman, J. M., and R. L. Leibel. "Tackling a Weighty Problem." *Cell* 69 (1992): 217–20.

Fuh, M. M-T., S-M. Shieh, D-A. Wu, Y-D. I. Chen, and G. M. Reaven. "Abnormalities of Carbohydrate and Lipid Metabolism in Patients with Hypertension." *Arch Intern Med* 147 (June 1987): 1035–38.

Fujimoto, S. "Studies on the Relationships between Blood Trace Metal Concentrations and the Clinical Status of Patients with Cerebrovascular Disease, Gastric Cancer, and Diabetes Mellitus." *Hokkaido Igaku Zasshi* 62, no. 6 (1987): 913–32.

Galvan, A. Q., E. Muscelli, C. Catalano, A. Natali, G. Sanna, A. Masoni, B. Bernar-

REFERENCES

dini, A. Barsacchi, and E. Ferrannini. "Insulin Decreases Circulating Vitamin E Levels in Humans." *Metabolism* 45, no. 8 (1996): 998–1003.

Garg, A., A. Bonanome, S. M. Grundy, Z. Zhang, and R. H. Unger. "Comparison of a High-Carbohydrate Diet with a High–Monounsaturated-Fat Diet in Patients with Non–Insulin-Dependent Diabetes." *New England Journal of Medicine* 319 (1988): 829–34.

Garg, A., S. M. Grundy, and R. H. Unger. "Comparison of Effects of High and Low Carbohydrate Diets on Plasma Lipoproteins and Insulin Sensitivity in Patients with Mild NIDDM." *Diabetes* 41, no. 10 (1992): 1278–85.

Garg, A., J. H. Helderman, M. Koffler, R. Ayuso, J. Rosenstock, and P. Raskin. "Relationship between Lipoprotein Levels in Vivo Insulin Action in Normal Young White Men." *Metabolism* 37, no. 10 (1988): 982–87.

Geiselman, P. J. "Sugar-Induced Hyperphagia: Is Hyperinsulinemia, Hypoglycemia, or Any Other Factor a 'Necessary' Condition?" *Appetite* 11, suppl. 1 (1988): 26–34.

Geiselman, P. J., and D. Novin. "The Role of Carbohydrates in Appetite, Hunger and Obesity." *Appetite: J Intake Res* 3 (1982): 203–23.

Ginsberg, H., J. M. Olefsky, G. Kimmerling, P. Crapo, and G. M. Reaven. "Induction of Hypertriglyceridemia by a Low-Fat Diet." *Journal of Clinical Endocrinological Metabolism* 42 (1976): 729–35.

Goldfine, A. B., D. C. Simonson, F. Folli, M. E. Patti, and C. R. Kahn. "Metabolic Effects of Sodium Metavanadate in Humans with Insulin Dependent and Non–Insulin Dependent Diabetes Mellitus in Vivo and in Vitro Studies." *Journal of Clinical Endocrinological Metabolism* 80, no. 11 (1995): 3311–20.

Gong, E. J., and F. P. Heald. "Diet, Nutrition, and Adolescence." In *Modern Nutrition in Health and Disease*, 7th ed., edited by M. E. Shils and V. R. Young, 969–81. Philadelphia: Lea & Febiger, 1988.

Grimaldi, A., C. Sachon, F. Bosquet, and R. Doumith. "Intolerance to Carbohydrates: The Seven Questions." *Rev Med Interne* 11, no. 4 (1990): 297–307.

Groop, L. C., and J. G. Eriksson. "The Etiology and Pathogenesis of Non–Insulin-Dependent Diabetes." *Ann Med* 24, no. 6 (1992): 483–89.

Grugni, G., G. Moreni, G. Guzzaloni, A. Ardizzi, C. De Medici, A. Sartorio, and F. Morabito. "No Correlation between Insulinemic Levels and Arterial Hypertension in Obese Females." *Minerva Endocrinol* 15, no. 2 (1990): 141–43.

Gupta, R. "Lifestyle Risk Factors and Coronary Heart Disease Prevalence in Indian Men." *J Assoc Physicians India* 44, no. 10 (1996): 689–93.

Gupta, R., H. Prakash, V. P. Gupta, and K. D. Gupta. "Prevalence and Determinants of Coronary Heart Disease in a Rural Population of India." *J Clin Epidemiol* 50, no. 2 (1997): 203–9.

Gwinup, G., and A. N. Elias. "Hypothesis: Insulin Is Responsible for the Vascular Complications of Diabetes." *Medical-Hypotheses* 34, no. 1 (1991): 1–6.

Haenel, H. "Phylogenesis and Nutrition." *Nahrung* 33, no. 9 (1989): 867–87.

Haffner, S. M., E. Ferrannini, H. P. Hazuda, and M. P. Stern. "Clustering of Cardiovascular Risk Factors in Confirmed Prehypertensive Individuals." *Hypertension* 20, no. 1 (1992): 38–45.

Haffner, S. M., M. P. Stern, H. P. Hazuda, B. D. Mitchel, and J. K. Patterson. "Cardiovascular Risk Factors in Confirmed Prediabetic Individuals: Does the Clock for Coronary Heart Disease Start Ticking before the Onset of Clinical Diabetes?" *Journal of the American Medical Association* 263, no. 21 (1990): 2893–98.

———. "Incidence of Type II Diabetes in Mexican Americans Predicted by Fasting Insulin and Glucose Levels, Obesity, and Body-Fat Distribution." *Diabetes* 39 (1990): 283–88.

Hallfrisch, J. "Metabolic Effects of Dietary Fructose." *Federation of American Societies for Experimental Biology Journal* 4, no. 9 (1990): 2652–60.

Heaton, K. W., S. N. Marcus, P. M. Emmett, and C. H. Bolton. "Particle Size of Wheat, Maize, and Oat Test Meals: Effects on Plasma Glucose and Insulin Responses and on the Rate of Starch Digestion in the Liver." *American Journal of Clinical Nutrition* 47, no. 4 (1988): 675–82.

Heber, G. L. "The Endocrinology of Obesity." In *Treatment of Obesity: A Multidisciplinary Approach*, edited by G. L. Blackburn, P. N. Benotti, and E. A. Mascioli. Presented through the Department of Education at Harvard Medical School, November 7–9, 1991.

Heller, R. F., and R. F. Heller. "Dietary Carbohydrates: The Frequency Factor." Paper presented at the annual meeting of the American Institute of Nutrition, April 30, 1993.

———. "Hunger and Cravings in the Overweight: A Physical Cause." Paper presented at the annual meeting of the American Institute of Nutrition, April 27, 1994.

———. "Hunger and Cravings in the Overweight: Correcting a Physical Cause." Paper presented at the annual meeting of the American Institute of Nutrition, April 27, 1994.

———. "Hyperinsulinemic Obesity and Carbohydrate Addiction: The Missing Link Is the Carbohydrate Frequency." *Medical Hypotheses* 42 (1994): 307–12.

———. "Hypertension in the Normal-Weight and Overweight: Correcting a Physical Cause." Paper presented at the annual meeting of the American Institute of Nutrition, April 13, 1995.

———. "Hypertriglyceridemia in the Normal-Weight and Overweight: Correcting a Physical Cause." Paper presented at the annual meeting of the American Institute of Nutrition, April 13, 1995.

———. "Profactor-H (Elevated Circulating Insulin): The Link to Health Risk Factors and Diseases of Civilization." *Medical Hypotheses* 45 (1995): 325–30.

REFERENCES

Hermann, W. J., K. Ward, and J. Faucett. "The Effect of Tocopherol on High-Density Lipoprotein Cholesterol." *American Journal of Clinical Pathology* 72, no. 5 (1979): 848–52.

Himsworth, H. P. "Diabetes Mellitus: Its Differentiation into Insulin-Sensitive and Insulin-Insensitive Types." *Lancet* (1936): 127–30.

Himsworth, H. P., and R. B. Kerr. "Insulin-Sensitive and Insulin-Insensitive Types of Diabetes Mellitus." In *Clinical Science Incorporating Heart*, vol. 4, edited by Thomas Lewis, 119–52. London: Shaw and Sons, 1939.

Hollenbeck, C., A. M. Coulston, and G. M. Reaven. "Effects of Sucrose on Carbohydrate and Lipid Metabolism in NIDDM Patients." *Diabetes Care* 12, no. 1 (1989): 62–66.

Hollenbeck, C., and G. M. Reaven. "Variations in Insulin-Stimulated Glucose Uptake in Healthy Individuals with Normal Glucose Tolerance." *Journal of Clinical Endocrinological Metabolism* 64 (1987): 1169–73.

Hrnciar, J., K. Jakubikova, and J. Okapcova. "How Should We Implement the Basic Principles of Treatment of Type 2 Diabetes Mellitus from the Aspect of the Hormone-Metabolic Syndrome X (5H)?" *Vnitr Lek* 38, no. 8 (1992): 729–37.

Hu, F. B., M. J. Stampfer, J. E. Mason, E. Rim, G. A. Colditz, B. A. Rosner, C. H. Hennekens, and W. C. Willet. "Dietary Fat Intake and the Risk of Coronary Heart Disease in Women." *New England Journal of Medicine* 337 (1997): 1491–99.

Hubner, G., H. H. Von Dorsche, and H. Zuhlke. "Morphological Studies of the Effect of Chromium-III-Chloride on the Islet Cell Organ in Rats under the Conditions of High and Low Fat Diets." *Anat Anz* 167, no. 5 (1988): 389–91.

Hud, J. A., Jr., J. B. Cohen, J. M. Wagner, and P. D. Cruz Jr. "Prevalence and Significance of Acanthosis Nigricans in an Adult Obese Population." *Arch Dermatol* 128, no. 7 (1992): 941–44.

Hughes, C. E. "Prayer and Healing: A Case Study." *J Holist Nurs* 15, no. 3 (1997): 318–24.

Ishiguro, T., Y. Sato, Y. Oshida, K. Yamanouchi, M. Okuyama, and N. Sakamoto. "The Relationship between Insulin Sensitivity and Weight Reduction in Simple Obese and Obese Diabetic Patients." *Nagoya J Med Sci* 49 (1987): 61–69.

Ishizuka, J., R. J. Bold, C. M. Townsend Jr., and J. C. Thompson. "In Vitro Relationship between Magnesium and Insulin Secretion." *Magnes Res* 7, no. 1 (1994): 17–22.

Janka, H. U., A. G. Ziegler, E. Standl, and H. Mehnert. "Daily Insulin Dose as a Predictor of Macrovascular Disease in Insulin Treated Non–Insulin-Dependent Diabetics." Part 2. *Diabetes Metab* 13, no. 3 (1987): 359–64.

Jeejeebhoy, K. N., R. C. Chu, E. B. Marliss, G. R. Greenburg, and A. Bruce-Robertson. "Chromium Deficiency, Glucose Intolerance and Neuropathy

Reversed by Chromium Supplementation in a Patient Receiving Long Term Total Parenteral Nutrition." *American Journal of Clinical Nutrition* 30 (1977): 531–38.

Jenkins, D. J. A. "Nutrition and Diet in Management of Diseases of the Gastrointestinal Tract: (D) Colon." In *Modern Nutrition in Health and Disease*, 7th ed., edited by M. E. Shils and V. R. Young, 1023–66. Philadelphia: Lea & Febiger, 1988.

Jenkins, D. J. A., N. Shapira, G. Greenberg, A. L. Jenkins, G. R. Collier, C. Poduch, T. M. Wolever, R. A. Anderson, and L. M. Blendis. "Low Glycemic Index Foods and Reduced Glucose, Amino Acid, and Endocrine Responses in Cirrhosis." *Am J Gastroenterol* 84, no. 7 (1989): 732–39.

Jern, S. "Effects of Acute Carbohydrate Administration on Central and Peripheral Hemodynamic Responses to Mental Stress." *Hypertension* 18, no. 6 (1991): 790–97.

Johansson, G. "Four Years' Experience with Magnesium Hydroxide in Renal Stone Disease." *Magnesium Bulletin* (February 1981).

Kakar, F., S. D. Hursting, M. M. Henderson, and M. D. Thornquist. "Dietary Sugar and Breast Cancer: Epidemiologic Evidence." *Clinical Nutrition* 9 (1990): 68–71.

Kakar, F., M. D. Thornquist, M. M. Henderson, R. D. Klein, S. M. Kozawa, G. A. Santisteben, S. D. Hursting, and N. D. Urban. "The Effect of Dietary Sugar and Dietary Antioxidants on Mammary Tumor Growth and Lethality in BALB/C Mice." *Clinical Nutrition* 9 (1990): 62–67.

Kannel, W. B., P. W. Wilson, and T. J. Zhang. "The Epidemiology of Impaired Glucose Tolerance and Hypertension." Part 2. *American Heart Journal* 121, no. 4 (1991): 1268–73.

Kaplan, N. M. "The Deadly Quartet: Upper-Body Obesity, Glucose Intolerance, Hypertriglyceridemia, and Hypertension." *Arch Intern Med* 149 (1989): 1514–20.

Kazumi, T., G. Yoshino, K. Matsuba, M. Iwai, I. Iwatani, M. Matsushita, T. Kasama, T. Hosokawa, F. Numano, and S. Baba. "Effects of Dietary Glucose or Fructose on the Secretion Rate and Particle Size of Triglyceride-Rich Lipoproteins in Zucker Fatty Rats." *Metabolism* 40, no. 9 (1991): 962–66.

Kemp, K. "Carbohydrate Addiction." *Practitioner* 190 (1963): 358–64.

Klurfeld, D. M., L. M. Lloyd, C. B. Welch, M. J. Davis, O. L. Tulp, and D. Kritchevsky. "Reduction of Enhanced Mammary Carcinogenesis in LA/N-Cp (Corpulent) Rats by Energy Restriction." *Proc Soc Exp Biol Med* 196, no. 4 (1991): 381–84.

Koop, C. E. *The Surgeon General's Report on Nutrition and Health*. U.S. Department of Health and Human Services, publication no. 88-50210, 1988.

Koppel, J. D. "Nutrition, Diet, and the Kidney." In *Modern Nutrition in Health and Disease*, 7th ed., edited by M. E. Shils and V. R. Young, 1230–68. Philadelphia: Lea & Febiger, 1988.

Kornhuber, H. H., J. Kornhuber, W. Wanner, A. Kornhuber, and C. H. Kaiserauer. "Alcohol, Smoking and Body Build: Obesity as a Result of the Toxic Effect of 'Social' Alcohol Consumption." *Clin Physiol Biochem* 7, nos. 3–4 (1989): 203–16.

Kozlovksy, A. S., P. B. Moser, S. Reisner, and R. A. Anderson. "Effects of Diets High in Simple Sugars on Urinary Chromium Losses." *Metabolism* 35, no. 6 (1986): 515–18.

Kumpulainen, J. T., W. R. Wolf, C. Veillon, and W. Mertz. "Determination of Chromium in Selected United States Diets." *J Agric Food Chem* 27, no. 3 (1979): 490–94.

Lääkso, M., H. Sarlund, R. Salonen, M. Suhonen, K. Pyörälä, J. T. Salonen, and P. Karhapää. "Asymptomatic Atherosclerosis and Insulin Resistance." *Atheroscler and Thromb* 11 (1991): 1068–76.

Landin, K. "Treating Insulin Resistance in Hypertension with Metformin Reduces Both Blood Pressure and Metabolic Risk Factors." *Journal of Internal Medicine* 229, no. 2 (February 1991): 181–87.

Landsberg, L. "Insulin Resistance, Energy Balance and Sympathetic Nervous System Activity." *Clin Exp Hypertens* 12, no. 5 (1990): 817–30.

———. "Obesity, Metabolism, and Hypertension." *Yale J Biol Med* 62, no. 5 (1989): 511–19.

Lange, J., J. Arends, and B. Willms. "Alcohol-Induced Hypoglycemia in Type 1 Diabetes." *Medizinische Klinik* 86, no. 11 (1991): 551–54.

Lefebvre, P. J., and A. J. Scheen. "Hypoglycemia." In *Diabetes Mellitus, Theory and Practice*, edited by H. Rifkin and D. Porte Jr., 896–910. 1990.

Leibel, R. "Obesity and Nutrient Metabolism." Paper presented at the American Association for the Advancement of Science, May 26, 1984.

Leiter, E. H. "Control of Spontaneous Glucose Intolerance, Hyperinsulinemia, and Islet Hyperplasia in Nonobese C3H.SW Male Mice by Y-Linked Locus and Adrenal Gland." *Metabolism* 37, no. 7 (1988): 689–96.

Leutenegger, M. "Theoretical Aspects of the Relationship between Diabetic Macroangiopathy and Hyperinsulinism." *Presse Med* 21, no. 28 (1992): 1324–29.

Levin, J. S. "How Prayer Heals: A Theoretical Model." *Altern Ther Health Med* 2, no. 1 (1996): 66–73.

Lillioja, S., D. M. Mott, B. V. Howard, P. H. Bennett, H. Yki-Jarvinen, D. Freymond, B. L. Nyomba, F. Zurlo, B. Swinburn, and C. Bogardus. "Impaired Glucose Tolerance as a Disorder of Insulin Action: Longitudinal and Cross-Sectional Studies in Pima Indians." *New England Journal of Medicine* 318 (1988): 1217–25.

Linder, M. C., ed. *Nutritional Biochemistry and Metabolism with Clinical Applications*. New York: Elsevier, 1985.

Lindin, K., L. Tengborn, and U. Smith. "Treating Insulin Resistance in Hypertension with Metformin Reduces Both Blood Pressure and Metabolic Risk Factors." *Journal of Internal Medicine* 229, no. 2 (1991): 181–87.

Linscheer, W. G., and A. J. Vergroesen. "Lipids." In *Modern Nutrition in Health and Disease*, 7th ed., edited by M. E. Shils and V. R. Young, 72–107. Philadelphia: Lea & Febiger, 1988.

Lithell, H. "Insulin Resistance and Cardiovascular Drugs." *Clin Exp Hypertens* 14, nos. 1–2 (1992): 151–62.

Liu, G., A. Coulston, C. Hollenbeck, and G. Reaven. "The Effect of Sucrose Content in High and Low Carbohydrate Diets on Plasma Glucose, Insulin, and Lipid Responses in Hypertriglyceridemic Humans." *Journal of Clinical Endocrinological Metabolism* 59, no. 4 (1984): 636–42.

Losonczy, K. G., T. B. Harris, and R. J. Havlik. "Vitamin E and Vitamin C Supplement Use and Risk of All-Cause and Coronary Heart Disease Mortality in Older Persons: The Established Populations for Epidemiologic Studies of the Elderly." *American Journal of Clinical Nutrition* 64, no. 2 (1996): 190–96.

Lutz, W. "Life Expectancy—The Japanese Experience." *Wein Med Wochenschr* 141, no. 7 (1991): 148–50.

Macdonald, I. "Carbohydrates." In *Modern Nutrition in Health and Disease*, 7th ed., edited by M. E. Shils and V. R. Young, 38–51. Philadelphia: Lea & Febiger, 1988.

Mahler, R. J. "Diabetes and Hypertension." *Horm Metab Res* 22, no. 12 (1990): 599–607.

Malinow, M. R., P. B. Duell, D. L. Hess, P. H. Anderson, W. D. Kruger, B. E. Phillipson, R. A. Gluckman, P. C. Block, and B. M. Upson. "Reduction of Plasma Homocyst[e]ine Levels by Breakfast Cereal Fortified with Folic Acid in Patients with Coronary Heart Disease." *New England Journal of Medicine* 338, no. 15 (1998): 1009–15.

Marshall, S., W. T. Garvey, and R. R. Traxinger. "New Insights into the Metabolic Regulation of Insulin Action and Insulin Resistance: Role of Glucose and Amino Acids." *Federation of American Societies for Experimental Biology Journal* 5 (1991): 3031–36.

Marston, R. W., and B. B. Peterkin. "Nutrient Content of the National Food Supply." *Natl Food Rev* 9 (1980): 21–25.

McCarty, M. F. "Complementary Vascular-Protective Actions of Magnesium and Taurine: A Rationale for Magnesium Taurate." *Med Hypotheses* 46, no. 2 (1996): 89–100.

Melchoir, J. C., D. Rigaud, N. Colas-Linhart, A. Petiet, A. Girard, and M. Apfelbaum. "Immunoreactive Beta-Endorphin Increases after an Aspartame

REFERENCES

Chocolate Drink in Healthy Human Subjects." *Physiol Behav* 50, no. 5 (1991): 941–44.

Mizushima, S., Y. Nara, M. Sawamura, and Y. Yamori. "Effects of Oral Taurine Supplementation on Lipids and Sympathetic Nerve Tone." *Adv Exp Med Biol* 403 (1996): 615–22.

Modan, M. and H. Halkin. "Hyperinsulinemia or Increased Sympathetic Drive as Links for Obesity and Hypertension." *Diabetes Care* 14, no. 6 (1991): 470–87.

Modan, M., H. Halkin, S. Almog, A. Lusky, A. Eshkol, M. Sheft, A. Shitrit, and Z. Fuchs. "Hyperinsulinemia: A Link between Hypertension, Obesity and Glucose Intolerance." *Journal of Clinical Investigation* 75 (1985): 809–17.

Modan, M., H. Halkin, A. Lusky, P. Segal, Z. Fuchs, and A. Chetrit. "Hyperinsulinemia Is Characterized by Jointly Distributed Plasma VLDL, LDL, and HDL Levels: A Population Study." *Atheroscler* 8, no. 3 (1988): 227–36.

Molnar, D. "Insulin Secretion and Carbohydrate Tolerance in Childhood Obesity." *Klin Padiatr* 202, no. 3 (1990): 131–35.

Morgan, J. B., D. A. York, A. Wasilewska, and J. Portman. "A Study of the Thermic Responses to a Meal and to a Sympathomimetic Drug (Ephedrine) in Relation to Energy Balance in Man." *Brit J Nutr* 47 (19XX): 21–32.

Mosca, L., M. Rubenfire, C Mandel, C. Rock, T. Tarshis, A. Tsai, and T. Pearson. "Antioxidant Nutrient Supplementation Reduces the Susceptibility of Low Density Lipoprotein to Oxidation in Patients with Coronary Artery Disease." *J Am Coll Cardiol* 30, no. 2 (1997): 392–99.

Mountjoy, K. G., and I. M. Holdaway. "Effect of Insulin Receptor Down Regulation on Insulin-Stimulated Thymidine Incorporation in Cultured Human Fibroblasts and Tumor Cell Lines." *Cancer Biochem Biophys* 12, no. 2 (1991): 117–26.

Nader, S. "Polycystic Ovary Syndrome and the Androgen-Insulin Connection." *American Journal of Obstetrics and Gynecology* 165, no. 2 (1991): 346–48.

National Research Council, Food and Nutrition Board, Commission on Life Sciences. *Recommended Dietary Allowances*, 10th ed., 241–43. Washington, D.C.: National Academy Press, 1989.

Niijima, A., T. Togiyama, and A. Adachi. "Cephalic-Phase Insulin Release Induced by Taste Stimulus of Monosodium Glutamate (Umami Taste)." *Physiol Behav* 48, no. 6 (1990): 905–8.

Nobels, F., and D. Dewailly. "Puberty and Polycystic Ovarian Syndrome: The Insulin/Insulin-Like Growth Factor I Hypothesis." *Fertil Steril* 58, no. 4 (1992): 655–66.

Noble, E. P., R. E. Noble, T. Ritchie, K. Syndulko, M. C. Bohlman, L. A. Noble, Y. Zhang, R. S. Sparkes, and D. K. Grandy. "D2 Dopamine Receptor Gene and Obesity." *Int J Eat Disord* 15, no. 3 (1994): 205–17.

Noberasco, G., P. Odetti, D. Boeri, M. Maiello, and L. Adezati. "Malondialdehyde (MDA) Level in Diabetic Subjects: Relationship with Blood Glucose and Glycosylated Hemoglobin." *Biomed Pharmacother* 45, nos. 4–5 (1991): 193–96.

O'Dea, K. "Westernization and Non–Insulin-Dependent Diabetes in Australian Aborigines." *Ethn Dis* 1, no. 2 (1991): 171–87.

———. "Westernization, Insulin Resistance and Diabetes in Australian Aborigines." *Med J Aust* 155, no. 4 (1991): 258–64.

O'Donnell, M. J., and P. M. Dodson. "The Non-Drug Treatment of Hypertension in the Diabetic Patient." *J Hum Hypertens* 5, no. 4 (1991): 287–94.

OH, W., N. L. Gelardi, and C. J. Cha. "Maternal Hyperglycemia in Pregnant Rats: Its Effect on Growth and Carbohydrate Metabolism in the Offspring." *Metabolism* 37, no. 12 (1988): 1146–51.

Ohlson, L. O., B. Larsson, P. Bjorntorp, H. Eriksson, K. Szardsudd, L. Welin, G. Tibblin, and L. Wilhelmsen. "Risk Factors for Type 2 (Non–Insulin-Dependent) Diabetes Mellitus: Thirteen and One-Half Years of Follow-Up of the Participants in a Study of Swedish Men Born in 1913." *Diabetologia* 31, no. 11 (1988): 798–805.

Olefsky, J. M. "Obesity." In *Harrison's Principles of Internal Medicine*, 12th ed., edited by J. D. Wilson, D. Braunwald, K. J. Isselbacher, R. G. Petersdorf, J. B. Martin, A. S. Fauci, and R. K. Root, 411–17. McGraw-Hill, Health Professions Division, 1991.

"Oral Contraceptives." Mead Johnson Laboratories. OVCON®50 and OVCON®35 (Norethindrone and Ethinyl Estradiol tablets, UPS). A Bristol-Meyers Squibb Company, Evansville, Indiana, 1990.

Paolisso, G., and E. Ravussin. "Intracellular Magnesium and Insulin Resistance: Results in Pima Indians and Caucasians." *Journal of Clinical Endocrinological Metabolism* 80, no. 4 (1995): 1382–85.

Paolisso, G., M. R. Tagliamonte, R. Marfella, G. Verrazzo, F. D'Onofrio, and D. Giugliano. "L-Arginine but Not D-Arginine Stimulates Insulin-Mediated Glucose Uptake." *Metabolism* 46, no. 9 (1997): 1068–73.

Passwater, R. A. *Supernutrition for Healthy Hearts.* New York: Dial, 1978.

Patel, P., M. A. Mendall, D. Carrington, D. P. Strachan, E. Leatham, N. Molineaux, J. Levy, C. Blakeston, C. A. Seymour, A. J. Camm, et al. "Association of *Helicobacter Pylori* and *Chlamydia Pneumoniae* Infections with Coronary Heart Disease and Cardiovascular Risk Factors." *British Medical Journal* 311, no. 7007 (1995): 711–14.

Pedersen, O. "Insulin Resistance—A Pathophysiological Condition with Numerous Sequelae: Non–Insulin-Dependent Diabetes Mellitus (NIDDM), Android Obesity, Essential Hypertension, Dyspipidemia and Atherosclerosis." *Ugeskr Laeger* 154, no. 20 (1992): 1411–18.

Peterson, C. M., and L. Jovanovic-Peterson. "Randomized Crossover Study of 40% vs. 55% Carbohydrate Weight Loss Strat with Previous Gestational Diabetes

REFERENCES

Mellitus and Non-Diabetic Women of 130%–200% Ideal Body Weight." *J Amer Coll Nutr* 14, no. 4 (1995): 369–75.

Petrides, A. S., and R. A. Defronzo. "Glucose Metabolism in Cirrhosis." *H Hepatol* 8, no. 1 (1989): 107–14.

Piatti, P. M., A. E. Pontirol, A. Caumo, G. Santambrogio, L. D. Monti, S. Costa, F. Garbetta, L. Baruffaldi, C. Cobelli, and G. Pozza. "Hyperinsulinemia Decreases Second-Phase but Not First-Phase Arginine-Induced Insulin Release in Humans." *Diabetes* 43, no. 9 (1994): 1157–63.

Pi-Sunyer, F. X. "Obesity." In *Modern Nutrition in Health and Disease*, 7th ed., edited by M. E. Shils and V. R. Young, 795–816. Philadelphia: Lea & Febiger, 1988.

Pollare, T., B. Vessby, and H. Lithell. "Lipoprotein Lipase Activity in Skeletal Muscle Is Related to Insulin Sensitivity." *Arterioscler Thromb* 11, no. 5 (1991): 1192–1203.

Pontremoli, R., I. Zavaroni, S. Mazza, M. Battezzati, F. Massarino, A. Tixianello, and G. M. Reaven. "Changes in Blood Pressure, Plasma Triglyceride and Aldosterone Concentration, and Red Cell Cation Concentration in Patients with Hyperinsulinemia." Part 1. *American Journal of Hypertension* 4, no. 2 (1991): 159–63.

Poulter, N. R. "Treatment of Hypertension: A Clinical Epidemiologist's View." *Journal of Cardiovascular Pharmacology* 18, suppl. 2 (1991): S35–38.

Prelevic, G. M., M. I. Wurzburger, L. Balint-Peric, and J. Ginsberg. "Twenty-Four-Hour Serum Growth Hormone, Insulin, C-Peptide and Blood Glucose Profiles and Serum Insulin-Like Growth Factor-I Concentrations in Women with Polycystic Ovaries." *Horm Res* 37, nos. 4–5 (1992): 125–31.

Princen, H. M., W. Van Duyvenvoorde, R. Buytenhek, A. Van Der Laarse, G. Van Poppel, J. A. Gevers Leuven, and V. W. Van Hinsbergh. "Supplementation with Low Doses of Vitamin E Protects LDL from Lipid Peroxidation in Men and Women." *Arterioscler Thromb Vasc Biol* 15, no. 3 (1995): 325–33.

Proctor, C. A., T. B. Proctor, and B. Proctor. "Etiology and Treatment of Fluid Retention (Hydrops) in Meniere's Syndrome." *Ear Nose Throat J* 71, no. 12 (1992): 631–35.

Proudler, A. J., C. V. Felton, and J. C. Stevenson. "Ageing and the Response of Plasma Insulin, Glucose and C-Peptide Concentrations to Intravenous Glucose in Postmenopausal Women." *Clinical Science* 83 (1992): 489–94.

Pyörälä, M., H. Miettinen, M. Laakso, and K. Pyörälä. "Hyperinsulinemia Predicts Coronary Heart Disease Risk in Healthy Middle-Aged Men: The 22-Year Follow-Up Results of the Helsinki Policemen Study." *Circulation* 98 (1998): 398–404.

Randolph, T. G. "The Descriptive Features of Food Addiction." *Quart J Studies Alcohol* 17 (1956): 198–224.

———. "Masked Food Allergy as a Factor in the Development and Persistence of Obesity." *J Lab Clin Med* 32 (1947): 1547–49.

Randolph, T. G., and R. W. Moss. *An Alternative Approach Allergies.* New York: Lippincott and Crowell, 1980.

Randolph, J. F., S. Kipersztok, J. W. Ayers, R. Ansbacher, H. Peegel, and K. M. Menon. "The Effect of Insulin on Aromatase Activity in Isolated Human Endometrial Glands and Stroma." *American Journal of Obstetrics and Gynecology* 157, no. 6 (1990): 1534–39.

Ravussin, E. "Energy Metabolism in Obesity: Studies in the Pima Indians." *Diabetes Care* 16, no. 1 (1993): 232–38.

Ravussin, E., and C. Bogardus. "Energy Expenditure in the Obese: Is There a Thrifty Gene?" *Infusionstherapie* 17 (1990): 108–12.

Reaven, G. M. "Insulin Resistance and Compensatory Hyperinsulinemia: Role in Hypertension, Dyslipidemia, and Coronary Heart Disease." Part 2. *American Heart Journal* 121, no. 4 (1991): 1283–88.

———. "Insulin Resistance, Hyperinsulinemia, and Hypertriglyceridemia in the Etiology and Clinical Course of Hypertension." *American Journal of Medicine* 90, no. 2A (1991): 7S–11S.

———. "Relationship between Insulin Resistance and Hypertension." *Diabetes Care* 14, suppl. 4 (1991): 33–38.

———. "Role of Insulin Resistance in Human Disease." *Nutrition* 131, no. 1 (1997): 65.

Reaven, G. M., and B. B. Hoffman. "Hypertension as a Disease of Carbohydrate and Lipoprotein Metabolism." *American Journal of Medicine* 87, no. 6A (1989): 2S–6S.

Reiser, S., M. C. Bickard, J. Hallfrisch, O. E. Michaelis IV and E. S. Prather. "Blood Lipids and Their Distribution in Lipoproteins in Hyperinsulinemic Subjects Fed Three Different Levels of Sucrose." *Journal of Nutrition* 111 (1981): 1045–57.

Reiser, S., A. S. Powell, D. J. Scholfield, P. Panda, K. C. Ellwood, and J. J. Canary. "Blood Lipids, Lipoproteins, Apoproteins, and Uric Acid in Med Fed Diets Containing Fructose or High-Amylose Cornstarch." *American Journal of Clinical Nutrition* 49, no. 5 (1989): 832–39.

Ri, K. "Study on Insulin Resistance in Rats Treated with Estrogen and Progesterone—Assessment with Euglycemic Clamp Technique." *Nippon Naibunpi Gakkai Zasshi* 63, no. 6 (1987): 798–808.

Riales, R. "Effect of Chromium Chloride Supplementation on Glucose Tolerance and Serum Lipids Including High-Density Lipoprotein of Adult Men." *American Journal of Clinical Nutrition* 34, no. 12 (1981): 2670–78.

Rimm, I. J., and A. A. Rimm. "Association between Juvenile Onset Obesity and Severe Obesity in 73,532 Women." *American Journal of Public Health* 66 (1976): 479–81.

Robertson, D., J. C. Frolich, R. K. Carr, J. T. Watson, J. W. Hollifield, D. G. Shand,

REFERENCES

and J. A. Oates. "Effects of Caffeine on Plasma Renin Activity, Catecholamines and Blood Pressure." *New England Journal of Medicine* 298, no. 4 (1978): 181–86.

Rodin, J. "Insulin Levels, Hunger, and Food Intake: An Example of Feedback Loops in Body Weight Regulation." *Health Psychol* 4 (1985): 1–18.

Rohner-Jeanrenaud, F., and B. Jeanrenaud. "A Role for the Vagus Nerve in the Etiology and Maintenance of the Hyperinsulinemia of Genetically Obese Fa/Fa Rats." *International Journal of Obesity* 9, suppl. 1 (1985): 71–75.

Rombauer, I. S., and Becker M. Rombauer. *Joy of Cooking*. New York: New American Library, 1964.

Rönnemaa, T., M. Laakso, K. Pyörälä, V. Kallio, and P Puukka. "High Fasting Plasma Insulin Is an Indicator of Coronary Heart Disease in Non–Insulin-Dependent Diabetic Patients and Nondiabetic Subjects." *Arterioscler-Thromb* 11, no. 1 (1991): 80–90.

Rosolova, H., O. Mayer Jr., and G. Reaven. "Effect of Variations in Plasma Magnesium Concentration on Resistance to Insulin-Mediated Glucose Disposal in Nondiabetic Subjects." *Journal of Clinical Endocrinological Metabolism* 82, no. 11 (1997): 3783–85.

Rossi-Fanelli, F., A. Cascino, and M. Muscaritoli. "Abnormal Substrate Metabolism and Nutritional Strategies in Cancer Management." *J Parenter Enteral Nutr* 15, no. 6 (1991): 680–83.

Ruderman, N. "Exercise in Therapy and Prevention of Type II Diabetes: Implications for Blacks." *Diabetes Care* 13, no. 11 (1990): 1163–68.

Rupp, H. "Insulin Resistance, Hyperinsulinemia, and Cardiovascular Disease: The Need for Novel Dietary Prevention Strategies" (editorial). *Basic Res Cardiol* 87, no. 2 (1992): 99–105.

Saad, M. F., W. C. Knowler, D. J. Pettitt, R. G. Nelson, D. M. Mott, and P. H. Bennett. "The Natural History of Impaired Glucose Tolerance in the Pima Indians." *New England Journal of Medicine* 319 (1988): 1500–6.

Salomaa, V. V., J. Tuomilehto, M. Jaucianien, H. J. Korhonsen, J. Stengard, M. Uusitupa, M. Pitkanen, and I. Penttilla. "Hypertriglyceridemia in Different Degrees of Glucose Intolerance in a Finnish Population-Based Study." *Diabetes Care* 15, no. 5 (1992): 657–65.

Sanchez, A., and R. W. Hubbard. "Plasma Amino Acids and the Insulin/Glucagon Ratio as an Explanation of the Dietary Protein Modulation of Atherosclerosis." *Medical Hypotheses* 35, no. 4 (1991): 324–29.

Sato, Y., S. Shiraishi, Y. Oshida, T. Ishiguro, and N. Sakamoto. "Experimental Atherosclerosis-Like Lesions Induced by Hyperinsulinism in Wistar Rats." *Diabetes* 38 (1989): 91–96.

Saudia, T. L., Mr. R. Kinney, K. C. Brown, and L. Young-Ward. "Health Locus of Control and Helpfulness of Prayer." *Heart Lung* 20, no. 1 (1991): 60–65.

Scallet, A. C., P. L. Faris, M. C. Beinfeld, and J. W. Olney. "Hypothalamic Neurotoxins Alter the Contents of Immunoreactive Cholecystokinin in Pituitary." *Brain Res* 407, no. 2 (1987): 390–93.

Schneider, D. J., and B. E. Sobel. "Augmentation of Synthesis of Plasminogen Activator Inhibitor Type 1 by Insulin and Insulin-Like Growth Factor Type I: Implications for Vascular Disease in Hyperinsulinemic States." *Proc Natl Acad Sci USA* 88, no. 22 (1991): 9959–63.

Schroeder, H. A. "The Role of Chromium in Mammalian Nutrition." *American Journal of Clinical Nutrition* 21, no. 6 (1968): 230–44.

Schumann, D. "Post-Operative Hyperglycemia: Clinical Benefits of Insulin Therapy." *Heart-Lung* 19, no. 2 (1990): 165–73.

Schwarz, K., and W. Mertz. "A Glucose Tolerance Factor and Its Differentiation from Factor 3." *Arch Biochem Biophys* 72 (1957): 515–18.

Sechi, L. A., A. Melis, A. Pala, A. Marigliano, G. Sechi, and R. Tedde. "Serum Insulin, Insulin Sensitivity, and Erythrocyte Sodium Metabolism in Normotensive and Essential Hypertensive Subjects with and without Overweight." *Clin Exp Hypertens* [A] 13, no. 2 (1991): 261–72.

Sharma, A. M., K. Ruland, K. P. Spies, and A. Distler. "Salt Sensitivity in Young Normotensive Subjects Is Associated with a Hyperinsulinemic Response to Oral Glucose." *J Hypertens* 9, no. 4 (1991): 329–35.

Shelepov, V. P., V. A. Chekulaev, and G. R. Pasha-Zade. "Effect of Putrescine on Carbohydrate and Lipid Metabolism in Rats." *Biomed Sci* 1, no. 6 (1990): 591–96.

Shelmet, J. J., G. A. Reichard, C. L. Skutches, R. D. Hoeldtke, O. E. Owen, and G. Boden. "Ethanol Causes Acute Inhibition of Carbohydrate, Fat, and Protein Oxidation and Insulin Resistance." *Journal of Clinical Investigation* 81, no. 4 (1988): 1137–45.

Shils, M. E. "Enteral (Tube) and Parenteral Nutrition Support." In *Modern Nutrition in Health and Disease*, 7th ed., edited by M. E. Shils and V. R. Young, 1023–66. Philadelphia: Lea & Febiger, 1988.

Sicree, R. A., P. Z. Zimmet, H. O. M. King, and J. S. Coventry. "Plasma Insulin Response among Nauruans: Prediction of Deterioration in Glucose Tolerance over 6 Yr." *Diabetes* 36 (1987): 179–86.

Sidey, F. M. "Role of the Adrenal Medulla in Stress-Induced Hyperinsulinemia in Normal Mice and in Mice Infected with *Bordetella Pertussis* or Treated with Pertussis Toxin." *Journal of Endocrinology* 118, no. 1 (1988): 135–40.

Simons, L. A., M. Von Konigsmark, and S. Balasubramaniam. Aust. "What Dose of Vitamin E Is Required to Reduce Susceptibility of LDL to Oxidation?" *N Z J Med* 26, no. 4 (1996): 496–503.

Simonson, D. C. "Hyperinsulinemia and Its Sequelae." *Horm Metab Res* 22, suppl. (1990): 17–25.

REFERENCES

Singer, P., and R. Baumann. "Glucose-Induced or Postprandial Hyperinsulinemia in Mild Essential Hypertension—An Underestimated Biochemical Risk Factor." *Medical Hypotheses* 34, no. 2 (1991): 257–164.

Skouby, S. O., O. Andersen, K. R. Petersen, L. Molsted-Pedersen, and C. Kuhl. "Mechanism of Action of Oral Contraceptives on Carbohydrate Metabolism at the Cellular Level." Part 2. *American Journal of Obstetrics and Gynecology* 163, no. 1 (1990): 343–48.

Skouby, S. O., O. Andersen, N. Saurbrey, and C. Kuhl. "Oral Contraception and Insulin Sensitivity: In Vivo Assessment in Normal Women and in Women with Previous Gestational Diabetes." *Journal of Clinical Endocrinological Metabolism* 64 (1987): 519–26.

Smith, U., S. Gudbjornsdottir, and K. Landin. "Hypertension as a Metabolic Disorder—An Overview." *Journal of Internal Medicine* 735, suppl. (1991): 1–7.

Somogyi, J. C., and U. Nageli. "Antithiamine Effect of Coffee." *Int J Vit Nutr Res* 46, no. 2 (1976): 149–53.

Sowers, J. R. "Is Hypertension an Insulin-Resistant State? Metabolic Changes Associated with Hypertension and Antihypertensive Therapy." Part 2. *American Heart Journal* 122, no. 3 (1991): 932–35.

Sowers, J. R., P. R. Standley, J. L. Ram, M. B. Zemel, and L. M. Resnick. "Insulin Resistance, Carbohydrate Metabolism, and Hypertension." Part 2. *American Journal of Hypertension* 4, no. 7 (1991): 46S–472S.

Spring, B., J. Chiodo, M. Harden, M. J. Bourgeois, J. D. Mason, and L. Lutherer. "Psychobiological Effects of Carbohydrates." *Journal of Clinical Psychiatry* 50, no. 5, suppl. (1989): 27–33.

Spustova, V. "Insulin Resistance as a Risk Factor in Atherosclerosis." *Vnitr Le* 38, no. 11 (1992): 1105–10.

Statistical Bulletin. "Diabetes Mortality Update." *Statistical Bulletin* (October–December 1989): 24–35.

———. "Hypertension in the United States: 1960 to 1980 and 1987 Estimates." *Statistical Bulletin* (1989): 13–17.

———. "Life Expectancy Remains at Record Level." *Statistical Bulletin* (1989): 26–30.

Staub, H. W., G. Reussner, and R. Thiessen Jr. "Serum Cholesterol Reduction by Chromium in Hypercholesterolemic Rats." *Science* 165 (1969): 746–47.

Stern, M. P., and S. M. Haffner. "Body Fat Distribution and Hyperinsulinemia as Risk Factors for Diabetes and Cardiovascular Disease." *Atheroscler* 6 (1986): 123–30.

Stern, M. P., J. A. A. Knapp, H. P. Hazuda, S. M. Haffner, J. K. Patterson, and B. D. Mitchell. "Genetic and Environmental Determinants of Type II Diabetes in Mexican Americans. Is There a 'Descending Limb' to the Modernization/Diabetes Relationship?" *Diabetes Care* 14, no. 7 (1991): 649–54.

Stock, S., L. Granstrom, L. Backman, A. S. Matthiesen, and K. Uvnas-Moberg. "Elevated Plasma Levels of Oxytocin in Obese Subjects before and after Gastric Banding." *International Journal of Obesity* 13, no. 2 (1989): 213–22.

Stolar, M. W. "Atherosclerosis in Diabetes: The Role of Hyperinsulinemia." *Metabolism* 37, no. 2, suppl. 1 (1988): 1–9.

Stoll, B. A. "Nutrition and Breast Cancer Risk: Can an Effect via Insulin Resistance Be Demonstrated?" *Breast Cancer Res Treat* 38, no. 3 (1996): 239–46.

Stoll, B. A., and G. Secreto. "New Hormone-Related Markers of High Risk to Breast Cancer." *Ann Oncol* 3, no. 6 (1992): 435–38.

Storlien, L. H., E. W. Kraegen, A. B. Jenkins, and D. J. Chisholm. "Effects of Sucrose vs. Starch Diets on in Vivo Insulin Action, Thermogenesis, and Obesity in Rats." *American Journal of Clinical Nutrition* 47, no. 3 (1988): 420–27.

Storlien, L. H., N. D. Oakes, D. A. Pan, M. Kusunoki, and A. B. Jenkins. "Syndromes of Insulin Resistance in the Rat: Inducement by Diet and Amelioration with Benfluorex." *Diabetes* 42, no. 3 (1993): 457–62.

Stout, R. W. "Insulin and Atherogenesis." *Eur J Epidemiol* 8, suppl. 1 (1992): 134–35.

———. "Insulin and Atheroma: 20-Year Perspective." *Diabetes Care* 13, no. 6 (1990): 631–54.

———. "Overview of the Association between Insulin and Atherosclerosis." *Metabolism* 34, no. 12 (1985): 7–12.

Striffler, J. S., M. M. Polansky, and R. A. Anderson. "Dietary Chromium Improves IVGTT Insulin and Glucose Responses in Sucrose-Fed Cr-Deficient Rats." Abstract 6285 in *Federation of American Societies for Experimental Biology Journal* 4/5–4/9 (1992): A2022.

Suadicani, P., H. O. Hein, and F. Gyntelberg. "Serum Selenium Concentration and Risk of Ischaemic Heart Disease in a Prospective Cohort Study of 3000 Males." *Atherosclerosis* 96, no. 1 (1992): 33–42.

Sugiyama, Y. "The Role of Insulin in Reproductive Endocrinology and Perinatal Medicine." *Nippon Sanka Fujinka Gakkai Zasshi* 42, no. 8 (1990): 791–99.

Takeshita, A., Y. Hirooka, and T. Imaizumi. "Role of Endothelium in Control of Forearm Blood Flow in Patients with Heart Failure." *J Card Fail* 2, no. 4, suppl. (1996): S209–15.

Telander, R. L., S. A. Wolf, P. S. Simmons, D. Zimmerman, and M. W. Haymond. "Endocrine Disorders of the Pancreas and Adrenal Cortex in Pediatric Patients." *Mayo Clin Proc* 61, no. 6 (1986): 459–66.

Tepperman, J., and H. Tepperman. *Metabolic and Endocrine Physiology*. 5th ed. Chicago: Year Book Medical Publishers, 1987.

Thomas, D. E., J. R. Brotherhood, and J. C. Brand. "Carbohydrate Feeding before Exercise: Effect of Glycemic Index." *International Journal of Sports Medicine* 12, no. 2 (1991): 180–86.

Thomas, S. R., J. Neuzil, and R. Stocker. "Inhibition of LDL Oxidation by

REFERENCES

Ubiquinol-10: A Protective Mechanism for Coenzyme Q in Atherogenesis?" Source *Mol Aspects Med* 18, suppl. (1997): S85–103.

Thomassen, A., T. T. Neilsen, J. P. Bagger, and P. Henningsen. "Effects of Intravenous Glutamate on Substrate Availability and Utilization across the Human Heart and Leg." *Metabolism* 40, no. 4 (1991): 378–84.

Toepfer, E. W., W. Mertz, E. E. Roginski, and M. M. Polansky. "Chromium in Foods in Relation to Biological Activity." *J Agr Food Chem* 21, no. 1 (1973): 69–73.

Troisi, R. J., S. T. Weiss, D. R. Parker, D. Sparrow, J. B. Young, and L. Landsberg. "Relation of Obesity and Diet to Sympathetic Nervous System Activity." *Hypertens* 17, no. 5 (1991): 669–77.

Tseng, C. H., and T. V. Tai. "Risk Factors for Hyperinsulinemia in Chlorpropamide-Treated Diabetic Patients: A Three-Year Follow-Up." *J Formos Med Assoc* 91, no. 8 (1992): 770–74.

Tufts University Diet and Nutrition. Vol. 11, no. 5, July 1993.

Tweng, C. H., and T. Y. Tai. "Risk Factors for Hyperinsulinemia in Chloropropamide-Treated Diabetic Patients: A Three-Year Follow-Up." *J Formos Med Assoc* 91, no. 8 (1992): 770–74.

Uhde, T. W., J. P. Boulenger, D. C. Jimerson, and R. M. Post. "Caffeine: Relationship to Human Anxiety, Plasma MHPG and Cortisol." *Psychopharmacol-Bull.* 20, no. 3 (1984): 426–30.

Unterberger, P., A. Sinop, W. Noder, M. R. Berger, M. Fink, L. Edler, D. Schmahl, and H. Ehrhart. "Diabetes Mellitus and Breast Cancer: A Retrospective Follow-Up Study." *Onkologie* 13, no. 1 (1990): 17–20.

Urdl, W., G. Desoye, B. Schmon, H. M. Hoffmann, and G. Ralph. "Interaction between Insulin and Insulin-Like Growth Factor I in the Pathogenesis of Polycystic Ovarian Disease." *Ann NY Acad Sci* 626 (1991): 177–83.

U.S. Department of Agriculture, Department of Health and Human Services. *USDA Dietary Guidelines.* Home and Garden Bulletin no. 232, December 1995.

Vaaler, S. "Carbohydrate Metabolism, Insulin Resistance, and Metabolic Cardiovascular Syndrome." *Journal of Cardiovascular Pharmacology* 20, suppl. 8 (1992): S11–14.

Vagnini, F. J., S. Hill, and J. Puvolgel. "The Use of High Resolution Arterial Imaging to Assess Arteriosclerosis." *Angiology, J Vasc Dis* 48, no. 12 (1997): 1023–30.

Vaisman, N., D. Sklan, and Y. Dayan. "Effect of Semi-Starvation on Plasma Lipids." *International Journal of Obesity* 14, no. 12 (1990): 989–96.

Valensi, P. "Pathogenic Role of Hyperinsulinism in Macroangiopathy: Epidemiological Data." *Presse Med* 21, no. 28 (1992): 1307–11.

Van Der Walt, J. G., and M. J. Linington. "A Review of Energy Metabolism in Producing Ruminants." Part 2, "Control of Nutrient Partitioning." *J S Afr Vet Assoc* 61, no. 2 (1990): 78–80.

Van Itallie, T. B. "Health Implications of Overweight and Obesity in the United States." Part 2. *Annals of Internal Medicine* 103, no. 6 (1985): 983–88.

Van Soeren, M., T. Mohr, M. Kjaer, and T. E. Graham. "Acute Effects of Caffeine Ingestion at Rest in Humans with Impaired Epinephrine Responses." *J Appl Physiol* 80, no. 3 (1996): 999–1005.

Velek, J., L. Karasova, T. Pelikanova, T. Sosna, and J. Skibova. "Blood pressure and Insulin Resistance in Type 2 Diabetics." *Vnitr Lek* 37, nos. 9–10 (1991): 752–60.

Weaver, J. U., P. G. Kopelman, and G. A. Hitman. "Central Obesity and Hyperinsulinemia in Women Are Associated with Polymorphism in the 5' Flanking Region of the Human Insulin Gene." *European Journal of Clinical Investigation* 22, no. 4 (1992): 265–70.

Webster's New Twentieth Century Dictionary. 2d ed., unabridged. New York: World Publishing Co., 1975.

Wendorf, M. "Archeology and the 'Thrifty' Non Insulin Dependent Diabetes Mellitus (NIDDM) Genotype." *Adv Perit Dial* 8 (1992): 201–7.

———. "Diabetes, the Ice Free Corridor, and the Paleoindian Settlement on North America." *Am J Phys Anthropol* 79, no. 4 (1989): 503–20.

Wendorf, M., and I. D. Goldfine. "Archeology of NIDDM: Excavation of the 'Thrifty' Genotype." *Diabetes* 40, no. 2 (1991): 161–65.

White, P. J., K. A. Cybulski, R. Primus, D. F. Johnson, G. H. Collier, and G. C. Wagner. "Changes in Macronutrient Selection as a Function of Dietary Tryptophan." *Physiology and Behavior* 43 (1988): 73–77.

Wicklmayr, M., K. Rett, H. Baldermann, and G. Dietze. "The Kallikrein/Kinin System in the Pathogenesis of Hypertension in Diabetes Mellitus." Part 2. *Diabete Metab* 15, no. 5 (1989): 306–10.

Woods, S. C., D. Porte Jr., E. Bobbioni, E. Ionescu, J. F. Sauter, F. Rohner-Jeanrenaud, and B. Jeanrenaud. "Insulin: Its Relationship to the Central Nervous System and to the Control of Food Intake and Body Weight." *American Journal of Clinical Nutrition* 42 (1985): 1063–71.

Woteki, C. E., S. O. Walsh, N. Raper, et al. "Recent Trends and Levels of Dietary Sugars and Other Caloric Sweeteners." In *Metabolic Effects of Utilizable Dietary Carbohydrates,* edited by S. Reiser, 1–27. New York: Marcell Dekker, 1982.

Yale, J. "Taming the Hunger Hormone: Is Insulin the Key to Weight Control?" *American Health,* January–February 1984.

Yam, D., A. Fink, I. Nir, and P. Budowski. "Insulin-Tumor Interrelationships in Thymoma Bearing Mice: Effects of Dietary Glucose and Fructose." *Br J Cancer* 64, no. 6 (1991): 1043–46.

Young, I. S., J. J. Torney, and E. R. Trimble. "The Effect of Ascorbate Supplementation on Oxidative Stress in the Streptozotocin Diabetic Rats." *Free Radic Biol Med* 13, no. 1 (1992): 41–46.

REFERENCES

Zavaroni, I., E. Bonora, M. Pagliara, E. Dall'Aglio, L. Luchetti, G. Buonanno, P. A. Bonati, M. Bergonzani, L. Gnudi, M. Passeri, and G. Reaven. "Risk Factors for Coronary Artery Disease in Healthy Persons with Hyperinsulinemia and Normal Glucose Tolerance." *New England Journal of Medicine* 320, no. 11 (1989): 702–6.

Zimmet, P. Z. "Hyperinsulinemia—How Innocent a Bystander?" *Diabetes Care* 16, suppl. 3 (1993): 56–70.

INDEX

Abdominal obesity, 56–58
A'cbay, O., 228
Activity, 121, 187–194
    and consistency, 189–191
    frequency of, 191, 193
    increasing, 193, 194
    intensity of, 193–194
    lack of, 67
    light, 191–192
    moderate, 192
    and schedule, 189
    selection of, 190
    vigorous, 192
Activity Level, 107
Adachi, A., 141
Alcoholic beverages, 124, 137, 140, 310
American Cancer Society, 123, 258, 312
American Dietetic Association (ADA), 308–309
American Heart Association (AHA), 9, 53, 54, 123, 177–179, 247, 249, 253, 258, 280, 310–312
American Institute of Nutrition, 75, 90
American Journal of Clinical Nutrition, 173
Anderson, R. A., 157
Annals of the New York Academy of Science, 53

Antacid tablets and liquids, 203, 204
Anti-inflammatories, 202, 204, 214
Antioxidant supplementation, 167–176, 230
Appetizers:
    high-carbohydrate, Reward Meal recipes, 283–286
        exquisite deviled eggs, 285–286
        marinated beef strips, 283–284
        salmon and cheese canapés, 284
        stuffed avocado halves, 285
    low-carbohydrate recipes, 267–269
        deviled eggs, 268
        filled mushrooms, tangy, 267
        stuffed celery, 268–269
L-arginine, 234
Argument escalation, avoidance of, 207
Aspirin, 174, 202, 204, 214
Atherosclerosis, 9, 48, 57, 93, 97
Avocado(s):
    with fettucine and "beef," 301–302
    halves, stuffed, 285

Balanced nutrition (*see* Nutritional guidelines)
Balanced supplementation (*see* Supplementation)

Balancing carbohydrates in Reward Meals, 124–127
BASIC Plan, 119–194
  overview, 121
  steps in (*see* Activity; Nutritional guidelines; Supplementation)
  water consumption, 146–147
Beans and vegetarian "sausage," 305
Bearon, L. B., 239
Beck-Nielsen, H., 95
Beef:
  strips, marinated, 283–284
  and tomato stew, 292
  "Beef" with avocados and fettucine, 301–302
Beresford, Shirley, 176–177
Beta-carotene, 230–231
Beverages (alcoholic), 124, 137, 140, 310
Beverages (non-alcoholic):
  caffeine-rich, 214
  diet drinks, 145–150
  high-carbohydrate, 137
  low-carbohydrate, 135
Bioflavinoids, 174
Birth control pills, 174, 230–231
Black, H. R., 77
Blood clots, 94
Blood-clotting abnormalities, 13
Blood fat levels, 55, 66, 67, 75, 79–81
  confusion about, 79
  and high insulin levels, 52
  and Insulin Resistance Syndrome, 56, 57, 59
  new directions in research on, 221
  and saturated dietary fats, 80–81
Blood salt levels, 78
Blood sugar levels, 56–60, 75, 88–91
Blood tests, 100–103
Brain cells, 56
Breaded fish fillets, 293–294
Breads:
  French whole-wheat toast, 283
  list of, 135
  whole-wheat toast broil, 281

Breakfast:
  high-carbohydrate, Reward Meal recipes, 281–283
    French wheat toast, 283
    pancakes supreme, 282
    whole-wheat toast broil, 281
  low-carbohydrate recipes, 138–139, 261–263
    freedom frittata, 261
    high-fiber stuffed mushrooms, 261–262
    quiche sans crust, 262–263
    turkey sausage treat, 263
  skipping, 217
Breakthroughs in research (*see* Research, emerging breakthroughs in)
Breath fresheners, 203
Broccoli and carrot soup, cream of, 290
Broth, 141
Burgers, tofu, 275–276
Butter, 134

Cabbage:
  delight, 270
  with tofu and mushrooms, 276
Caesar's salad, 289–290
Caffeine reduction, 212–214
Caffeine withdrawal, 213
Canapés, salmon and cheese, 284
Carbohydrate act-alikes, 139–146
Carbohydrate-Addicted Kids (Heller and Heller), 250
Carbohydrate Addict's Cookbook, The (Heller and Heller), 250
Carbohydrate Addict's Diet, The (Heller and Heller), 250
Carbohydrate Addict's Gram Counter (Heller and Heller), 250
Carbohydrate Addict's Healthy Heart Program:
  and adult-onset diabetes, 91
  case study, 82–87
  and *Dietary Guidelines for Americans*, 123
  essential points, 122–123
  and heart disease, 97–98

INDEX

overview, 121–122
and physician's recommendations, 120
stages of (*see* BASIC Plan; Heart Health-Enhancing Options)
Carbohydrate Addict's Heart Health Quiz, 104–116
 Activity Level, 107
 Family and Personal Medical History, 105–106
 Heart Disease Risk Profile, 111–116
 Heart Disease Risk Score analysis, 109–110
 Nutritional Profile, 106–107
 scoring, 108–109
 Stress Level, 107–108
 subscores, 114–115
Carbohydrate Addict's Lifespan Program (Heller and Heller), 250
Carbohydrate Addict's Official Website, 247–248, 249–250
Carbohydrate Addict's Program for Success (Heller and Heller), 250
Carbohydrate consumption frequency, 61–63, 74–75
Carbohydrate content of foods (*see* High-carbohydrate foods; Low-carbohydrate foods)
Carbohydrate-craving, 60–61
Carbohydrates, complex, 209–212
Cardiovascular Wellness, 249, 252
Cardiovascular Wellness Centers, The, 248–249, 251–252
L-carnitine, 232
Carotenoids, 230
Carrot and broccoli soup, cream of, 290
Celery, stuffed, 268–269
Cereals:
 high-fiber, 165
 list of, 135
Cheese, 133
 and salmon canapés, 284
 see also names of cheeses
Chewing gum, 138, 145
Chicken:
 peppered fillet of, 271–272
 and rice casserole, 293
"Chicken":
 loaf, 304–305
 sautéed, 279
Cholesterol, 13, 52, 53, 78, 79, 97–98, 171
 and coronary artery disease, 93–94
 and fructose, 210
 "good" *vs.* "bad," 226
 new directions in research on, 221
 and omega-3 oils, 229
 recommended intake of, 310
Chromium picolinate, 160
Chromium supplementation, 157–162, 184–186
Circulation, 54
Clam(s):
 dip, tangy, 266
 fried, 295
Clinical Nutrition, 53
Coconut oil, 224
Coenzyme Q-10, 233–234
Coffee, 138
Cold medications, 204, 214
Combined Heart Disease Risk Score, 108–114
 analysis of, 109–110
 and Heart Disease Risk Profile, 111–114
Comings, D. E., 60–61
Complex carbohydrates, 209–212
Concentration difficulties, 56, 59
Coronary artery disease, 92–95
Coronary heart disease, 92, 95
Cortisol, 213
Cottage cheese, 133
Cough remedies, 202–204, 214
Cream, 133, 138*n*
Cream cheese dip, tangy, 265
Cream of broccoli-carrot soup, 290
Creamy dressing, sumptuous, 266
Crepes, easy, 299–300

Dairy:
 high-carbohydrate, 135
 low-carbohydrate, 130, 132–133
D2 dopamine receptor gene (DRD2), 60–61

Deadly Quartet, The (*see* Blood fat levels; Diabetes, adult-onset; High blood pressure; Weight gain)
DeFronzo, R. A., 52, 95–96
Del Prato, S., 95
Department of Nutrition, School of Public Health, Loma Linda, 220
Depression, 59
Desserts, 297–301
　easy crepes, 299–300
　fruity dumplings, 300–301
　key lime pie, 297–298
　mixed fruit(s):
　　compote, 298
　　with honey-lemon dressing, 300
　Deviled eggs, 268
　　exquisite, 285–286
Diabetes, 51
Diabetes, adult-onset, 9, 13, 52, 58, 59, 60, 66, 67, 89–91, 145, 170
Dietary fats:
　low-fat alternatives, 258, 259, 280, 308–309
　low-fat diets, 69, 77, 79, 81, 223
　low-fat recommendations, 259, 280, 310, 311
　new directions in research on, 221–226
　polyunsaturated, 222–225
　saturated (*see* Saturated fats)
　unsaturated, 80–81, 134, 221–222
Dietary guidelines, health agency, 123, 258, 259, 307–312
Dietary Guidelines for Americans, 123
Diet drinks, 145–150
Diets, 69, 71, 77, 79, 81, 223
Dips:
　high-carbohydrate, Reward Meal recipe: spinach yogurt, 287–288
　low-carbohydrate recipes, 265–266
　　clam, tangy, 266
　　cream cheese, tangy, 265
　　spinach, spicy, 266
Disraeli, Benjamin, 246
Diuretics, 182

Djuhuus, M. S., 182
Doubtful risk profile, 111
Dressings (*see* Salad dressings)
Duke University Medical Center, 170
Dumplings, fruity, 300–301
Durnin, J. V., 72

Egg(s), 133
　breakfast quiche sans crust, 262–263
　deviled, 268
　　exquisite, 285–286
　foo yung, 273
　freedom frittata, 261
Emerging breakthroughs in research (*see* Research, emerging breakthroughs in)
Enhancing Options (*see* Heart Health-Enhancing Options)
Essential hypertension (*see* High blood pressure)
Excitotoxin, 141
Exquisite deviled eggs, 285–286

Fasting hypoglycemia, 89*n*
Fasting insulin test, 100–102
Fats (*see* Blood fat levels; Dietary fats)
Fatty acids, 223–224
Feraille, E., 79
Ferrannini, E., 52, 95–96
Fettucine with "beef" and avocados, 301–302
Fiber supplementation, 162–167
Fibrin, 94
Fibronogen, 67
Fish:
　broiled, 274
　canned tuna (*see* Tuna, canned)
　fillets, breaded, 293–294
　low-carbohydrate, list of, 132–133
Flake tuna salad with dressing, 269
Folic acid supplementation, 176–180
Folsom, A. R., 80
Food balance, 74–75
Food frequency reduction, 214–218
Food lists:
　high-carbohydrate, 135–138

INDEX

high-fiber, 165–167
low-carbohydrate, 132–135
Fowl (*see* Poultry)
Fox Weekend on Health, 16
Franklin, Ben, 152, 235
Freedom frittata, 261
Free glutamates, 139–143, 220
Free Medline, 248, 249, 253
Free radicals, 168, 173
French wheat toast, 283
Frittata, freedom, 261
Fructose, 210–211
Fruit:
  dumplings, 300–301
  high-fiber, 165
  and insulin levels, 210–211
  list of, 136
  mixed:
    compote, 298
    with honey-lemon dressing, 300
Fruit juices:
  elimination from diet, 211
  list of, 136

Galvan, A. G., 169–170
Garg, A., 96
Garlic dressing, basic, 264
Gastric inflammation, and *Helicobacter pylori*, 226–229
Geiselman, Paula, 73–74
Genetics, 60–61, 113
Glucagon, 49–50
Glucose challenge, 103
Glucose intolerance, 57
Glucose levels (*see* Blood sugar levels)
Glucose tolerance factor (GTF) chromium, 159–162
Glutamates, 139–143, 220
Goldfine, A. B., 232
Goodall, E., 74
Grains, list of, 135
Green garden mayonnaise dressing, 265
Green pepper and tomato salad with dressing, 289

Grimaldi, A. C., 95
Gum disease, and *Helicobacter pylori*, 226–229

Hallfrisch, J., 210
Ham and cauliflower supreme, 272
HDL cholesterol, 52, 53, 98, 171, 221, 226, 229
Headaches, 59
Health agency dietary guidelines, 123, 258, 259, 307–312
Healthy for Life (Heller and Heller), 250
Heart attack, 95, 97
Heart disease, 67, 92–98
Heart disease risk factors, 9, 13, 63, 65–91, 96–97
  and Insulin Resistance Syndrome, 56, 57
  see also Blood fat levels; Diabetes, adult-onset; High blood pressure; Weight gain
Heart Disease Risk Profile, 111–116
Heart Disease Risk Score analysis, 109–110
Heart Health–Enhancing Options, 197–245
  adding, 199–200
  caffeine reduction, 212–214
  choosing, 197–199
  complex carbohydrates, 209–212
  food frequency reduction, 214–218
  over-the-counter remedy timing, 201–204
  overview, 121–122
  pacing of changes, 200–201
  stress reduction, 205–209
Heart Health Quiz (*see* Carbohydrate Addict's Heart Health Quiz)
Heart Show, The, 16, 249, 252
Helicobacter pylori, 226–229
High blood pressure, 9, 13, 48, 55, 66, 67, 76–79
  and caffeine, 212
  and high insulin levels, 52, 53, 77–79
  and other heart disease risk factors, 76
  as symptom, 79
  traditional treatment of, 76–77

High-carbohydrate, Reward Meal recipes, 279–304
  appetizers, 283–286
    exquisite deviled eggs, 285–286
    marinated beef strips, 283–284
    salmon and cheese canapés, 284
    stuffed avocado halves, 285
  breakfasts, 281–283
    French wheat toast, 283
    pancakes supreme, 282
    whole-wheat toast broil, 281
  desserts, 297–301
    easy crepes, 299–300
    fruity dumplings, 300–301
    key lime pie, 297–298
    mixed fruit compote, 298
    mixed fruits with honey-lemon dressing, 300
  dip, spinach yogurt, 287–288
  guidelines, 279–281
  proteins, 292–297
    batter-fried scallops, 297
    beef and tomato stew, 292
    breaded fish fillets, 293–294
    chicken and rice casserole, 293
    classic fried clams, 295
    potted pork roast, 294
    veal medallions with mushrooms and herbs, 296
  salad dressings, 286–288
    oil and vinegar, 287
    Russian, simple homemade, 286
    spicy vinaigrette, 286
  salads, 288–290
    Caesar's, 289–290
    green pepper and tomato with dressing, 289
    spinach, vitamin-rich, with dressing, 288
  soups, 290–291
    cream of broccoli-carrot, 290
    split-pea, old-fashioned, 291
  vegetarian (nonmeat) alternatives
    "beef" with avocados and fettucine, 301–302
    "chicken" loaf, 302–303

    macaroni with tomatoes, 304
    "sausage" and beans, 303
High-carbohydrate foods:
  balancing with low-carbohydrate foods, 124–127
  list of, 135–138
High-fiber foods, 165–167
High-fiber stuffed mushrooms, 261–262
"High-protein" power bars, 136
High risk profile, 113–114
Himsworth, H. P., 50–51
Homocysteine, 176–180
Hormonal balance, 49
Hormonal imbalance, 9
  see also Hyperinsulinemia
Hu, Frank B., 80, 222
Hughes, C. E., 237
Hydrogenated fats, 221–222
Hydrolyzed protein, 141
Hyperinsulinemia, 9–12
  and heart disease, 67, 92–96
  and heart disease risk factors (*see* Heart disease risk factors)
  and Insulin Resistance Syndrome (*see* Insulin Resistance Syndrome)
  personal stories of discovery of, 21–47
  research on, 11–14, 50–54, 63–64
Hypertension (*see* High blood pressure)
Hypoglycemia, 57, 89–91, 216

Ideal individualized nutrition, 155–156
Ignatowski, Vladislov, 220
Insoluble fiber, 163
Insulin release, 9
  and blood sugar, 88–91, 144
  and carbohydrate consumption frequency, 61–62
  excess (*see* Hyperinsulinemia)
  and folic acid, 176
  function of, 49
  and *Helicobacter pylori*, 226–229
  impact of, 48
  relationship with chromium, 157–158
  relationship with glucagon, 49–50
  and soy protein, 220

INDEX

and stress, 205
thrifty gene (carbohydrate-craving gene), 60–61
and vanadium, 231
waves of, 128–130
Insulin resistance, 9, 10, 12, 51–53, 55
see also Insulin Resistance Syndrome
Insulin Resistance Syndrome, 51–53, 54–63, 97
and Combined Heart Disease Risk Score, 110–113
and fasting insulin test, 101, 102
first stage, 56, 58–59
fourth stage, 58, 59
and frequency of carbohydrate consumption, 61–62
second stage, 56, 58–59
third stage, 57, 59
and thrifty gene (carbohydrate-craving gene), 60–61
Irritability, 56, 59
Ischemic heart disease, 92

Jeejeebhoy, K. N., 158
Joslin Diabetes Center, 232
Journal of Clinical Endocrinological Metabolism, 53
Journal of Holistic Medicine, 237
Journal of the American College of Cardiology, 175
Journal of the American Medical Association (JAMA), 53, 177, 178

Key lime pie, 297–298
Koenig, H. G., 239
Kozlovsky, A. S., 158

Laboratory procedures, traditional, 99–103
Lamb chops, broiled, 275
Lancet, 50, 53
Landin, K., 79
Landsberg, L., 78
LDL cholesterol, 98, 175, 221, 226, 229
Lee, Mu-En, 177
Legumes:

high-fiber, 165
list of, 136
Leibel, R., 72
Light-headedness, 56
Lipoic acid, 233
Lithell, H., 95
Liver, 58, 89
Losonczy, K. G., 173
Low-carbohydrate foods:
balancing with high-carbohydrate foods, 124–127
list of, 132–135
Low-carbohydrate meals and snacks, 130–139
Low-carbohydrate recipes, 257–278
appetizers, 267–269
deviled eggs, 268
filled mushrooms, tangy, 267
stuffed celery, 268–269
breakfast, 261–263
freedom frittata, 261
high-fiber stuffed mushrooms, 261–262
quiche sans crust, 262–263
turkey sausage treat, 263
dips, 265–266
clam, tangy, 266
cream cheese, tangy, 265
spinach, spicy, 268
guidelines, 257–259
and microwave ovens, 260
proteins, 271–275
broiled fish, 274
cauliflower and ham supreme, 272
classic roast pork, 273–274
egg foo yung, 273
peppered fillet of chicken, 271–272
salad dressings, 264–265
creamy, sumptuous, 264
garlic, basic, 264
green garden mayonnaise dressing, 265
salads, 269–271
cabbage delight, 270
flake tuna with dressing, 269
seafood, 269–270
sprout 'n' chef, 271

Low-carbohydrate recipes (*cont.*)
    vegetarian (nonmeat) alternatives, 275–278
        sautéed "chicken," 277
        "steak" casserole, 277–278
        tofu with cabbage and mushrooms, 276
        ultimate tofu burgers, 275–276
Low-fat alternatives, 258, 259, 280, 308–309
Low-fat diets, 69, 77, 79, 81, 223
Low-fat recommendations, 259, 280, 310, 311
Low-salt alternatives, 258, 259, 280, 309
Low-salt diets, 77
Low-salt recommendations, 259, 280
Low-saturated fat alternatives, 258, 259, 280, 308–309
Low-saturated fat recommendations, 259, 280
Luncheon meats, 132
Lunches, low-carbohydrate, 139

Macaroni with tomatoes, 304
Magnesium supplementation, 180–184, 231
Malinow, Manuel R., 179
Marinated beef strips, 283–284
Marshall, Barry, 227
Marshall, J. A., 80
Mayer, E. J., 80
Mayonnaise, 134, 259–260
Mayonnaise dressing, green garden, 265
Meats, low-carbohydrate:
    list of, 132
    see also names of meats
Medical History, 105–106
Mercury contamination, 229–230
Metabolic Syndrome (*see* Insulin Resistance Syndrome)
Metabolism, 169
Microwave ovens, 260
Mild risk profile, 111–112
Milk, 133, 138*n*
Miller, D. S., 71
Mints, 138, 145
Mixed fruit(s):
    compote, 298
    with honey-lemon dressing, 300
Moderate risk profile, 112–113

Monosodium glutamate (MSG), 138, 141–143
Monounsaturated fats, 222–225
Mood swings, 59
Morgan, J. P., 71–72
Mosca, L., 175
Mumford, P., 71
Mushrooms:
    and herbs with veal medallions, 296
    stuffed, high-fiber, 261–262
    with tofu and cabbage, 276

National Institute of Mental Health, 213
National Institutes of Health, 227
National Research Council, 161
New England Journal of Medicine, 53, 178, 179, 212, 222
Noble, E. P., 61
Nonsteroidal anti-inflammatory medications, 202, 204, 214
Noodles, 136
Novin, David, 73–74
Nutritional counseling, 248, 251
Nutritional guidelines:
    avoidance of carbohydrate act–alikes, 139–146
    daily Reward Meal, 123–127
    low-carbohydrate meals and snacks, 130–139
    Reward Meal duration, 127–130
Nutritional Profile, 106–107
Nutritional recommendations, health agency, 123, 258, 259, 307–312
Nutritional supplementation (*see* Supplementation)
Nuts, list of, 136

Oakley, Godfrey, Jr., 180
Obesity, 55–58, 66, 67, 68–76
    abdominal, 56–58
    and amount consumed, 71–73
    and high insulin levels, 53
    hyperinsulinemia as cause of, 69–70
    and other heart disease risk factors, 68–69
    see also Weight gain

INDEX

Oil(s), 134, 224
   Omega-3, 229–230
   and vinegar dressing, 287
Old-fashioned split-pea soup, 291
Olive oil, 261
Omega-3 oils, 229–230
Oral glucose tolerance test with insulin sampling, 103
Over-the-counter remedy timing, 201–204
Oxidation, 167–168

Palm oil, 224
Pancakes supreme, 282
Passwater, Richard A., 158
Pasta, 136, 167
   fettucine with "beef" and avocados, 301–302
   macaroni with tomatoes, 304
Pauling, Linus, 172
Peppers, green, and tomato salad with dressing, 289
Perfectionism, 200
Peripheral vascular disease, 48
Physicians, 4–6
Phytoestrogens, 220
Pie, key lime, 297–298
Plaque, 78, 93–95
Polycystic ovarian syndrome (PCOS), 9, 58
Polyunsaturated fats, 222–225
Pork:
   cauliflower and ham supreme, 272
   roast, classic, 273–274
   roast, potted, 294
Portion size, 124–125, 131
Postprandial reactive hypoglycemic response, 89, 101
Potted pork roast, 294
Poultry:
   chicken and rice casserole, 293
   low-carbohydrate, 132
   peppered fillet of chicken, 271–272
   turkey sausage, 263
Power bars, "high-protein," 136
Power drinks, 136

Prayer, power of, 235–245
Preventive medicine, 15–17, 249
Primary hypertension (*see* High blood pressure)
Princen, H. M., 172
Profactor, 97
Profactor-H (*see* Hyperinsulinemia)
Protein:
   high-carbohydrate, Reward Meal recipes
      batter-fried scallops, 297
      beef and tomato stew, 292
      breaded fish fillets, 293–294
      chicken and rice casserole, 295
      classic fried clams, 295
      potted pork roast, 294
      veal medallions with mushrooms and herbs, 296
   in low-carbohydrate meals and snacks, 130, 131
   low-carbohydrate recipes, 271–275
      broiled fish, 274
      cauliflower and ham supreme, 272
      classic roast pork, 273–274
      egg foo yung, 273
      peppered fillet of chicken, 271–272
   in reward Meals, 124–126
Protein powders, 136

Quiche sans crust, breakfast, 262–263

Reaven, G. M., 51
Recipes (*see* High-carbohydrate, Reward Meal recipes; Low-carbohydrate recipes)
Recommendations; Folic Acid and Cardiovascular Disease (AHA), 178
Remedies (over-the-counter) timing, 201–204
Research, emerging breakthroughs in, 219–234
   beta-carotene, 230–231
   L-carnitine, 232
   coenzyme Q-10, 233–234

Research, emerging breakthroughs in (cont.)
  Helicobacter pylori, 226–229
  lipoic acid, 233
  omega-3 oils, 229–230
  selenium, 232–233
  soy protein, 220–221
  taurine, 231
  vanadium, 231–232
Resources, 246–254
  American Heart Association, 249, 253
  Carbohydrate Addict's Official Website, 247–248, 249–250
  Cardiovascular Wellness, 249, 252
  The Cardiovascular Wellness Centers, 248–249, 251–252
  Free Medline, 248, 249, 253
  Heart Show, The, 249, 252
Reward Meals:
  and complex carbohydrates, 210
  daily, 123–127
  duration, 127–130
  and fiber supplementation, 164
  over-the-counter remedies taken during, 203
  recipes (see High-carbohydrate, Reward Meal recipes)
  reducing size of, 216
Reynolds, Helenbeth Reiss, 180
Rice, 136, 167
  and chicken casserole, 293
Robertson, D., 212
Rodin, Judith, 74
Russian dressing, simple homemade, 286

Salad dressings, 134
  high-carbohydrate, Reward Meal recipes, 286–287
    oil and vinegar, 287
    Russian, simple homemade, 286
    spicy vinaigrette, 286
  low-carbohydrate recipes, 264–265
    creamy, sumptuous, 264
    garlic, basic, 264
    green garden mayonnaise dressing, 265

Salads:
  and fiber supplementation, 164
  high-carbohydrate, Reward Meal recipes, 288–290
    Caesar's, 289–290
    green pepper and tomato with dressing, 289
    spinach, vitamin-rich, with dressing, 288
  with low-carbohydrate breakfasts, 139
  low-carbohydrate recipes, 269–271
    cabbage delight, 270
    flake tuna with dressing, 269
    seafood, 269–270
    sprout 'n' chef, 271
  in Reward Meals, 124–126
Salmon and cheese canapés, 284
Salt:
  low-salt alternatives, 258, 259, 280, 309
  low-salt diets, 77
  low-salt recommendations, 259, 280
  retention of, 78
Saturated fats, 67, 69, 80–81, 88, 134, 224
  low-saturated fat alternatives, 280, 308–309
  low-saturated fat recommendations, 259, 280
Sausage, turkey, 263
"Sausage" and beans, 302–303
Scallops, batter-fried, 297
Seafood:
  batter-fried scallops, 297
  classic fried clams, 295
  salad, 269–270
  tangy clam dip, 266
  see also Fish
Seeds, list of, 136
Selenium, 232–233
Sharma, A. M., 79
Sigerist, Henry E., 65
Silverstone, T., 74
Simons, L. A., 172
Simonson, D. C., 52, 74, 95
Simple sugars, 209
Sims, E. A. H., 71

INDEX

Skipping meals, 131, 215–216
Snacks:
  high-fiber, 167
  low-carbohydrate, 130–139
Soluble fiber, 163
Soups, 290–291
  cream of broccoli-carrot, 290
  split-pea, old-fashioned, 291
Sour cream, 133
Soy protein, 220–221
Soy protein powder, 136
Spicy:
  spinach dip, 268
  vinaigrette, 286
Spinach:
  dip, spicy, 268
  salad, vitamin-rich, with dressing, 288
  and yogurt dip, 287–288
Split-pea soup, old-fashioned, 291
Sprout 'n' chef salad, 271
Stampfer, Meir, 177
Starches, 209–212
State of Deficiency school of thought, 152–154
State of Therapeutics school of thought, 154–155
"Steak" casserole, 277–278
Stew, beef and tomato, 292
Stolar, M. W., 97
Stool softeners, 203, 204
Stout, R. W., 77, 95
Stout, Robert W., 52–53
Stress, 67
Stress Level, 107–108
Stress reduction, 205–209
Stress signals, 206–207
Stuffed:
  avocado halves, 285
  celery, 268–269
  mushrooms, high-fiber, 261–262
Sugars:
  reducing intake of, 309
  simple, 209
Sugar substitutes, 137, 138, 140, 143–146
Sumptuous creamy dressing, 264

Supplementation, 121, 152–186
  chromium, 157–162, 184–186
  conflicting viewpoints concerning, 153–155
  fiber, 162–167
  folic acid, 176–180
  and ideal individualized nutrition, 155–156
  magnesium, 180–184
  resource for supplements, 252
  vitamin C, 172–176
  vitamin E, 167–172
Surgeon General's Report on Nutrition and Health, The, 53, 103
Sweet, Leonard I., 219
Sweet-tasting over-the-counter medications, 202–203
Syndrome X (*see* Insulin Resistance Syndrome)

Tangy:
  clam dip, 266
  cream cheese dip, 265
Taurine, 231
Tea, 138
Testing, 248–249, 251
  Carbohydrate Addict's Heart Health Quiz (*see* Carbohydrate Addict's Heart Health Quiz)
  traditional laboratory procedures, 99–103
Textured vegetable protein, 133
  in low-carbohydrate meals and snacks, 130
  in Reward Meals, 130
  sautéed "chicken," 277
  "steak" casserole, 277–278
Thrifty gene (carbohydrate-craving gene), 60–61
Tofu:
  burgers, ultimate, 275–276
  with cabbage and mushrooms, 276
Togiyama, N. A., 141
Tomato(es):
  and beef stew, 292
  and green pepper salad with dressing, 289
  with macaroni, 304

Trans fatty acids, 79, 80, 221–222, 225
Treatment, 248–249, 251
Triglyceride levels, 52, 53, 210
Tropical oils, 224
Tuna, canned, 141
   salad with dressing, 269
Turkey sausage treat, breakfast, 263

Ultimate tofu burgers, 275–276
Unsaturated fats, 80–81, 134, 221–222
U.S. Department of Agriculture, 157
U.S. Department of Health and Human Services, 123, 247, 258, 280
U.S. Food and Drug Administration, 179

Vanadium, 231–232
Veal medallions with mushrooms and herbs, 296
Vegetables:
   high-carbohydrate, 137
   high-fiber, 165
   low-carbohydrate, 125, 130, 131, 133–134
   see also names of vegetables
Vegetarian (nonmeat) alternatives, 301–304
   high-carbohydrate, Reward Meal recipes
      "beef" with avocados and fettucine, 301–302
      "chicken" loaf, 302–303
      macaroni with tomatoes, 304
      "sausage" and beans, 303
   low-carbohydrate recipes, 275–278
      sautéed "chicken," 277
      "steak" casserole, 277–278
      tofu with cabbage and mushrooms, 276
      ultimate tofu burgers, 275–276
Vinaigrette, spicy, 286
Vinegar and oil dressing, 287
Vitamin C supplementation, 172–176
Vitamin E supplementation, 168–172

Ward, K. D., 80
Warren, John Robin, 227
Water consumption, 146–147
Weight gain, 48, 55
   and heart disease, 67
   and insulin release, 73–75
   and Insulin Resistance Syndrome, 56–59
   and thrifty gene (carbohydrate-craving gene), 60–61
   see also Obesity
Weight loss, 14, 69
Whole-wheat:
   French toast, 283
   toast broil, 281

Yogurt and spinach dip, 287–288

ABOUT THE AUTHORS

For more than a decade, RICHARD F. HELLER, M.S., PH.D., and RACHAEL F. HELLER, M.A., M.PH., PH.D., each held two professorial appointments and conducted research at Mount Sinai School of Medicine in New York City and in the Department of Biomedical Sciences in the Graduate School of the City University of New York. They are coauthors of many books, including the bestselling *The Carbohydrate Addict's Diet* and *The Carbohydrate Addict's Life Span Program.*

DR. FREDERIC J. VAGNINI, M.D., F.A.C.S., is the medical director of The Cardiovascular Wellness Centers of New York. He has served as assistant clinical professor of surgery at Cornell University for more than twenty-five years. Dr. Vagnini is the author and coauthor of many research papers and articles on cardiovascular and heart disease, preventive medicine, and the role of nutrition in heart health. He is the host of *The Heart Show* on WOR-AM in New York.